Remote Medicine

A Textbook for Trainee and Established Remote Healthcare Practitioners

Other Related Titles from World Scientific

Hazmat Medical Life Support: A Basic Provider Manual
by Hock Heng Tan, Mark Leong, R Ponampalam, Chun Yue Lee and
Jimmy Goh
ISBN: 978-981-4583-15-2 (pbk)

Textbook of Occupational Medicine Practice
Fourth Edition
edited by David Koh and Tar-Ching Aw
ISBN: 978-981-3200-69-2

Health Hazards of Environmental Arsenic Poisoning:
From Epidemic to Pandemic
edited by Chien-Jen Chen and Hung-Yi Chiou
ISBN: 978-981-4291-81-1

Remote Medicine

A Textbook for Trainee and Established Remote Healthcare Practitioners

editors

Nelson Norman
Emeritus Professor of Environmental Medicine, University of Aberdeen, UK

Malcolm Valentine
Former General Medical Practitioner and Occupational Physician, Aberdeen, UK

World Scientific

NEW JERSEY · LONDON · SINGAPORE · BEIJING · SHANGHAI · HONG KONG · TAIPEI · CHENNAI · TOKYO

Published by

World Scientific Publishing Europe Ltd.

57 Shelton Street, Covent Garden, London WC2H 9HE

Head office: 5 Toh Tuck Link, Singapore 596224

USA office: 27 Warren Street, Suite 401-402, Hackensack, NJ 07601

Library of Congress Cataloging-in-Publication Data
Names: Norman, Nelson, editor. | Valentine, Malcolm Jack, editor.
Title: Remote medicine : a textbook for trainee and established remote healthcare practitioners /
    editors, Nelson Norman, Malcolm Jack Valentine.
Description: New Jersey : World Scientific, [2020] | Includes bibliographical references and index.
Identifiers: LCCN 2019049826 | ISBN 9781786347503 (hardcover)
Subjects: MESH: Telemedicine | Health Services Accessibility | Emergency Medical Services |
    Rural Health Services | Wilderness Medicine | Occupational Health Services |
    Extreme Environments
Classification: LCC R859 | NLM W 83 | DDC 362.10285--dc23
LC record available at https://lccn.loc.gov/2019049826

British Library Cataloguing-in-Publication Data
A catalogue record for this book is available from the British Library.

Cover Acknowledgements
Top: Telemedicine. Shirley Mackilvenny reading a research paper in the UAE for delivery
in at a meeting in Glasgow.
Middle right: A remote industrial site in Siberia and an episode of casualty handling.
Middle left: The image on the right shows practical first-aid training in the Arabian Desert.
Bottom: A caboose situated near Halley bay, some 800 miles from the South Pole. Scientists
lived there while studying Emperor Penguins.

For any available supplementary material, please visit
https://www.worldscientific.com/worldscibooks/10.1142/Q0222#t=suppl

Contents

About the Editors

Professor Nelson Norman MB ChB, PhD, MD, DSc, FRCS (Edin & Glasg), FFOM, FRSB, CB is a graduate of the Universities of Glasgow and Aberdeen. He is President of the International Remote Healthcare Association and a Senior Research Fellow at Glasgow University. Former posts held were President of the Institute of Remote Healthcare, Director of the British Antarctic Survey Medical Unit, Professor of Community Medicine at the UAE University, Medical Director RGIT Survival Centre Ltd., Director RGIT Centre for Offshore Health, Professor of Environmental Medicine, University of Aberdeen and Consultant Surgeon, Grampian Health Board.

Dr Malcolm J Valentine MB ChB, MD, FRCGP, DRCOG is a graduate of the University of Aberdeen. He researched causes of medical evacuations from offshore installations, practiced Hyperbaric Medicine, was a HSE Appointed Radiation Doctor and Occupational Health Doctor — parallel to his career-long role as a General Practitioner. He was for a number of years Editor of the *Journal of the IRHC*.

About the Authors

Professor David A Alexander MA (Hons), CPsychol, PhD, (Hon) DSc, FBPS, FRSM, (Hon) FRCPsych is Emeritus Professor of Mental Health in Aberdeen. Formerly, he was a Professor of Mental Health in the Faculty of Medicine, Aberdeen University; Consultant in Charge of the Regional Traumatic Stress Clinic and Director of the Aberdeen Centre for Trauma Research. He has worked with the Scottish Police for over 20 years, and is an Associate Member of both the Scottish Institute for Policing Research and the Scottish Police College. He has also been deployed operationally to local, national and international incidents of a serious nature. He is one of three Principal Advisors to the UK police services for the most serious incidents. Over a seven- year-period he was a Visiting Consultant at HMP Peterhead, when it was Scotland's maximum-security prison.

Professor Sergey Antipov PhD, Professor of Siberian State Medical University, General Director of CCM LLC (Russia). From 1992–1999 Dr Antipov worked as a surgeon in the Research Institute of Oncology of Tomsk Scientific Center, Siberian Branch of Russian Academy of Medical Sciences. Since 1996 he has been holding a teaching fellow position with the Department of Oncology at Siberian State Medical University. He has published more than 85 scientific papers with much of his research focused on the early diagnosis, prevention and treatment of gastric cancer. Sergey Antipov obtained a Doctor of Medical Sciences (PhD) degree in 2012 and was appointed as a Professor in the Department of Surgery and Oncology in 2013.

Dr Antipov is particularly interested in innovations and investments in healthcare services. In 2006 he founded a company specializing in providing occupational medicine services. By 2014 Dr Antipov had founded several companies that were consolidated by the managing company CCM LLC. Today CCM LLC provided various industrial medicine and healthcare services in Russia and abroad.

Erzhena Badmaeva PhD student, Siberian State Medical University. She works as the Head of the Health Department of the Tomsk region. Erzhena has been involved in telemedicine research for over 5 years. She's currently conducting a joint research with the Association of Remote Healthcare (Russia) on remote healthcare issues.

Dr Alison Carroll has been working with the Oil and Gas industry for almost 30 years, following an initial career in standard psychiatry she has managed several cases of acute psychiatric illness over the years, both in the UK offshore sector and worldwide. She has particular interest in psychiatric disorders in the workplace and post-traumatic stress disorder.

Dr Finlay D Dick MD, FRCP, FFOM, MRCGP is an occupational physician based in Scotland. He has over 25 years of experience in occupational medicine across a range of public and private sector organisations including in the upstream oil and gas industry. He has published 30 scientific papers, been a contributing author to four textbooks of occupational medicine and co-edited the Oxford Handbook of Occupational Health.

Dr Thomas French MB, ChB, MRCP (UK) graduated from Glasgow University in 2011. He has worked in various placements and specialties throughout the west coast of Scotland, eventually settling on acute medicine as his chosen specialty. He has broad interests in internal medicine aside from the acutely unwell patient in stroke medicine and vascular access. Outside the clinical environment, he has been appointed as Chief Medical Officer to Trust Ruby International, and is a qualified rugby referee officiating at both amateur and professional levels.

Harry Horsley RGN, graduated in Modern Languages, switched careers and trained in Aberdeen to become a Registered Nurse in 1981. After a few years of staffing, he was recruited by Professor Norman to join the British Antarctic Survey (BAS), overwintering in 1984 on the Faraday base. His subsequent career has involved coordinating the BAS Medical Unit in Aberdeen, a lectureship in occupational health nursing at the Robert Gordon University, and finally 12 years working in the offshore oil and gas industry.

Professor Andrei Karpov PhD, MD, Professor of Siberian State Medical University, President of Association of Remote Healthcare (Russia) worked at Tomsk Cancer Research Institute of the Russian Academy of Science (1982–2001) and developed the programs for screening and preventing the most important diseases (cancer, cardiovascular diseases, thyroid gland pathology, osteoporosis). He also introduced the strategy for protecting and improving the health of the working population, including programs for personnel of oil and gas, mining and nuclear industries.

Since 2001, Dr Karpov has conducted research on radiation risk assessment of cancer and non-cancer diseases in people exposed to chronical occupational irradiation at Seversk Biophysical Research Center of the Russian Federal Medical and Biological Agency.

In 2017, he became President of the Association of Remote Healthcare (Russia) and leads the development of educational programs for remote healthcare practitioners and elaboration of remote healthcare standards in Russia.

Graham Page ChM, FRCS (Ed), FRCEM, FFOM was Professor of Emergency Medicine at Aberdeen Royal Infirmary for 30 years. He was heavily involved in the management of the Piper Alpha disaster in 1988. He has long been interested in remote healthcare and involved in emergency medical cover for remote installations in the North Sea and worldwide. He also has experience of the medical management of diving emergencies, particularly in saturation divers.

Dr Will Ponsonby FFOM is a senior occupational physician who has much experience in remote industrial worksites such as the North Sea Offshore industry, the industrial areas of the Middle East, Russia, Kazakhstan and Azerbaijan. He has held senior medical posts in Shell and Rio Tinto and is currently President of the Society of Occupational Medicine.

Brian Wells BSc (Pharm), PhD FRPharm S began as a community pharmacist and went on to become a proprietor providing medical supplies to offshore installations, thus leading to the founding of Wells Offshore. He undertook oil company sponsored research into the pharmaceutical aspects of offshore health provision. This led to a PhD in 1990 and subsequent offshore and remote healthcare related work in addition to the supply role, including pharmaceutical advice, assistance with formulary development and medic training. Currently he is Offshore Pharmaceutical Consultant for Wells Offshore (now part of the Day Lewis Group) as well as Pharmaceutical Advisor to United Healthcare Global Medical (UK) Ltd.

Foreword

This book details the evolution of Remote Medicine from a niche interest of a few intrepid explorers to an emerging specialty affecting the lives of increasing numbers of workers, travellers and even ordinary citizens. The editors, Professor Nelson Norman and Dr Malcolm Valentine, are not only recognized experts in the field but write clearly and lucidly from their own experiences of medical practice in a number of remote environments. Their interest in the subject, first stimulated by the time one of them spent with the British Antarctic Survey, was fortified by the challenges of oil exploration in the dangerous conditions of the North Sea. Over the years, as the workforce not only increased greatly but grew older, clinical practice had to cope with the medical problems of an ageing population as well as acute trauma. The editors rapidly realized that healthcare workers had to be properly trained to deal with these changes which were replicated in many different parts of the world.

As oil exploration and mining moved into ever more remote and hostile terrain, medical services in many different countries faced similar challenges. While practitioners saw the need for shared research and communications to help solve common problems, medical and academic authorities have been slow to provide the necessary faculty support. That may now be changing with an increasing appreciation that techniques developed for truly remote locations may be applied to rural and even urban situations with improvements in patient care. As a population ages, the need to monitor many aspects of medical and social care inevitably grows more rapidly than the healthcare workforce. Hence the increasing interest in applying remote medicine solutions in different situations.

The editors were amongst the first to appreciate the importance of the evolving specialty of Remote Medicine. This readable volume will interest all considering how best clinical care can be delivered in the future. We have much to learn from Remote Medicine wherever we live and work.

Professor Sir Graeme Catto

Preface and Acknowledgements

Remote Healthcare is an emerging and rapidly advancing specialty of medicine. Much research and discussion is still needed before its tenets are finally agreed upon and accepted. This book provides a statement of its present position as a text for the knowledge and skill requirements to produce a competent remote healthcare practitioner, based on the system of healthcare which was first introduced in the 1970s for the offshore oil industry in the North Sea and which is now being evaluated for international use by collaborative critical research, with a view to the emergence of fully competent, qualified and registered Remote Healthcare Practitioners for global industry and also those general communities which live in remote places with hostile environments worldwide.

The development of the concept and the tenets of remote medicine over the years has been contributed to by a number of agencies and key individuals; and those mainly involved are acknowledged here. They include industrial and academic groups, service groups such as the military and police, together with those involved with environmental problems and hazards such as the hyperbaric environment in diving and environmental heat and cold.

Initial industrial development was by the medical directors of the oil industry such as Colin Jones of British Petroleum, Ronald Houston of Shell and William Leese of Mobil and they were ably supported by Matt Linning, then General manager of BP Pet Dev. The Robert Gordon University in Aberdeen was a key initial academic collaborator under the leadership of its Principal, Peter Clark, but with medical input from John Brebner and Valerie Maehle. George Smith established the Institute of Environmental and Offshore Medicine in Aberdeen University and Kenneth Donald provided input from Edinburgh University. The UAE University in Abu Dhabi was also much involved from the early days under the influence of Iain Ledingham, Owen Lloyd, Mohammed El-Sadig and with Graeme Nicol and Saleh Al-Mesaabi from ADNOC. The Grampian Health Board provided considerable service input under the guidance of its CAMO, Bruce Howie and with special involvement by David Proctor and Graham Page. The Grampian Police were in charge of preparations and action for emergencies and disasters and collaborated closely with medical groups. Key figures here were John Nicol, Ian Oliver and John Duff on mountain rescue. This led to the development of associated emergency services in the UAE police directorate in Abu Dhabi, under the direction of Mohammed Al-Keilli and Mustapha Shahab and also with Omer Sakaaf of the police ambulance service in Dubai.

Initial training courses were devised by Colonel James Adam of the RAMC while Royal Naval involvement related to saturation diving and hypothermia, directed by its MDG, Vice-admiral Sir John Rawlins and Commander David Elliott. The British Antarctic Survey was closely involved from the outset in defining the problems of medical provision in the ultimate remote situations and with extreme environmental hostility. The key contributors here were then Director Richard Laws, Eric Salmon, on logistics and personnel selection and David Walton on research.

The early development of remote healthcare was thus led by a wide variety of medical agencies and distinguished contributors. Current development is by an international consortium of universities- Glasgow University, led by Matthew Walters, the UAE University, led by: Michal Grivna and Mohammed El Sadig, the Siberian State Medical University, led by Andrey Karkov and the Camerino University of Italy, led by Francisco Amanta and Frano Mika. The academic group will be directed by two industrial companies led by Sergey Antipov in Russia and Nahyan Helal in the UAE. Finally, we express our grateful acknowledgment for excellent administrative support from Sarah-Jane Mackie.

This book is intended to provide the academic knowledge base for the professional development of the Remote Healthcare Practitioner. Hopefully there is also sufficient material in the book to promote self-awareness of the practitioners' knowledge level and thus the pursuit of further sources of information with consequent professional development.

Nelson Norman and Malcolm Valentine

https://doi.org/10.1142/9781786347510_0001

Chapter 1

Remote Medicine: History, Development of the Concept and Research

J Nelson Norman

Introduction

Remote healthcare was probably practised initially by armies marching through lands distant from their origins and it is significant that advances in medicine are often made in association with war. Indeed, the Romans are said to have had good healthcare as they marched through Gaul and Britannia. In more recent times, however, the motivating factors have been the need for the oil and gas industry to care for its personnel as they seek energy sources in increasingly remote and hostile places, as well as the problems facing Governments worldwide in providing healthcare for those who live and work in remote and rural areas of their nations. Medical communications is a key technology in all aspects of remote healthcare. Modern advances in that area originated in the space industry (NASA) as the world prepared to visit and explore the moon.

Development of Remote Medicine in the North Sea

In the early days of energy exploration, the oil companies merely took their required medical resources with them and even established fully equipped hospitals in the remote areas of exploration and production. This also provided well needed and appreciated medical support for many remote, backward and — at that time — poor states such as Kuwait, Abu Dhabi and Oman. Although the oil industry may have preferred to remain self-sufficient, that approach was not tenable when the action moved to the North Sea. This region posed huge new engineering problems of establishing the necessary massive structures — midway between Norway and Scotland — in deep cold water and it is one of the most hostile environments on earth. Health services were already well advanced in the nations surrounding the area and the media reported constantly on the horrendous accidents resulting from an inexperienced industry struggling with new and extremely challenging problems in both engineering and in the management of the healthcare of its rapidly increasing workforce.

The concept of offshore medicine thus came into being in the mid-1970s as a new branch of medicine which was sufficiently specialised to warrant special development. It subsequently became known as remote healthcare to indicate its global significance and its breadth outside the pure practice of medicine. The problems posed by offshore healthcare became so intense and challenging by the mid-1970s that the industrial, health and academic authorities in Aberdeen came together to solve the problem. First base in the successful solution of any complex problem is to arrive at a clear statement of the central problem. This was the time and distance which separates the sick or injured man from the facilities he may need for his care or even survival. This was the central tenet of remote healthcare at that time and remains the central problem for solution in its various aspects to this day.

There is also no doubt that the main central area tenet of medicine is diagnosis, for effective management of a medical condition requires the establishment of a clear diagnosis. Thus, following the clear recognition of the basic problem of remote healthcare it was possible to establish a system of medicine to manage the problem. The system which emerged after much discussion has five related and essential components (Norman and Brebner, 1987; Cox, 1987; Brebner, 1990):

1. Immediate care training for the whole population at risk
2. Development of increasingly sophisticated communications
3. Establishment of medical co-ordination and advisory site
4. An appropriate system of evacuation
5. Continuing research and audit

The first requirement is the training of the population at risk in immediate care to cover that vital time interval before definitive care can be provided. This is most effective if it is associated with the most sophisticated communications available so that advice can be readily provided by medical authorities at a distance — the third component. The fourth component is the availability of appropriate evacuation facilities. That can create major problems on its own in hostile environmental conditions and extreme remote situations. Equally, care of the sick during the extended time that evacuation may take can cause very challenging situations. The fifth and final priority of research and audit should probably be placed first because research must be at the beginning of any new initiative since it is the fastest way to provide the information to allow sensible development and solution of the problems which will inevitably arise in any new system of medicine.

As a research project, this approach had the disadvantage of being based purely on the opinions of those conducting the study. While a rigorous project with the collection and analysis of hard data would have been preferable, there just there just was not enough time to do this and activity by then was well established by commercial expectations, even if the morbidity and mortality rates in the early days were unacceptable. The system was thus established and developed and fortunately it suited the needs of the industry well.

First-Aid Training

This is essentially a special type of first-aid for laymen which takes into account the particular environmental problems of the work-site or the community. In addition to the usual first-aid areas, particular emphasis must be placed on communication skills for the quality of the description of the problem will reflect directly on the quality of advice provided by the remote doctor. Also, much emphasis must be placed on the accurate clinical measurement of certain basic parameters, such as pulse, respiratory rate, temperature and possibly blood pressure and they must be related to time. The importance of careful note keeping with time also needs to be emphasised together with eventually sending the notes with the patient in the ambulance.

A secondary but important function for trained first-aiders in any remote location is their deployment in a major incident especially if there is only one doctor or medic. Casualty handling teams should be trained and kept up to speed by regular innovative exercises so that they can immediately spring into useful action in an emergency.

Since evacuation and transportation may take many hours or even days, it is also important to give the trainees some clinical information on the basic clinical problems they may meet rather than the usual protocol type of training. This will allow the first-aider to make modifications to standard management in special circumstances such as the introduction of oral fluids during long or delayed evacuations and in hot weather. It will also allow for better management if evacuation is delayed and the first-aider is in charge for a more extended period than usual (Norman *et al.*, 2004).

Communications

A main part of an effective system of remote healthcare is the transmission of advice to and from the remote site. While the practitioner at the site needs to be able to use his initiative, it is clear that the senior staff at the home site must bear primary responsibility for the management of the patient once again in much the same way as the hospital consultant is responsible for the actions of his registrar. The responsibility issue is rather more complex when the primary consideration of time and distance comes into play. While the senior man at base cannot be blamed for non-attendance if the remote practitioner is several hundred miles away, it must be regarded as his responsibility to ensure that the remote practitioner is adequately trained to care for the particular population for which he is responsible. In commercial situations, the responsibility to ensure that the remote practitioner is adequately trained and equipped for his task should be held in large part by the authority employing him — usually in these days the provider of medical services since major companies have often out-sourced their medical services. In these days of litigation, the absence of regulation and registration of remote practitioners causes concern particularly for the practitioners themselves since they are often self-employed and thus vulnerable.

Voice communications can be misunderstood due to both poor technology and also to unusual accents, etc. and should always be followed by confirmatory written statements or instructions by fax or e-mail. Modern medical communications technology is developing all the time and it is necessary for both the doctors and the headquarters co-ordinating site to understand and practise the use of the equipment. It is also advisable for doctors to avoid the use of technical terms in dealing with lesser medical mortals (Leese, 1977).

Medical Co-Ordinating Centre

It is usual for a company to have a dedicated group of doctors to provide advice for their remote practitioners and these are usually local practitioners who have a special knowledge of the environmental conditions and particular occupational hazards of the area but there may be a sudden need for more specialised advice — as in an outbreak of an unusual infection or diagnostic problem and there is a case for the existence of a group of consultants who can be called upon for a second opinion or for special knowledge not immediately available to the local group. This needs to be set up in advance because it takes time to identify an appropriate consultant and once again, to be of value, he must be familiarised with the tenets of remote healthcare and communications technology if he is to be in a position to provide good advice.

In medical communications the best results will be obtained if the supervising doctor has been involved personally in training the remote population since he should then have a knowledge of the capabilities of the remote group and the resources at their disposal. He will thus be able to avoid giving instructions beyond the understanding or capability of the remote group. He will also be able to develop the type of relationship which in hospital practice develops between a consultant and his registrar and provides the safest and most effective patient care. This requires practice on both sides (Proctor, 1976).

Evacuation

Evacuation creates particular problems when it is required from remote places in hostile environments. The problem with distance during evacuation is the same as the central problem of remote healthcare — the time and distance taken to deliver the casualty to the hospital facilities he may need for his care. The clinical management of the casualty during transport over a long distance is thus an important aspect. In the North Sea this was initially approached by training escorts who were advanced first aid personnel. In serious cases however, they often became very stressed and also the approach did not fulfil the legal requirements in such areas as the Middle East offshore structures. Attention is now being directed towards the instrumentation of ambulances and helicopters with increasingly sophisticated measuring equipment to allow personnel at a distant hospital to follow progress and to offer advice to the ambulance personnel. The ultimate is the visualisation of the casualty. This also of course implies the need to provide training for ambulance personnel so that they can operate the equipment and respond to the instructions of the doctor at a distance (Leese, 1984; Wright *et al.*, 1988).

Trained ambulance personnel have reached a very high standard in military situations, particularly those associated with war zones in Afghanistan and Iraq where groups of ambulance personnel have actually swooped down on a battle scene from a helicopter, rescued casualties and provided emergency care on the return journey to hospital.

The training of ambulance personnel in the use of modern equipment and in communicating with hospital is similar to that required for remote medical practitioners communicating with a distant doctor. This suggests that ambulance personnel should be trained in the same establishment as the emerging remote healthcare practitioners. There are special circumstances where urgent diagnosis is important during transportation as medical knowledge advances. Such a case is stroke where cerebral thrombosis must be distinguished from haemorrhage if thrombolysins are to be used within the recommended three-hour period. In helicopter evacuation, consideration also needs to be given to the problems caused by such cases as epilepsy and acute psychiatric emergencies where safety of the helicopter is as or more important than the casualty.

Research and Audit

The fifth and final component in the system of remote healthcare is research and audit. There is little doubt that this should have come first because the development of any new system of medicine must be preceded by research if the most successful way forward is to be achieved. The five-point system was developed largely by discussion between academics and oil company doctors, together with specialists in the various areas involved — diving medicine, occupational medicine, military medicine, etc. The conclusions reached were further discussed at the various committees which emerged such as the Diving Medical Advisory Committee and the Council of the Institute of Environmental and Offshore Medicine, the medical sub-committee of the UK Offshore Operators Association (UKOOA) etc. The system was thus established by default since it suited the needs of the industry well.

The first real research in the area was in fact published as late as 1988 when hard data on the reasons for evacuations from offshore structures in the North Sea was collected in a joint research project between nine oil operating companies in the North Sea and the universities in Aberdeen. This revealed many surprises, such that one of the main reasons for evacuation was toothache! Also, a majority of evacuations were required for the normal spread of conditions which flesh is heir to rather than specific occupational medical problems. The pattern was different from that found in the general population since the offshore population had been medically screened, but the pattern changed with time due to the gathering experience of the industry and the emergence of safety and training departments. Initially, over 90% of the evacuations were required for accidents and traumatic events while very few were required for illness. As time passed and the population aged, the experience and actions taken by industry resulted in the gradual decline of traumatic events and the gradual increase in illness as the ageing population began to suffer from cardiac events, cholecystitis and obesity, etc. (Norman *et al.*, 1988).

In order to test the validity of the system, advantage was taken of the need at that time for medical cover by the British Antarctic Survey (BAS). Difficulty had been experienced in recruiting doctors for service on the Antarctic stations and since this was an area of extreme remoteness and environmental hostility there was a perceived developing crisis in Antarctic exploration and development. An experiment was thus developed between the British Antarctic Survey and the Institute of Environmental and Offshore Medicine at Aberdeen University to determine whether the system of healthcare established for the industry in the North Sea would work for the support of the groups of scientists working in isolated parts of the Antarctic.

Development of Remote Healthcare for the Antarctic

This study started slowly and proceeded over several years as doctors were recruited to take part in it. The problem had been that although there was no shortage of young doctors who would find a spell of work in the Antarctic attractive, it did not fit well with planning advice on training and career development given at that time by the leaders of the medical profession. It was, however, established with the Survey that following a tour in the Antarctic and the prosecution of a research project established by the University that the doctor would be given a paid year in which to write up his research and possibly obtain a higher degree. Equally, while in the Antarctic there was plenty of time for the doctor to study for higher qualifications in medicine in his chosen specialty. The final year of the tour would also allow him to make appropriate contacts and find support in the prosecution of his chosen specialty, (Norman and Laws, 1988).

On the aspect of medical service for the Antarctic Survey, exactly the same system as had been established in the North Sea was established for the Antarctic personnel. Medical standards of selection were conducted on exactly the same criteria as was being developed for the North Sea. Wintering in the Antarctic required a particularly high standard of medical fitness and the highest standard used in the North Sea was that for saturation divers so that was the standard required for those who wintered in the Antarctic.

The same first component of education and training for the population at risk was used and the Aberdeen personnel provided the course in immediate care used in the North Sea and the Middle East for all who visited the Antarctic under the British flag including the personnel on the expedition ships. Equally, the doctors were instructed on teaching techniques for maintaining these skills in the field and provided with appropriate teaching aids. This gave those exploring polar areas on their own or in small groups confidence and provided assurance that the doctors would have readily available assistance in the event of a major incident. All this of course mirrored the developments taking place for the North Sea and the Middle East. The medics of ADMA and ADCO, the operating oil companies of the ADNOC group in Abu Dhabi, had also been instructed on the development of casualty handling teams to assist them in the event of a major incident.

In addition, a special course was designed and given to the doctors for six weeks before deployment. This essentially consisted of areas which were not part of the standard medical curriculum such as how to take an x-ray rather than how to interpret it. Special advice was also given on medical communication, emergency dentistry, environmental medicine and first-aid. It is interesting to note that on evaluation the doctors unanimously stated that the part of the course they found most useful was the first-aid course which had not been part of their undergraduate course! In many ways this six-week course, which eventually merited the award of a diploma by the Robert Gordon University, could be regarded as the forerunner of the international qualifying course for Remote Healthcare Practitioners being developed today (Norman, 1985).

The second component of communication was equally difficult initially in the Antarctic, as it was in the North Sea, and was based on radio signals at appropriate times of the day. This was of course sorted out with time as telecommunications developed and after the Falklands war the UK Government provided finance so that there was telephone communication between the bases and medical support in Aberdeen. This also facilitated the supervision of the research work being conducted.

The third component of availability of distant medical advice was provided from Aberdeen. Three consultants were involved so that one was on call 24 hours of the day for the Antarctic. The whole consultant corps of the Aberdeen hospitals collaborated in this experiment and provided advice in their specialties when requested by the on-call consultants. This resulted in a very high standard of available medical advice for the Antarctic doctors and thus a high standard of medicine was practised by this means in the Antarctic — albeit many thousand miles south of Aberdeen.

It is worth noting that the consultants in Aberdeen also took part in the pre-expedition training of the Antarctic doctors. This facilitated the ability of the latter to obtain advice and that of the consultants to provide advice since they were already aware of the training and level of the doctors they were advising. Many of these points have been used over the years in the development of the system not only for the industry but for the whole area of healthcare provision for those who live and work in remote places associated with hostile environments.

The next component to be addressed was that of evacuation and during the Antarctic winter this was always very difficult and frequently impossible. Ships are only available during the summer months. Equally, it was found that the medical decisions on evacuation sometimes differ markedly from those which would apply in less extreme situations and this has implications for the training of those responsible for such decisions in other hostile areas.

Case Study 1

A twenty-two-year-old man who sustained a head injury while serving on an Antarctic base some 40 miles from the coast where there was a ship which could evacuate him. An x-ray had been taken but was of poor quality. It suggested, however, the possibility of depressed fracture of the skull and the local medical recommendation was for evacuation. This was rejected by the consultant in Aberdeen, however, and thereafter, some discussion ensued between the BAS logistics people in Cambridge and the intervening medical authorities in the Falkland Islands. Eventually, the Aberdeen consultant was told that he had only one day to make his final decision, for the ship was in danger of foundering and required to leave immediately. He did not alter his advice and his reasoning was that he was doubtful of the diagnosis in the first place since the patient was conscious and in apparent good health. Equally, he was under the care of a doctor provided with the full range of medical supplies. Evacuation for a start would require the casualty to be loaded onto a sledge and transported over the humps and bumps of the ice shelf terrain of the Antarctic for the 40 miles to the ship where he would come under the care of a doctor of equal training and experience to that on the base but with very much less medical equipment. It could then take around six weeks for the ship to reach the Falkland Islands and a small hospital after passing through the 'roaring forties and the screaming fifties' of latitude. An air journey to Montevideo would then be required to access the nearest neurosurgeon!

The Aberdeen consultant's view was that it was better for the patient to be left in his warm bunk on the station under the care of a doctor with good communications and equipment and in the event that elevation of a fragment of skull was required, this would be under the direction of an experienced neurosurgeon in UK and on a stable warm base rather than on the high seas in a gale and with greatly inferior equipment and by a doctor with precisely the same level of experience as his colleague on the Antarctic station.

Aside from making an important point on decision taking about evacuation, an equally important point is the need for readily available advice from an experienced senior authority at a distance for the junior remote practitioner.

The next case provides another example illustrating this principle.

Case Study 2

While an expedition ship was being anchored to the sea ice by burying the anchor in an area carved from the sea ice, one of the seamen, aged forty, had a heart attack and suffered cardiac arrest. Since all those deployed to the Antarctic under the British flag had the benefit of the first-aid resuscitation training from Aberdeen, his heart was successfully restarted and he was returned to the ship and placed under the care of the new doctor who duly reported the incident to Antarctic headquarters in Cambridge. The logistics headquarters personnel contacted the duty consultant in Aberdeen, described the incident and suggested that he only needed to inform the seamen's relatives because arrangements had been made for a plane to land on the sea ice to transport the casualty to New Zealand for treatment. The opinion immediately expressed by the consultant was that taking the casualty from the warm sickbay on the ship, lowering him over the side to a sledge, transporting him over the ice to a plane, followed by many hours flight to New Zealand would result in the possible early demise of the patient. Instead he advised that the casualty should be left where he was under the care of the doctor who had been provided with an ECG machine and a defibrillator. The ECG tracings were then telemetered to the desk of a consultant cardiologist in Aberdeen who assumed control and advised the remote doctor on further management in much the same way as a consultant advises his registrar or nurses in a coronary care unit. Eventually, the ship returned to the Falkland Islands and after consultation with a cardiologist there he was flown to Aberdeen where he had an angioplasty, recovered well and eventually went back to work.

These cases illustrate important points for the whole area of global remote healthcare. When a man on one of the stations developed appendicitis, the Aberdeen consultant advised conservative management by the system which had not been in fashion for many years and it worked well. Subsequently, a similar case took place in the North Sea in a saturation diving chamber and was similarly successfully managed. Several others followed and appendicitis is now routinely managed conservatively in urban surgical practice showing that the lessons learned in remote healthcare can sometimes be translated even into routine urban practice!

From a slow start the experiment worked well for the British Antarctic Survey since the initial recruits performed well in later life, obtained higher degrees and professional qualifications in good time and demonstrated advantages in career prospects rather than the disadvantages suggested by senior members of the medical establishment. The British Antarctic Survey now has no shortage of applicants for Antarctic service and many important points emerged in the development of remote healthcare (Norman and Brebner, 1988; Norman, 1989).

The experiment validated the original establishment of the system of healthcare established for the North Sea in the 1970s. Its success has provided confidence for further development in the international areas now being explored by the oil industry and also for all those who live in remote communities worldwide where healthcare is less developed than in urban areas where doctors prefer to work and specialists must to maintain their skills.

Research formed the basis for the development of the early courses for rig medics and they were designed by the Aberdeen Universities following the experience gained from the research both in the North Sea and in the Antarctic. The initial course was good in that it involved the hospital consultants who would care for the casualties when they were evacuated. Thus, the surgeon in charge of the burns unit was able to advise on the immediate care of burns and how he would like them to be managed before being delivered to his unit and the neurosurgeon was able to advise on the immediate care of head injuries before being delivered to his unit. This worked well in the prescribed area of the North Sea and its supporting hospitals but would be more difficult as the industry moves to ever more remote areas in its search for further energy sources.

In any event, responsibility for rig medic education was given to the Health and Safety Executive in the North Sea in the latter part of the 1980s (Health and Safety Executive, Offshore Division, 2002). Shortly thereafter the Aberdeen universities opted out and directed their efforts elsewhere. In effect that ended the period of independent academic medical research by the associated universities and the further development of the education of rig medics was continued by a series of providers and largely on a commercial basis. Ten years or so later, however, a university-based study was undertaken on the current problems faced and complained of by rig medics and this showed that their complaints were of professional isolation, lack of professional identity, lack of ability to identify appropriate educational courses and the absence of any system of regulation or registration (Horsley, 2005).

The Institute of Remote Healthcare was established in 2008 and accepted the challenge with a mission statement on improvement of healthcare for those who live and work in remote areas associated with hostile environments. This was an independent academic institution which had no funding apart from that provided by its members (both individual and corporate) who were interested in supporting its aims. It proceeded to establish a series of seminars and conferences in an attempt to answer problems raised by the medics, whom it now termed remote healthcare practitioners. It also established a website and a journal to further encourage discussion and consultation. Lack of funding, however, meant that research was slow to develop. Education for the developing remote healthcare practitioners still seemed the main area requiring attention and a major conference was held in Bergen where a large number of stakeholders from universities, oil companies and the providers of medical services came together in an attempt to determine what a fully competent remote healthcare practitioner should know and what skills he should possess. In many ways this resembled the 1970s approach when industry and academia came together to solve a problem. This resulted in the publication of a consensus opinion document in the journal of the Institute of Remote Healthcare (2016). This followed further consultations and conferences and it was approved by 129 stakeholders after the extent of consensus had been tested by a Delphi study.

The way forward seemed clear: for the educational institutions to develop appropriate courses; but if remote healthcare practitioners were to develop into the new medical specialty towards which they were aiming, it was important that the final courses developed were based on rigorous international research to determine what knowledge and skills one actually needed to be internationally competent, bearing in mind the different disease patterns, environments legal systems and dangers and since the consensus document was based on opinion rather than hard data. The Institute of Remote Healthcare closed in 2018 but since then industry has found it useful and the answer to this fundamental research question was regarded as important for the further development of remote healthcare in general and the emergence of fully competent remote healthcare practitioners as the industry penetrated into increasingly remote areas in the search for further energy sources. Equally, many governments have become conscious of difficulty in providing healthcare for their remote communities and oil industry medics were now seen as a useful and distinct medical resource, particularly in areas of vast remoteness as in Russia and certain parts of the Middle East and Africa. This was discussed at a conference in Tomsk, Siberia during which it was agreed to establish a purely research based association initially backed by four universities — Glasgow, the UAE University in Abu Dhabi, the Siberian State Medical University in Tomsk and the University of Camerino in Italy. The international Remote Healthcare Association was thus set up in 2019 and the foundation research project was the final determination of the educational and skill requirements to produce a fully competent remote healthcare practitioner initially for the international oil and gas industry based on data from medics practising in the North Sea, the oilfields of the ADNOC group in Abu Dhabi and those of Russia. The establishment of academic collaboration between the four universities will ensure research rigour and their close association with credible centres of accreditation and examination, such as a Royal College of Medicine and Surgery or a national centre of registration. Once again, as in the 1970s this research is required by industry in the form of the ADNOC group together with a main provider of oilfield medical support services in Russia — CCM. This will hopefully ensure its successful support and completion.

When this data is collected to a common protocol, analysed, and published, it will be possible for the institutions interested in education to elaborate on and provide appropriate research-based curricula. It is equally important, however, that the courses should be accredited and the trainees examined and awarded with appropriate certificates of competence by a credible centre recognized for this purpose such as a Royal College of Medicine and Surgery or a National Centre recognised for the purpose of regulation and registration.

This should finally allow the remote healthcare practitioner to become a recognized healthcare specialist in his own right and to seek appropriate registration, develop a career strategy not only in the oil and gas industry but also in those areas of community healthcare in the remote areas which interest him.

In order to establish the educational process on a firm footing it seems clear that an appropriate text is required and that is the function and aim of this book.

References

Brebner JA. 1990. The provision of healthcare in remote hostile environments Robert Gordon University, Aberdeen: PhD thesis.

Consensus Document. 2016. Competency and training for health care practitioners. *J Remote Healthcare* **7**: 31–51.

Cox RAF. 1987. *Offshore Medicine*. London: Springer Verlag.

Health and Safety Executive (HSE). 2002. Offshore Division. Operations Notice 55. Suitable secondary roles for offshore medics. Available at www.hse.gov.uk/offshore/notices/on_55.htm.

Horsley HD. 2005. An exploration of the role, practice and educational needs of offshore medics in the United Kingdom Continental Shelf. University of Aberdeen: MSc dissertation.

Leese WLB. 1977. Some medical aspects of North Sea oil industry. *Scot Med J* **22**: 258–266.

Leese WLB. 1984. Helicopter evacuation. *Travel Med Int*: 232–234.

Norman JN. 1985. Proposed diploma in remote health care. In: *The Rig Medic in Exploration Medicine. Proc. Int. Conf.*, RGIT, Aberdeen, 7.1,1: 1–4.

Norman JN. 1989. Medical care and human biological research in the British Antarctic Survey Medical Unit. *Arct Med Res* **48**: 103–116.

Norman JN, Al-Mesabi SH and El-Sadig MA. 2004. *Emergency First-Aid for Industrial and Remote Settings*. Victoria, Canada: Trafford.

Norman JN, Ballantine BN, Brebner JA, Brown B, Gauld SJ, Mawdsley J, Roythorne C, Valentine MJ and Wilcock EM. 1988. Medical evacuations from offshore structures. *Br J Ind Med* **45**: 619–623.

Norman JN and Brebner JA. 1987. *The Offshore Health Handbook*. London: Martin Dinitz.

Norman JN and Brebner JA. 1988. The establishment of an occupational health service for the British Antarctic Survey. *Arct Med Res* **47** Suppl 1: 365–367.

Norman JN and Laws RM. 1988. Remote health care for Antarctica: the BAS medical unit. *Polar Record* **24**: 317–320.

Proctor DM. 1976. Medicine and the North Sea — hospital support in offshore emergencies. *J Soc Occup Med* **26**: 50–52.

Wright IH, McDonald JC, Rogers PN and Ledingham IMcA. 1988. Provision of facilities for secondary transport of seriously ill patients in the United Kingdom. *Br Med J* **296**: 543–545.

https://doi.org/10.1142/9781786347510_0002

First-Aid for Industrial and Remote Settings

Chapter 2

J Nelson Norman

Introduction

The remote healthcare practitioner requires a good knowledge of first-aid since he will often be the only medical practitioner present at the scene of an accident or sudden illness and he may need to cope with the situation for a considerable time before the casualty can be evacuated to definitive care. Also, since the first component of remote healthcare is first-aid training for the whole population at risk he should be in a position to provide good first-aid instruction to the population for which he is responsible and maintain their skills. It is also highly recommended that he should train an advanced group of casualty handlers to assist him in the event of a major incident in a remote place before help from a distance can arrive. This chapter is thus designed not only to provide basic first-aid knowledge for the remote healthcare practitioner but also to provide information which will be of value in designing first-aid training courses for him. This can be challenging if not considered in advance since it implies the provision of useful information on the functions of major systems and parts of the body and maintainence of the interest of laymen. If interest cannot be aroused in trainees and complex questions answered readily, they will not learn and thus be of little help when the emergency arises.

There are three main phases in the management of a casualty in any situation but they are of particular importance in remote areas. They are:

- Immediate care
- The evacuation phase
- The definitive phase in hospital

Each of these phases is equally important and the best result will be achieved if each component works in sympathy with the others. The timing of evacuation is of importance and should take place only after stabilisation of the casualty has been undertaken at the site and in the full knowledge of the hazards of a particular journey, its duration, the mode of transport to be used and the personnel in the transport modality. The thinking and decision making will be different in remote situations from the golden hour of severe trauma management stressed in road traffic accidents. Equally, the decision to evacuate a casualty from a remote site is best made after consultation between the remote practitioner and the doctor at a medical centre.

There are three main aims of first-aid:

- Preserve life
- Prevent worsening
- Promote recovery

The first aim is the most important and you must remember whose life is most important to preserve. It is your own life. In the initial panic of an accident it is very easy to rush into a dangerous situation without thought for safety and to lose your own life. Is the casualty still connected to the high-voltage wire which electrocuted him? Are you about to rush into a gas field area without a breathing set? Has the traffic been controlled in a road traffic accident? If you do not remember to think about safety as you approach an accident area you will not be much use to the casualty — or to anyone else — if you die!

The first-aider at the remote site is part of a chain of care — albeit an important link — and his immediate actions may not only determine the survival of the casualty, but the possibility of causing permanent disability if he does not handle him correctly. Careless handling of a casualty with a minor fracture of a spinal bone could result in the conversion of a simple injury to a state of permanent paralysis. This is one reason why the second aim of first-aid is to prevent worsening. Incompetent first-aid can be more damaging to the casualty than none at all. It is important always to remember that an unconscious casualty does not feel pain, for example.

The third aim is to promote recovery. This is placed third in line deliberately because the preservation of life and the prevention of worsening must always come first. The promotion of recovery follows and allows the first-aider to use his judgement and knowledge, when the initial priorities have been dealt with, to determine the best course of action but that part is more fully dealt with in the definitive hospital phase.

Emergencies usually arise unexpectedly and always cause a degree of confusion if not downright panic in those close by and upon whom the casualty may be relying to save his life. Panic is responsible for the majority of wrong actions and careless handling and it is difficult to determine what can be done about it. A certain degree of panic will initially be present in even the most experienced and knowledgeable first-aider. This is probably because most will rarely be presented with real emergencies which are unexpected. Panic will always cloud the issue and make it difficult to think in a clear and logical manner. Since the necessary immediate actions to preserve life and to prevent worsening must be undertaken rapidly that phase is best learned as a drill (see below) and when that has been followed and the panic has settled the first-aider can then use his mind to determine the next best steps to promote recovery.

Determining Priorities

The most natural response to observing another human in serious trouble is to rush to his aid. The first and key duty of the first-aider is to preserve life but it is very important to emphasise once more that the most important life to preserve is your own.

Case Study 1

Many years ago, in the onshore workings of a well-known Middle East oil company a man was working on a gas pipe joint in a depression when it suddenly leaked. The high concentration of hydrogen sulphide in the gas ensured that he lost consciousness and stopped breathing after a few breaths. His friend saw what had happened and rushed to his aid only to be overcome by the gas just as rapidly. A third and then a fourth man ended up in the same condition. In all seven men succumbed until the eighth stopped, thought through and assessed the situation. He sounded the alarm, sought out a breathing apparatus and dealt with the emergency. Several lives were lost from thoughtlessness and panic.

An important function of the remote healthcare practitioner is training the population for which he is responsible in immediate care, together with the institution of training of casualty handling teams to provide support for himself in a major incident situation until help from a distance arrives. A useful way to explain how the body works is to explain that it consists of millions of cells, each of which can be compared to a chemical factory which takes in raw materials (food and drink) and a produces a product. Like any other factory the cells need a source of energy or fuel and there are waste products to be expelled. The fuel is oxygen and the main waste product is carbon dioxide. If the cells are provided with oxygen in lesser quantities than they need, their function is disturbed and if the oxygen deprivation is sufficiently prolonged and severe, the factory (cell) will cease to function altogether. Soon thereafter it will undergo irreversible damage and, finally, it will die. It is important to learn to recognise the signs of oxygen deprivation, realise the significance and urgency and restore the oxygen supply as rapidly as possible. This is the first priority.

Some cells are less sensitive to lack of oxygen than others and the body takes action to deviate the available blood and thus oxygen to the areas where it is most needed. These prospective responses of the body towards its own survival should be assisted where possible. The brain is the tissue most sensitive to oxygen lack and when the brain is totally deprived of oxygen it will only survive intact for between 4 to 6 minutes. When the brain becomes critically short of oxygen, consciousness is lost and the casualty falls to the ground. This has a protective effect of using gravity to improve the blood or oxygen supply to the brain, since it is much easier for the heart to pump blood on the level to the brain than uphill.

The heart comes next. When the heart is deprived of oxygen it will soon stop beating but it will not suffer irreversible damage for about 15 minutes. Equally, the kidneys may survive oxygen deprivation for half an hour or a little more. Muscle, on the other hand, will last for about two hours and skin for seven or eight hours. When a man dies in the evening and you look at the body the next morning, it may well need a shave — because the skin did not necessarily cease its function when the heart stopped and the brain died.

The brain, the heart and the kidneys are thus regarded as the vital organs because they are the most sensitive to oxygen lack. For that reason, the seriously ill or sick person is usually laid down to help ensure the best oxygen supply to these important organs. It is also a reasonable manoeuvre to raise the legs, thus assisting gravity once again to pour as much blood as possible into the torso area and away from the limbs where it is less vital to maintain oxygen delivery during the emergency. The whole body can even be tilted head down to help deviate the maximum blood volume to the head end and the vital organs. There are, of course, important exceptions to these generalisations such as chest and head injuries.

Approach to a Casualty

Whether you are a boy scout, a policeman, an ambulance paramedic or a consultant surgeon the best approach to a case of sudden illness or injury is the same. As you approach, call for help or ask someone else to do so. Keep as calm as possible and as you move in remember the importance of checking the scene to avoid rushing into the toxic atmosphere of a gas-filled room or switching off the power of the flex leading to the electrical apparatus the casualty is holding. This is difficult in the presence of panic and that is why a drill type of approach works best. The call for help may not be necessary if you are dealing with a very minor injury but will do no harm and if you need help and have not called it is difficult to interrupt a resuscitation process you have embarked upon to do so.

When you arrive at the safe and secure locus, the casualty may explain his problem and you can set about treating him. If he is not conscious, however, he cannot do so and the approach is different, bearing in mind the priorities described above and the vulnerability of the various tissues. Thus, a drill needs to be followed.

Unconsciousness

In unconsciousness the body is in its most vulnerable condition. The automatic reflexes are all lost including the swallowing reflex which protects the airway and the corneal reflex which protect the eyes. Pain and discomfort are important protective mechanisms and the loss of pain is very important to remember in casualty handling since clumsy handling can result in serious damage to an already damaged area and can convert a simple injury such as a closed fracture to a much more serious and complicated condition such as a bone end now protruding through the skin.

It has already been established that the first priority is to ensure the supply of oxygen to tissues and this means that the first action should be to secure a clear airway. In the conscious subject the tongue is normally parked in the roof of the mouth but when consciousness is lost the tongue is no longer controlled and if the casualty is lying on his back his tongue may fall back and block the airway. The first action is to ensure that the airway is open by placing a finger gently on the chin and dipping the head back. This will ensure that the tongue is clear of the airway. Thereafter the mouth should be opened and a finger passed through it to ensure that blockage is not caused by vomit or food.

Having ensured that the airway is open the next step is to determine whether the casualty is breathing and if not, to do something about it. This is done partly by observing the presence of chest or abdominal movement but mainly by placing a ear hard against the casualty's nose and listening for/feeling the movement of air. If breathing is not detected or you are not sure then deliver two mouth-to-mouth breaths and then determine whether the pulse is present. If the pulse is present continue with mouth-to-mouth breathing until spontaneous respiration is established. If there is no detectable pulse then cardiopulmonary resuscitation should be undertaken. These practical manoeuvres must be undertaken precisely to be effective and are best learned by attending a standard first-aid course after which they should be practised regularly to avoid skill decay.

You have now attended to the risks to the most vulnerable organs — brain and heart — which are the immediate priorities and you can now proceed to a more detailed examination of the body for other injuries which may need attention. A useful mnemonic to remind you of the first three essential actions is ABC:

- A for Airway
- B for Breathing
- C for Circulation

Now that possible immediate life-threatening problems are either confirmed not to be present or have been dealt with, the following processes can be dealt with more calmly and methodically. Examine the whole body systematically starting from the head and working towards the feet. You are looking for evidence of injury, bleeding or broken bones which may need to be attended to before you proceed to the next step. Blood is obvious on a white shirt but not so on jeans or boiler suits, which can just seem damp. Feel the limbs systematically and firmly. Swelling or deformity may suggest a fracture but remember there will be no pain or discomfort. If bleeding is detected it should be stopped and if you suspect a fracture immobilise the part appropriately. Finally, it is worth checking the casualty's pockets — this could identify him or his next-of-kin and he may be carrying a card affirming that he is suffering from a condition associated with episodes of unconsciousness — epilepsy or diabetes. Also, he may have something in his pocket which could injure him when moved — such as a screwdriver.

You are now left with an unconscious casualty lying on his back, whose airway can become compromised at any time. The tongue may fall back — he may vomit and it is not uncommon for people to vomit when consciousness begins to return. The next action is placing him a position where the airway is as safe as it can be. This is known as the recovery position.

Recovery position

- Kneel close to the casualty and turn him towards yourself — where you exert most control when turning. Before turning him, tuck the nearside arm under the body and place the far side arm over the chest. Also, cross the far side leg over the nearside and turn the head slightly towards yourself.
- With one hand on the hip, or with the thumb hooked around the belt, and the other on the shoulder, turn the casualty onto his side facing you and in a position of balance. At that point, transfer one hand to the casualty's shoulder and support his head and face with your other hand.
- Gradually move your knees back and allow the casualty to fall towards you by his own weight while supporting the head towards a slightly extended resting position gently.
- Flex the knee which is now nearest you to maintain stability and recover the arm which the casualty may be lying upon, to avoid pressure damage.

The casualty is now in the recovery position but vigilance should be maintained — he must not be left alone until help arrives or consciousness returns. Many of the causes of unconsciousness are progressive conditions and progression can proceed to arrest of breathing or the heart. The first-aider should stay close to the head end and keep talking to the casualty as he watches for evidence of a changing state of consciousness and continues to observe the rate of breathing and the pulse. If left alone and consciousness begins to return, the casualty may well roll over onto his back and obstruct the airway with his tongue. Returning consciousness is also the time when vomiting is most likely to occur.

If the casualty begins to vomit while you are examining him or turning him in a controlled manner this becomes a life-threatening emergency and demands immediate and urgent action. Heave the casualty onto his side — away from you — without further hesitation. Keep your knees close to his upper back and bend over him so that you are in a position to help clear the airway as effectively and quickly as possible.

It is sometimes argued that it is safer to leave a casualty on his back if you suspect the possibility of an injury to his back or neck. If, however, he should vomit whilst on his back he is likely to die. If it is necessary to adopt the emergency approach to the recovery position it is likely that much more damage will be done than if he is turned in a slow, controlled manner. The important thing is to avoid twisting of the back and to support the head and neck as much as possible. If a neck cuff is available it is worth applying it before turning the casualty but if not, newspaper secured with a piece of string offers some protection. For all these reasons, the unconscious casualty should always be placed in the recovery position — slowly, deliberately and gently and observed continuously until transferred to the next line of care.

While it is accepted that the cause of unconsciousness is not nearly so important for the first-aider as its correct management, he should always be on the lookout for clues which could help those responsible for diagnosis and definitive care and pass this information on — an empty bottle of tablets on a bedside table, a card stating the name of a disease, like diabetes for instance. There are, however, a few conditions associated with unconsciousness which require special knowledge of the first-aider and it seems reasonable to deal with them at this time. These conditions are fainting, epilepsy, diabetes, stroke and head injury.

Fainting

Fainting is a condition which occurs when the brain becomes critically short of oxygen. Consciousness is lost and the casualty falls to the ground. Gravity then restores the oxygen supply and consciousness returns. It often occurs in a hot, stuffy room, or when standing for long periods — as in soldiers on parade — when blood pools in the lower part of the body and fails to transport oxygen in sufficient quantities to the brain. It can also occur in severe emotional distress where it acts as a protective mechanism, presumably by causing spasm of the blood vessels supplying the brain and slowing the heart.

The subject usually feels dizzy and disorientated before fainting and often feels sick, becomes pale and breaks out in a sweat. If these signs occur, a faint can be avoided by laying the casualty down and loosening tight clothing. If the faint does occur, however, it should be treated like any other cause of unconsciousness through the routine described above. By the time the casualty has been placed in the recovery position consciousness will usually have returned. If consciousness does not return medical advice should be sought since the cause may not be fainting. If consciousness returns readily the casualty should be kept lying down for an hour or so until the balance of his heart and blood vessels recovers — otherwise he will just faint again. Fainting is usually associated with a slow pulse and this helps to distinguish it from more serious conditions which are usually associated with a fast pulse.

Epilepsy

If the brain is considered to consist of a large mass of insulated wires, an epileptic attack can be likened to a short circuit or sudden electrical fault where there is a massive release of energy resulting in loss of consciousness and violent uncoordinated muscle activity known as convulsions. Sometimes, epilepsy follows a birth injury, sometimes a head injury and sometimes the cause is obscure.

If the epileptic is approached as in any other unconscious casualty it will be found that he is not breathing and the airway cannot be examined since the jaw is clamped shut tightly. The mouth cannot be opened because the spasm is too fierce. There is a popular myth that epileptics bite their tongue and so must have some sort of gag placed between the teeth. In fact, epileptics rarely do this and attempts to place something between the teeth are best avoided; if the object used breaks, parts may end up inside the mouth where they are not easily removable. If it does not break, the teeth probably will. The first-aider stupid enough to place his fingers between the teeth, deserves all he gets! The spasm will relax.

Since the chest muscles are also in spasm, there will be no evidence of breathing and the casualty may develop a deepening blue colour. This is one occasion when the first-aider should not be concerned if the casualty is not breathing — he will breathe again and in any case there is nothing he can do about it. The important thing to remember about an epileptic attack is the basic problem of unconsciousness that the casualty is unable to protect himself. Main efforts must therefore be directed towards preventing the casualty from injuring himself. Furniture against which he may strike and damage his limbs should be moved and the limbs directed away from such objects. In particular the head should be protected by placing a cushion beneath or even between the first-aiders knees. On no account should attempts be made to restrain the casualty — this will only result in broken bones.

The convulsion will only last for a few minutes and then the casualty will relax and become flaxen. The more usual type of unconscious casualty results and needs to be dealt with according to the usual drill. He should be put in the recovery position until consciousness is regained. He will probably be confused and disorientated for a while thereafter, so he should not be left alone until the first-aider feels it is safe to do so.

Epileptic fits are not common because drugs are available to control them. Following an attack, the drug regime may need reappraisal. An epileptic fit in a helicopter can be very difficult to manage and could also compromise the safety of the whole helicopter and its crew. If the casualty is to be evacuated from a remote place by helicopter after a fit, medical advice should be sought about possible medication and precautions before the journey is commenced.

Diabetes

In diabetes there is a failure to produce insulin and following a meal the concentration of blood sugar rises to such levels that it spills out in the urine and is lost. Insulin directs the absorbed sugars to storage sites in the liver and muscles and maintains the blood sugar concentration at a standard level. When an energy source is needed, insulin releases sugar from the storage depots and provides it. In diabetes the storage depots are thus empty, and muscle and other tissues are broken down for fuel. The body gradually wastes away and would die if synthetic insulin were not now available.

The diabetic taking insulin must live a reasonably ordered life however. His morning dose of insulin is calculated to take account of the meals he expects to eat and the physical exertion he expects to have. If his schedule is disturbed and he misses his lunch or plays an unexpected game of tennis for example, he may have too much insulin and the level of blood sugar falls.

When the blood sugar falls to low levels, the diabetic becomes dizzy, disorientated and confused. He often breaks out into a sweat. His speech can become incoherent and he can become physically objectionable or even violent. The appearances are so like drunkenness that such casualties are often arrested and put in a prison cell where they may be found dead some hours later. If nothing is done, the confused state proceeds to unconsciousness and then on to death.

All that is needed is to give the casualty sugar to eat — a sweet or even a biscuit. If there is rapid improvement, he should be given more sugar and sent for medical advice. If there is a delay, however, and the first-aider does not take such action, the opportunity will be missed and the casualty may become unconscious. Under these circumstances, of course, nothing can be given by mouth and he will become seriously ill, requiring intravenous sugar injection. It is universally accepted that there are two types of diabetic emergencies — one when the sugar level is too low and the other when it is too high. The first-aider does not need to distinguish between these states. If the blood sugar is too high and the casualty is given sugar, there will be no improvement, but no harm will have been done. The basic message is that if someone is behaving strangely, who is known or suspected to be diabetic he should be given sugar and even more if he improves. If the diagnosis is wrong no harm would have been done but if it is right a dangerous episode of unconsciousness would have been avoided and the casualty's life may even have been saved.

Stroke

A stroke occurs when a blood vessel in the brain becomes blocked by a blood clot or when the blood vessel ruptures and bleeding takes place, damaging surrounding brain tissue and increasing the pressure in the skull which also damages the brain further.

Stroke may present as a sudden case of unconsciousness and should be dealt with using the standard drill followed by taking medical advice. It may however develop more slowly and manifest itself by developing weakness in a limb and particularly in the muscles of one side of the face. Speech may be disturbed or difficult. If any of these signs occur and a stroke is suspected this must be regarded as a very urgent medical emergency because with the advent of fibrinolysis, the clot can be dissolved and the casualty returned to normal, avoiding permanent paralysis. Accurate diagnosis is however required to avoid worsening in a case of cerebral haemorrhage. If the treatment is to be successful it must be administered within three hours, however, and this is a particular problem when the condition arises in a remote area. Research is currently active towards the diagnosis of stroke in remote areas but the message for the first-aider at this time if he suspects the possibility of a stroke is the organisation of the most rapid evacuation possible to hospital and urgent discussion with the medical adviser if that is not possible.

Head injury

The brain snuggles into a rigid, bony case — the skull. When it is damaged it may bleed and it may swell — as other tissues do when injured. The problem is that there is no extra room within the skull and bleeding or brain swelling causes pressure on other parts of the brain. This can result in widespread brain damage and death unless the pressure is relieved in good time by surgical means. After a head injury, it is not easy to determine whether bleeding or swelling of the brain are going to take place, so detailed observation of the casualty is vital for some time afterwards.

If the casualty has been unconscious — even for a very short time — he must be considered to have suffered a significant head injury and he should be observed for 24 hours thereafter and immediately transferred to hospital care if signs of deterioration take place. The most urgent and serious emergency occurs when a casualty who has been unconscious and recovers lapses back into unconsciousness. This casualty must be transferred with the greatest urgency to the care of a surgeon if his life is to be saved.

Following an episode of unconsciousness in a head injury the following steps must be taken every 30 minutes for the next 24 hours and every hour for the following 24 hours:

- Determine and record the level of consciousness
- Record the breathing rate and pulse rate
- Examine the eyes and record the findings

There are connections between the eyes and various parts of the brain which are associated with both eye movements and vision. Any changes in eye responses are important indicators of possible problems developing in localised parts of the brain. Some of these signs can only be observed if the casualty is conscious, but some can be observed if he is unconscious. The important danger signs in the eyes of the unconscious casualty are:

- Unequal size or shape of the pupils
- The pupil does not constrict when exposed to light

The real danger signs when observing a casualty who has been unconscious following a head injury are:

- A deepening level of unconsciousness
- Slowing of the pulse rate
- Any of the eye signs described above

If any or all of these signs develop, surgical advice must rapidly be sought. During transportation from a remote place further deterioration may take place — breathing may stop or his heart may stop. The escort must therefore be trained in mouth-to-mouth breathing and cardiopulmonary resuscitation techniques.

Levels of Unconsciousness

In the management of head injuries, assessment of the levels of unconsciousness provide important prognostic information and management information. This is important for both ambulance personnel and doctors managing brain injury in hospital. The Glasgow coma scale (Teasdale and Jennett, 1974) was developed for this purpose. It provides numerical values for various verbal, motor and eye signs. For the first-aider it is possibly more effective for him to define the levels of consciousness using his own words and criteria, writing down the state achieved against time at which the observation was made. Such a system could look something like this:

- Level 1.   Normal state of consciousness, alert and fully orientated
- Level 2.   Confused, disorientated. Appears to be asleep but wakes when spoken to. Readily drifts back to sleep
- Level 3.   Unconscious but responds to painful stimuli by withdrawing the part hurt. May make unintelligible remarks or noises
- Level 4.   Unconscious and not responsive to any stimulus, painful or otherwise

The importance of repeated assessments and recordings and the relation of these assessments to time is best illustrated by considering the position of a single assessment of a casualty at level 3 above. This could indicate rapid deterioration if he was at level I an hour before or significant improvement if he was at level 4 an hour previously. This is a further indication of the importance of time in the dynamic situation found in casualty management.

Respiration and Respiratory Failure

Respiration or breathing is the mechanism the body uses to transport oxygen from the air to the blood, which transports it to the cells of the body. The oxygen enters through the lungs which are contained within the chest. This is a closed box bounded by bone and muscle on all sides and below by a dome shaped sheet of muscle — the diaphragm. The box is perforated above by the windpipe which is in communication with the surrounding atmosphere. The lungs adhere to the inside of the chest wall where there is a negative pressure and they slide easily over that wall by the presence of a lubricating material. Respiration is controlled by a centre in the brain known as the breathing centre. This centre senses the concentration of oxygen in the blood passing through it and when it senses that oxygen is required it sends impulses down the nerves to the muscles surrounding the chest with makes them contract more forcefully and more frequently.

The ribs are angled downwards and when the muscles between them contract they are lifted up so that the diameter of the chest from before increases backwards; at the same time the diaphragm contracts and becomes a straight sheet of muscle rather than a dome directed upwards. This increases the diameter of the chest from above downwards. Since the lungs adhere to the chest wall, the capacity of the lungs is increased and air is passively drawn from the outside down into the lungs. When the breathing centre ceases sending its impulses the muscles relax, the ribs fall into the resting position and the diaphragm once again domes up into the chest. This reduces the capacity of the lungs and air is once again passively forced outwards. This is known as the mechanism of breathing which will stop if there is damage to the breathing centre in the brain. It will also become ineffective if there is severe damage to the chest as, for example, in a crush injury.

The lungs essentially consist of a vast, very thin membrane and if the lungs were removed and the membrane spread out each lung membrane would cover half of a tennis court. During breathing one side of this membrane is covered with blood and the other with air. Diffusion of the gases across this membrane takes place very rapidly, the blood entering one side of the membrane is short of oxygen and contains an excess of carbon dioxide. When it leaves again, it has equilibrated with the air so that it has gained oxygen and lost carbon dioxide which leaves the lungs when expiration takes place.

Air contains 20% of oxygen and when it leaves the lungs it contains 16% of oxygen. Only 4% of oxygen is extracted. Exhaled air thus contains 16% of oxygen and that is a very useful gas for someone who has no oxygen because he is not breathing. That is the scientific basis of mouth-to-mouth breathing in resuscitation.

Normal breathing is quiet and painless and takes place at a rate of 10 to 20 breaths per minute in the adult at rest and the average rate it is taken is 15 breaths per minute or one every four seconds. This suggests that when breathing is taken over for someone who has stopped breathing, he should be given one breath every four seconds.

Respiratory failure

The leading causes of respiratory failure are:

- Obstruction of the airway
- Poisoning
- Head injury
- Drowning
- Chest injury

All these conditions lead to damage to the breathing centre and that is why breathing ceases. In poisoning, the breathing centre can be affected by such agencies as a massive overdose of sleeping tablets or the inhalation of a high concentration of a gas such as hydrogen sulphide or carbon monoxide. In head injury, if the brain bleeds or swells the increasing pressure within the skull may damage that part of the brain containing the breathing centre and breathing will stop. Certain of these causes require individual attention and obstruction or choking, drowning and chest injury will next be considered.

Choking

If a few crumbs or some fluid accidentally enters the windpipe it results in a violent spasm of coughing and spluttering. This means that air is still entering and leaving. The first-aider should however be concerned if the casualty cannot speak, places his hand on his throat and silently appears to be trying to rid himself of something blocking his air passage. This usually takes place during a meal or in a restaurant and is embarrassing. The casualty often rushes from the room to the toilet. Under no circumstances must he be left alone at this time because if his windpipe is indeed blocked, he has only a few minutes to live unless something is done.

It is now accepted that backslapping wastes time, is unlikely to dislodge a blockage and may in fact lodge it further down. The correct action is known as the Heimlich manoeuvre. Heimlich argued that there is always a quantity of residual air in the lungs when the windpipe is blocked and if a sharp upward flow of air takes place it would dislodge the blockage. This is achieved by an up and under thrust of the diaphragm by standing behind the casualty placing a fist midway between the belt line and the chest, while anchoring the casualty's body against the first-aider's own. A sharp up and under thrust is then delivered and if that does not result in the ejection of the block it should be repeated until it does for it is the most likely means of removing the obstruction. For efficiency this manoeuvre should be practised under instruction at a first-aid course.

If the obstruction is not removed the casualty will soon become unconscious. Indeed, he may be unconscious by the time he is found. In these circumstances the Heimlich manoeuvre for the unconscious casualty should be adopted. The head should be turned to one side and the body straddled over by the first-aider who should place the heel of his hand supported by the other hand in the same position as before and undertake upward and under abdominal thrusts. After four thrusts the offending object can be scooped from the mouth with a finger.

In dealing with an infant or a young child it is probably better to lift them upside down and slap the back. For a larger child an attempt can be made to tilt him head down over the first-aider's knees while slapping the back. If these manoeuvres do not work the Heimlich manoeuvre should be employed.

When the obstruction has been removed the casualty may still not be breathing if damage has been caused to the breathing centre. It may still be necessary to undertake mouth-to-mouth breathing in order to obtain satisfactory restoration of breathing. When this has been achieved, he may still be unconscious and needs to be placed in the recovery position until help arrives.

Drowning

When water hits the back of the throat the windpipe often goes into tight spasm, preventing the entry of further water. Air is also excluded and the breathing centre is eventually compromised and ceases to function. There may be very little water in the lungs but however much there is, there is always room in the lung membrane for oxygen transfer and what the casualty needs is the restoration of oxygen provision to restore the function of the breathing centre.

Attempts to remove water from the lungs thus wastes time and it is unlikely that it can be removed in any case. In drowning the lungs only fill completely with water after death. Equally, attempts to remove water are likely to result in gastric contents containing acid to be aspirated into the lungs where it will cause serious damage. If the casualty is not breathing, his urgent need is for oxygen before the heart stops and there is always space for oxygen to pass across the lung membrane.

It is not easy to remove an adult from the water and serious damage can be caused during panic-stricken attempts to do so. In one instance, this resulted in a broken neck and the paralysis of the casualty for life — this was in the hands of a trained lifeguard! In a swimming pool if the casualty is not breathing the safest action may be to take him to the shallow end where mouth-to-mouth breathing can be administered and where the first-aider can stand. This takes care of the immediate priority — and should help to reduce panic. The casualty can be removed from the pool thereafter, carefully and with plenty of help.

The management of partial drowning essentially depends upon the stage at which care is provided. After being removed from the water, if the casualty is still conscious and breathing, nothing further needs to be done. If he is unconscious but breathing adequately, he should be placed in the recovery position to await the return of consciousness. If the casualty is not breathing, he needs mouth-to-mouth breathing until respiration is restored, followed by placement in the recovery position. If the heart is also not beating, there is a requirement for cardiopulmonary resuscitation, once again followed by placement in the recovery position.

A real problem in practice is the large number of bystanders who will shower the first-aider with urgent demands for action and advice. It can be difficult to do the right thing under these circumstances which is nothing — other than placing the casualty in the recovery position and fighting off those who would wish to undertake dangerous and unnecessary manoeuvres.

Case Study 2

Many years ago in Qatar, a nine-year-old girl who was an excellent swimmer jumped into a hotel swimming pool and was soon seen to be in trouble sinking to the bottom of the pool. She was fished out and found to be unconscious, not breathing but with a good pulse. Mouth-to-mouth breathing was commenced by a competent lifeguard encouraged by a host of concerned bystanders. Breathing was not restored and a short time later the pulse could not be felt either. At post mortem it was found that the cause of the problem was a boiled sweet lodged in and blocking the windpipe. The lifeguard may have been distracted by the panic-stricken observers because if the chest was not rising with each breath and he could not feel the air entering the lungs he should have investigated the problem. Children often do silly things like suck a sweet and then jump into a swimming pool!

There is a condition known as secondary drowning (Oliver *et al.*, 1978) which occurs at times after water has entered the lungs and caused inflammation of the lung membrane. This results in the swelling and a collection of fluid from the inflamed tissue. The fluid collects in the lungs — hence the term secondary drowning. There is nothing a first-aider can do about this which requires ventilation and appropriate drug therapy. The important thing is for the first-aider to recognise this possibility which usually follows successful resuscitation 12 to 24 hours before inflammation and it is particularly important when it occurs in a remote location. If successful resuscitation takes place in a remote location the casualty should be evacuated so as to be at least within easy access of intensive care facilities. If this does not take place the casualty may awake in the night breathless and in severe distress and urgent evacuation at this point may not be sufficient to save his life.

Chest injury

A chest injury may be caused by a crush fracturing the ribs or it may be a perforating injury from an external foreign body such as the spear of a sub-aqua fisherman. If there is air or blood issuing from the perforation it should be sealed with a handkerchief and covered by a polythene bag which is strapped in position.

It is very important in the management of chest injury that the casualty should be maintained in the correct position while awaiting help. Unlike other situations where there is shortage of oxygen and the casualty is laid head down the chest injury casualty is better sitting up since he is relying on the up and downward movements of the diaphragm for gaseous exchange and this may be limited by the gut if he is lying down. Equally, he should be tilted towards the side of the injury. This allows maximal function of the good lung to take place and if there is bleeding on the damaged side it will limit passage of blood towards the good lung thus compromising its function.

The casualty with a chest injury is thus cared for sitting up and leaning towards the site of the injury. If he becomes very distressed or even stops breathing during transportation mouth-to-mouth breathing will be required until he gets to hospital.

Mouth-to-Mouth Breathing

Before commencing mouth-to-mouth breathing it is of course essential to determine that the heart is still beating and that the airway is clear. Thereafter kneel beside the casualty, clip the nose with fingers, take in a deep breath, obtain a complete seal over the casualty's mouth with your mouth and blow sharply and firmly. The chest should be seen to rise and fall with each breath and the first-aider should feel the air going in. It is of course only necessary to compress the nose as each breath is provided. The rate is one breath every four seconds.

There is a tendency to breathe too quickly at first and this may limit the possibility of sustaining the activity for the duration required. The first-aider should therefore try to pace himself, conserving himself and giving about 0.8 litres each time and blowing no more than once every four seconds. In that way, it will be possible to carry on for the period of time which may be necessary.

If the mouth has been injured and if bleeding making it difficult to obtain a seal it is possible to close the mouth with a dressing, a handkerchief or with your hand and to provide mouth-to-nose breathing. This is just as effective. In an infant or young child, the mouth should be placed over both the nose and the mouth of the child and breaths should be given lightly and more rapidly than in the adult. The breathing rate of a baby may be around 40 breaths per minute. If you are concerned about the hygienic aspects of mouth-to-mouth breathing and the possible transmission of infection, you can use a Laerdal pocket mask, which covers the casualty's nose and mouth. As you blow tilt the jaw back with your fingers to keep the airway open.

The Heart, Circulation and Circulatory Failure

When oxygen passes across the lungs and into the blood it becomes loosely attached to the red pigment in the blood (haemoglobin) and as the blood flows past the cells it provides oxygen to them and receives the waste products together with the substances which the cells have manufactured. Gaseous waste is transported to the lungs, fixed waste to the kidneys and manufactured substances to appropriate parts of the body. This transportation mechanism is achieved by means of a pump which circulates the blood around the body. This pump is the heart which is merely an extremely efficient, small, mechanical pump.

The heart consists of a number of muscle fibres knitted together and within this muscle mass are four spaces or chambers. The first of these chambers (right atrium) is a collection chamber which receives blood which has been returned from the cells, spent of its oxygen and loaded with carbon dioxide. When the muscular wall of that chamber contracts the blood is forced onwards into chamber 2 (right ventricle). When this thick-walled chamber contracts it forces the blood into the lungs and spreads it very thinly over the vast lung membrane. Gaseous exchange by diffusion take place and the now fully oxygenated blood returns to the second collecting chamber (left atrium). When that chamber contracts fully oxygenated blood enters the fourth and last chamber (left ventricle). When this very thick-walled chamber contracts it sends the blood all the way around the body, past all the cells and back to the first chamber to repeat the process.

When each chamber contracts, the blood passes onwards and none backwards. This is because each chamber is fitted with a non-return valve. In valvular disease of the heart the involved valve either becomes too narrow (stenosis) or does not close properly (incompetence). In either case, the heart has to work much harder and eventually it fails.

Unlike the lungs, the heart largely controls its own rate and rhythm of contraction in order to supply the cells with the oxygen (fuel) in the precise quantities they require. If the leg muscles become active during exercise, the heart will beat faster to provide the extra source of energy (oxygen) required. The heart is not under the control of the brain although, like all other parts of the body, it is affected by influences from the brain and it will for example beat faster in times of emotional disturbance or fear. In general, the heart determines its own rate and force of contraction in response to a series of feedback mechanisms from the cells and it is coordinated by a pacemaker mechanism within itself. This nerve-like conducting tissue sends impulses to various parts of the heart, initiating contraction of the muscle chambers in a coordinated manner. In certain disease states this coordination is lost and the individual fibres contract on their own and in their own time. This is known as ventricular fibrillation. When this takes place, the effect is the same as heart stoppage.

The heart is a very robust and remarkable pump and one of the reasons it will stop beating is if it runs out of fuel or gas — oxygen. It is much more robust than the delicate brain and it will often carry on pumping for a minute or so after the breathing centre in the brain has ceased to function and breathing has stopped. That is why it is so important to examine the airway and breathing before determining whether a pulse is present. If oxygen is provided before the heart stops there is no reason for it to stop beating and the chances of ending up with a live casualty are much greater than if the heart has also stopped.

If there is no pulse after the statutory breaths have been given, cardiac massage must also be provided. There is obviously no point in doing so, however, if the blood is not oxygenated. The provision of oxygen must take precedence over everything else.

Circulatory failure

The causes of circulatory failure are the same as the causes of breathing failure but heart stoppage takes place after breathing stoppage when the heart runs out of gas. Under these circumstances cardio-pulmonary resuscitation (CPR) is required.

The only other reason for heart stoppage is disease within the heart itself. The disease is, however, confined to the coronary arteries within the heart which supply it with oxygen and which can become progressively narrowed by the formation of foreign material in the walls of the arteries. When the disease of the arteries reaches a level where sufficient oxygen cannot be provided to sustain the increased output required in times of exertion, pain in the heart is experienced in the same way as pain in the legs is experienced if exertion exceeds possible oxygen supply to the leg muscles. Heart pain is known as angina and it manifests itself as central chest pain which may radiate down one or both arms and up into the neck. The pain ceases when the exertion is reduced or stopped. Angina is not serious in itself but is an indication of developing heart disease and suggests the need for medical advice and a review of lifestyle and approach to risk factors. The risk factors include those which something can be done about and those which little can be done about:

- Heredity
- Age
- Gender

The age of appearance of symptoms is becoming progressively younger and is not uncommon in 40 and 50-year-olds nowadays. In the past, heart problems were more common in men than women but as time passes the incidence in females is catching up with males.

The risk factors about which something can be done are:

- Blood pressure
- Diet
- Exercise
- Stress
- Smoking

Of these risk factors, smoking is by far the most serious risk about which something can certainly be done.

Heart attack

When a heart attack takes place, pain experienced as angina comes on. It may not be associated with exertion but it does not cease at rest. The casualty may break out in a sweat, become pale and is extremely anxious. What has happened is that one of the narrowed coronary artery branches becomes completely blocked and that part of the muscle supplied by it is deprived of oxygen. The pain remains until that part of the heart muscle deprived of oxygen dies. If the part of muscle affected is small it is possible for recovery to take place and normal heart action to resume. If a large part of muscle is damaged or destroyed this may not allow for recovery and the casualty may die. The symptoms will be much the same whether the portion of heart muscle affected is large or small, however.

The first action when a heart attack is suspected is to put the casualty at rest both physically and psychologically. He should be placed in the position of greatest comfort either lying down or sitting up if he is breathless. He will be agitated and anxious. This will cause the heart to beat faster. The first-aider must remain calm and provide reassurance to combat this. Help should be summoned urgently since the level of progression cannot be easily foreseen. Close monitoring is required and the heart may be thrown into such confusion that it either stops beating or develops the abnormal rhythm known as ventricular fibrillation described above.

Heart stoppage and ventricular fibrillation show the same signs but if the problem is ventricular fibrillation the heart will not restart by cardiac massage alone and electrical defibrillation will be required. If a defibrillator is available and the first-aider is trained in its use, that provides a major advantage, but if not that is why help must be called for immediately. Until a defibrillator is available cardiac massage is essential but before undertaking it, it is also important to be sure that the heart has indeed stopped to avoid further damage to a heart which is weak. Three conditions must be met before cardiac arrest can be diagnosed:

- The casualty must be unconscious.
- There must be no breathing.
- There must be no detectable pulse.

When the conditions are met for the diagnosis of cardiac arrest, kneel on one side of the casualty and identify a position on the breastbone about two fingers above the notch between the ribs. Next, place the heel of the hand over that point and the heel of the other hand over it interlocking the fingers. Keep the arms straight, locking the elbows, and let the weight of the body depress the breastbone about 1 ½ inches. The compression should be repeated as close to 75 times per minute as can be achieved, bearing in mind that time has to be taken to provide breathing also. It is now considered, however, that compression alone will suck in air and should not be interrupted to provide breathing. If massage is adequate, a pulse will be felt in the neck during each compression.

The best ratio is 15 compressions followed by two breaths and after four sequences, pause to determine whether a pulse can be felt in the neck. If not carry on with a further four sequences until a pulse is felt. It may be necessary thereafter to carry on with mouth-to-mouth breathing until respiration is fully re-established.

Cardiac massage is hard work particularly in a warm climate. It is an advantage if two people carry out this manoeuvre, one on each side of the body, rapidly changing the positions of massage and breathing. It is important that they become able to develop a rhythm which does not involve interruption of the process. Two men are hardly sufficient, however, in really hot climates where two or three minutes of continuing cardiac massage are as much as can be sustained. The importance of providing shade is vital and there is much to be said for training a resuscitation team in these circumstances. The finesse is for the team to be practised in changing from one operator to another without interrupting the resuscitation procedure and that requires practice. If half a dozen people are involved, those not undertaking resuscitation should remain either in the vehicle with air-conditioning or in adjacent accommodation (Norman et al., 2004).

If recovery is going to take place it usually does so within 10 to 15 minutes but it has taken place following much longer. After the decision has been taken to begin, it has to be remembered that death can only be pronounced by a medical practitioner and in his absence the process must be continued until the First-aider is exhausted and unable to continue.

The main subjects of unconsciousness and resuscitation have now been considered. Before moving further, it is wise to revise the drill type measures which must be adopted when an unconscious casualty is approached:

- Check for safety and shout for help
- Determine that the casualty is unconscious and shout for help
- Check the airway
- Check for breathing. Give two breaths if not breathing
- Check pulse. If present continue mouth-to-mouth
- If pulse is absent, start CPR, confirm help is coming and get a defibrillator
- Apply defibrillator and shock as it will advise if automated. If ventricular fibrillation is not present but there is still no pulse, continue CPR until a pulse returns
- Check for other problems — fractures or bleeding, etc.
- Check pockets for identification or card indicating medical problems
- Recovery position
- Do not leave the casualty alone unless it is unlikely that help will come

The big immediate emergencies have now been covered together with the protocol type approach drill recommended to cover the immediate priorities in the face of possible panic. It is now time to consider the further examination of the casualty and the actions to take when other conditions are found. The most immediate of these is the management of bleeding and the care of wounds.

Wounds and Bleeding

The body contains about 5L of blood of which just over half is the red pigment containing red blood cells and the remainder is water with dissolved salts and proteins. If blood is lost from the circulation, the heart has to beat faster in order to deliver the same required quantity of oxygen to the cells as before. If the bleeding is not stopped progressively greater demands will be made on the heart and eventually it will fail. Immediate action is needed. There is only one good method to stop bleeding. This is based on the fact that when blood is not flowing, it will clot in between five and eight minutes. This is achieved by applying direct pressure to the bleeding point and maintaining the pressure for 10 minutes, allowing an extra two minutes over the physiological 5 to 8 minutes. When the 10 minutes has elapsed, the pad should not be removed. This may disrupt the clots formed. Merely apply a bandage to the pad to maintain the dressing and the clot in position and gently take the casualty to receive further medical help. When applying pressure, the best position for the bleeding part is to raise it as high above the heart as possible as this will reduce the flow making it more difficult for the heart to pump uphill.

After applying the firm bandage, the limb can be maintained in a high position by using a sling while awaiting medical attention. If the wound is dirty, no attempt should be made to clean it nor should it be examined at this point. If the bleeding recommences during transportation either apply a further firm bandage without removing the initial dressing or if it becomes excessive stop and once again, elevate the limb and apply pressure for a further 10 minutes. There is no hurry to get to a doctor — the greatest urgency is to stop the bleeding and to keep it from recurring.

The ring pad

There may be a problem in applying direct pressure in certain circumstances such as in a windscreen injury or head injury where glass or bone could be pressed into the brain. Another situation is that of an open fracture with a bone spicule sticking through skin. In both cases bleeding can be torrential and must be stopped. This can be achieved by using a ring pad. To form a ring pad, take a piece of material (a triangular bandage is ideal) and form it into a ring. Place this around the wound avoiding the area of concern and apply pressure until the bleeding stops.

Pressure points

There are areas where major arteries run close to bones. These are termed pressure points and sometimes bleeding can be arrested by compressing an artery against the bone thus reducing or arresting the bleeding beyond that point. The first-aider is unlikely to remember where these points are in the panic of major bleeding and should be advised to stick to the well-tried method of direct pressure and elevation. Equally, the use of a tourniquet is not recommended since it has frequently been forgotten during transportation to hospital causing severe problems for the limb below the band from oxygen deprivation.

Internal bleeding

Sometimes bleeding takes place internally, for example in a crush injury resulting in a tear of the liver. Blood is not seen but this can be suspected when the same general signs of blood loss occur. The pulse rate will increase as will the breathing rate since the breathing centre will sense a need for more oxygen. Nothing can be done but the bleeding may not be excessive and could stop spontaneously. That is why it is very important to handle the casualty with great gentleness. In this situation course, panic-stricken movements could cause much damage.

Bleeding from special sites

(a) Varicose veins can present as large dilated thin-walled veins usually seen around the ankle. They are very easily damaged by collision with a piece of furniture. They bleed profusely and the blood does not spurt out but flows out in a great pool of dark blood. The pressure in the vein is low and when the casualty is laid down and the limb raised the bleeding will stop immediately. Merely apply pressure and a firm bandage and maintain that position. Within 10 minutes the defect will be sealed by a clot.

(b) Nose bleeds can occasionally be copious and difficult to stop. Slide fingers downwards from the bone in the nose to the soft part immediately below and compress that part for 10 minutes as before with the head bent forwards. The head in this position allows determination of whether bleeding has been controlled. If the head is held backwards it is not possible to determine whether bleeding has been controlled and if blood runs into the throat and induces a paroxysm of coughing this will make matters worse. The position of the head is thus important.

(c) Tooth socket. When a tooth is extracted a clot forms in the socket arresting the bleeding. If bleeding recurs when an exploring tongue removes the clot it can always be stopped by placing a piece of gauze on both sides of the socket and applying pressure for 10 minutes. The reason why this is often said to be difficult is because of impatience and pressure not being maintained for the full 10 minutes.

(d) Bleeding from the ear is a situation where there is an exception to the rule of arresting bleeding. If bleeding is clearly coming from the ear canal following an accident the possibility of a fracture of the base of the skull is suggested. The damage to the brain which can be caused by bleeding within the cranial cavity has been described in head injuries. No attempt should be made stop bleeding clearly coming from the ear canal in case pressure is built up within the skull. Merely clean the ear and allow blood to escape. There will not be much blood loss.

Wounds

Wounds come in a variety of shapes and sizes and with a variety of specific problems but the two problems universal to all wounds are bleeding and infection. In a very deep and extensive wound the main problem is likely to be bleeding. If it is a limb and it can be elevated that will take care of the venous component and attention can then be directed towards the identification and arrest of the arterial component before binding it up with a firm bandage. No attempt should be made to clean such a wound at this juncture since the arrest of bleeding must be the main priority. Cleaning can take place in hospital.

An extensive deep wound will not necessarily be painful since the nerve endings are largely confined to the skin. On the other hand, an abrasion where the skin surface has been removed exposing the nerve endings can be extremely painful. Equally, an abrasion needs to be thoroughly cleaned before it is covered. Permanent disfigurement may result if road dirt has been included in the healing process. This can be difficult particularly dealing with a child — badly contaminated by tar for example — and may require a local anaesthetic.

Minor wounds can be easily treated by approximating the wound edges and maintaining the position while covering it with the dressing. Before this is done, it must be thoroughly cleaned, otherwise it will become infected, take a long time to heal and be painful. If it is thoroughly cleaned, it should heal by first intention very quickly and become pain-free very soon.

Puncture wound

This is probably the most dangerous wound of all since it looks innocuous and may not bleed much. The problem is that the depth is unknown and the puncturing agent may have driven road dirt or bits of clothing deeply under the surface and it may have penetrated an underlying structure. Puncture wounds can lead to very nasty infections — tetanus, gas gangrene, etc. Such a wound should be examined and possibly explored by a surgeon to determine whether an organ or joint space has been entered and appropriate action taken. If a surgeon is not available, communication with one is advisable.

Foreign bodies in wounds

This could be a knife in the chest or a piece of metal sticking into a finger. Anything sticking into the body should not be removed by the first-aider. It may have damaged the wall of a blood vessel, and pulling it out may damage it further causing internal bleeding that cannot be controlled. It may have partly divided a nerve and pulling it out may divide it completely so that the surgeon cannot find the ends to join together. The first-aider should place ring pads or bandages around it to prevent it from moving and transfer the patient to hospital where the surgeon will x-ray the object before removing it and plan its removal in advance.

Case Study 3

A young man was thrown from a car in the country and he came to hospital with a fence stake impacted in his chest. He was still conscious and very much alive. At operation, it was found that the point of the stake lay between the great vessels leaving the heart, but it had not damaged them. An attempt to remove that stake at the scene would probably have resulted in his immediate death. Fortunately, he met with casualty handlers who recognised that it should not be moved and so he survived.

Accidental Amputation

A finger, a hand or even a foot is occasionally accidentally amputated. If the casualty can be delivered to hospital before the tissue dies, modern surgery can sometimes manage its successful reattachment. The amputated tissue should be wrapped in a clean cloth and placed within a polythene bag which is then placed within a bag of ice. If the tissue is placed straight into a bag of ice it will freeze and be useless on arrival at hospital.

By covering the management of bleeding and the associated wounds which often occur, the situations which must be dealt with most immediately have been covered — unconsciousness, breathing, circulatory failure and bleeding. It is now time to consider special types of wounds and how they should be managed. The first is wounds of skin — or burns. Thereafter wounds of bone, or fractures, will be discussed and finally eye injuries.

Burns

A burn is essentially a wound of skin and the skin has two main functions:

- To keep the water which forms 70% of the body inside the body
- To keep the germs in the environment outside the body

When the skin is damaged by fire, these functions are lost and the main problem against survival is thus loss of fluid on the one hand and infection on the other. When death takes place following extensive burns it usually occurs early from loss of fluid which has not been adequately replaced or much later from infection. Death from fluid loss can be prevented in a remote area particularly if those caring for the casualty are able to give fluid intravenously. If the burn victim survives this early fluid loss phase the next problem will come 2 or 3 weeks later when he may fail to cope with the bacterial invasion which takes place even with the assistance of antibiotics and a clean environment.

Skin consists of many layers of cells of which the deepest layer is the most important because these cells are constantly reproducing to replace the superficial cells which become flattened, die and are cast off by washing and the general process of living. When a burn takes place, if the destruction of skin cells falls short of the deepest layers the burn is classified as superficial or partial thickness. The skin will be replaced by cellular division of the deeper layer and healing will take place with little or no scarring. If all the skin cells are destroyed the burn is classified as full thickness or deep. The skin defect will not be replaced and skin grafting will be required. This type of burn will eventually heal with ugly scarring.

It can be difficult to distinguish a superficial from a deep burn in the early stages but a superficial burn is usually red, raw and painful since the nerve endings have not been destroyed while a deep burn often appears dry and is pain free since the nerve endings have been destroyed.

The risk to survival following a burn is more related to its extent — in terms of surface area — rather than its depth. A convenient method to estimate the extent of a burn was determined by Wallace who divided the surface of the body into a series of percentages of 9. He allocated 9% for the head and neck and 9% for each of the upper limbs. Each of the lower limbs was allocated 18%, and 18% for the front of the torso and a further 18% for the rear of the torso. That makes 99% and the remaining 1% was allocated to the perineum. This is a very helpful rule in determining roughly the extent of a burn. The determination of extent is assisted by the additional fact that the palm of the casualty's hand approximates to 1% of his body surface.

In a remote area it is important to be able to determine the seriousness of a burn and even more important the seriousness of a large number of burns to determine priorities of evacuation which will result in the largest numbers of survivors. A burn involving 1% is sufficient to require professional medical care. When 9% is reached transfer to hospital is essential for survival since the casualty will need intravenous fluids and special care against infection. When it reaches 30% survival is still possible provided urgent evacuation can be undertaken but when it reaches 65% and over survival is unlikely in remote areas.

Case Study 4

Following a blowout on an offshore oil installation there were five casualties incurring burns of 10%, 32%, 40%, 51% and 80%. The first helicopter to arrive could only accommodate three casualties and the three chosen where those with 32%, 40% and 51% burns. The 10% also requires urgent hospital treatment but the urgency was not so great as the other three. The casualty with 80% burns was considered unlikely to survive and thus was evacuated later with the lesser burns.

Immediate management of a burn

The aim of first-aid is to limit the burn(s) to the superficial variety and this is achieved by cooling the area with running cold water. Since attention must be directed to the survival of the deepest layer of cells, cooling should be maintained for about 10 minutes to allow maximum cooling to penetrate to the deep cells of the skin. Thereafter the area should be covered, preferably with a non-adherent dressing such as melanin. There is little value in applying creams before evacuation since they will be removed during a subsequent examination. Equally, attempts to remove burned clothing may cause further damage but jewellery such as rings should be removed since burned tissue will swell and render removal difficult or impossible later.

Blisters should not be burst since that will leave a painful raw area allowing more fluid to be lost and infection to enter. They provide protection while healing takes place beneath them. A polythene bag provides useful and easily applied protection for burned hands or feet and in the conflagration of a disaster, burned feet protected by a polythene bag can still walk into an ambulance or helicopter while burned hands protected by a polythene bag can still lift a stretcher.

Chemical burns

A chemical burn should be managed in the same way — with running cold water applied for around 10 minutes. In this case, however, clothing should be removed to prevent the chemical running down from it and affecting other parts.

Fractures

Bones have three main functions:

- They provide support for the organs and structures of the body.
- They provide protection.
- They allow movement.

Bones also provide the shape of the body and any change in body shape implies a bony problem. Since the human body is highly symmetrical, it is always important to compare one side with the other when considering a bony problem. This is particularly important in considering the common fractures of the wrist or ankle.

The skull provides protection for the brain, the ribs for the lungs and the vertebral column for the spinal cord. When these bones fracture, not only is the protection lost but additional injury can be caused to the structures they are intended to protect.

Movement is provided by the action of muscles passing from attachment with one bone to another bone across a joint, as in a system of levers. When a fracture takes place, these functions are lost — the shape of the part changes, protection is lost and movement can no longer take place.

When a fracture, which is a break in the continuity of a bone takes place, it usually results from direct violence at the point of impact. Thus, a fall on an outstretched hand usually results in a fracture of the wrist and a fall from a height landing on feet usually results in a fracture of the ankle. It is important to remember, however, that in some cases the force bypasses the point of impact and results in the fracture of a distant bone — by indirect violence. A fall in the outstretched hand will thus occasionally leave the wrist intact and result in a fracture of a bone around the shoulder such as the collar bone and a fall from a height may leave the ankle intact while the force passes up the long bones of the leg and results in a fracture of one of the vertebral bodies — often one of the most vulnerable in the neck. Fractures caused by indirect violence are uncommon and probably occur in less than in 10% of fractures but it is always wise to remember the possibility.

Fractures come in three main varieties:

- Closed
- Open
- Complicated

A closed fracture is a simple fracture with no associated wound and the bone remains within the intact skin.

An open fracture is one where there is an open wound associated with the fracture which can allow the transmission of organisms into the healing area. The bone ends may or may not stick out through the wound. This is a much more serious injury and it is easy to convert a simple, closed fracture to an open fracture by inappropriate and coarse casualty handling.

A complicated fracture is one where there is an additional or complicating injury. For example, in a fracture of the skull a piece of bone is stuck into the brain or a rib fracture which may be associated with damage to the lung. In a limb an artery may become trapped between the cut ends of a bone.

Classical features of a fracture

- A history of violence
- Pain
- Swelling
- Deformity
- Loss of function

In some cases of injury all of these signs will be present and obvious while in others there may be considerable soft tissue swelling and damage but no broken bones. When dealing with a fracture, and if there is any doubt the injury should be treated as a fracture. If a bone is not broken no harm will have been done but if a fracture is not recognised before the casualty is moved a simple fracture may be made worse by converting it to an open one.

Management of a fracture

Approach the casualty slowly for he will be in great pain and examine him carefully without attempting to move him. If there is a wound with bleeding, the bleeding must be stopped, possibly with the assistance of a ring pad, and the wound covered before proceeding to immobilise the fracture.

The purpose of immobilising a fracture is twofold. Firstly, to make it safe to move the casualty and secondly to relieve pain because effective immobilisation will greatly relieve the severe pain of a fracture. The aim is to prevent the bone ends moving in any plane and this is usually achieved by immobilising the joint above and the joint below the fracture in the limb and with the use of liberal padding. It is preferable to use some form of splint but the body itself can be used as a splint by bandaging one area to another such as the injured leg to the uninjured. If you do this, move the uninjured leg to align with the injured before binding them together with as much padding as is available. The use of inflatable splints can be helpful and are easily applied but remember the pressure changes which can take place in helicopter evacuation, and there may be pressure changes in the injured limb due to further bleeding or swelling. There are other useful splints available in industrial sites such as box splints or vacuum splints but a cervical splint is easy to apply and can be used to immobilise the neck. A piece of cardboard can suffice and is useful particularly in road traffic accidents because the neck bones are very delicate and the consequences of fracture can be dire.

Eye Injuries

The main problem which requires attention from first-aid is of course that of foreign bodies. They come in three varieties:

- Free-floating foreign bodies
- Embedded foreign bodies
- Penetrating foreign bodies

The part of the eye which covers the coloured portion is the window — the cornea. That part should never be touched when attempting to remove a foreign body.

A scratch on the cornea will heal with an opaque scar which will affect vision from then on. A free-floating foreign body is one which moves about freely and which can be flicked out with the edge of a handkerchief, provided it lies in the white part of the eye — sclera — or the red rim. Never touch it if it lies over the coloured portion of the eye. If it is free, it will move during blinking or can be washed off. If it will not move it is likely to be embedded.

Before attempting to remove a foreign body, however, it is necessary to examine the eye systematically. Before doing this, the casualty must be in a dust free atmosphere with a good light. Hold the eye open and examine its four quadrants in a systematic way, asking the casualty to look up, down, right and then left. The only bit unseen lies beneath the upper lid and that can be examined by grasping the eyelashes and turning the lid over a matchstick.

If a foreign body cannot be seen it is likely that it has already been removed even although the casualty still complains of feeling, "something in his eye". It has possibly caused some surface damage exposing a few nerve endings. This will become pain free in time.

If a foreign body such as a sliver of metal is embedded in the eye it should only be removed by a person who has had special training. For first-aid, simply ask the casualty to close his eye and place a pad over it with a piece of strapping until help is available.

Great care should be taken if the foreign body penetrates right into the substance of the eye. Every effort must be made to prevent its movement. A ring pad could be used or an object such as a plastic drinking cup held over it and attached with tapes. To prevent the injured eye from moving, the other eye must also be closed. This is because both eyes move together. Place a pad over that eye, secure it with strapping and remember that the casualty is now frightened and blind and should not be left alone.

Chemical burns of the eye

In acid splash of the eye first-aid action must be taken immediately and the chemical washed out with large quantities of water continuously for a full 10 minutes. The eye will be tightly closed and very painful and after the initial washing it will be necessary to hold it open by pouring water over it. In all cases it is essential to be very careful where the effluent goes. It is a tragedy if the other eye is damaged by allowing the effluent to run into it.

Welders flash and snow blindness

These are burns caused by intense UV light. The pain is intense, like a handful of sand being thrown into the eye. Pain does not usually happen until 12 to

24 hours after exposure to intense light. Place the casualty in a darkened room and apply cold compresses to the eyes. Pain will usually resolve within a further 24 hours.

Poisoning

There are several thousand toxic substances which on entering the body will harm it and may cause death. The remote healthcare practitioner should always be equipped with ready access to a poison centre for advice since he will not remember specific forms of treatment of each. It is important for him to do everything possible to identify the poisonous substance for the specialists to be able to provide the best management. The body has a remarkable ability for changing the chemical structure of toxic substances into a less poisonous form and then excreting them. Provided the body can be kept alive for long enough it will eventually alter and eliminate nearly all poisonous substances.

The effect which a poison has will largely be determined by four factors:

- Type of poison
- Dose of poison administered
- Time during which the poison is allowed to act on the tissue cells
- Route of entry

Since the dose and time of exposure of the cells to the poison are important, the obvious immediate action is to remove as much of the poison as possible and as fast as possible.

The mode of entry of poisons is either by:

- The gut following swallowing
- The lungs following inhalation, i.e. Gas poisoning
- Injection, e.g. Snake bite
- Absorption directly across the skin, e.g. lead in petrol

Swallowed poison

A swallowed poison passes down the vulnerable thin-walled oesophagus into the thick-walled stomach and only enters the body when it reaches the absorptive area of the small intestine. Depending upon whether the stomach was empty or contained a meal awaiting onward passage there is thus a variable time interval before the poison can be absorbed and how fast. Action can thus be taken to eliminate the poison by inducing vomiting. The best way to do this is to touch the soft palate with a finger. Care must be taken however to prevent aspiration of the poison or vomitus into the lungs during this procedure. For this reason, it has been suggested that it may be best to leave the poison undisturbed in the stomach until medical help is available. While this is reasonable in an urban situation the induction of vomiting should be considered in a remote situation where the time to access medical help may be considerable.

What is more important is the consideration of whether the substance swallowed was corrosive or bland. If it was corrosive it may well damage or even perforate the thin-walled oesophagus when swallowed and if it did not do so on the way down it may well do so on the way up. When a corrosive substance is swallowed it is best to leave it alone until medical help arrives. Some water can be given to wash out the mouth and the lining of the oesophagus and possibly also for the dilution of the poison in the stomach. Milk is even better since it is a buffer and will help to neutralise either acid or alkaline substances.

It is of course obvious that if the casualty is unconscious nothing other than placing him in the recovery position can be done. Any other action may result in aspiration of gastric contents into the longs with disastrous consequences.

Inhaled poison

The main difference between a swallowed and an inhaled poison is the speed with which the poison exerts its effects. If there is a contaminant gas in the air breathed the partial pressure of the contaminant gas in the blood will be the same as that in the air almost immediately. Equally, if the casualty is removed from the contaminated atmosphere to clean air the contaminant gases will diffuse back out again with equal rapidity, if breathing is adequate.

Gases which contaminate the atmosphere cause their effects by three main methods:

- The exclusion of oxygen
- Irritation
- A specific effect

Whatever the contaminant gas, it will take up space in the atmosphere normally occupied by oxygen and so reduce the quantity of oxygen available to the body. Thus, nitrogen which is a non-toxic carrier gas can cause this effect when cylinders in a store leak. If a casualty steps into a store largely contaminated by nitrogen, he may rapidly lose consciousness from lack of oxygen.

The acid and alkaline gases cause irritation when they dissolve in the body fluids, particularly those of the mouth and airway passages but including tears. It is important to remember that these gases will affect the eyes as well as the lungs. Such gases are chlorine which dissolves to form hydrochloric acid and sulphur dioxide which dissolves to form sulphuric acid.

Toxic gases also have specific effects. Carbon monoxide from exhaust fumes forms a stable compound with the red pigment in the blood rendering it unavailable for oxygen transport. This takes place slowly even in very low concentrations. Hydrogen sulphide is very different in that it has an affinity for nervous tissue. Thus, its typical smell of rotten eggs is soon lost as it inactivates the sense of smell. It's main danger however, is the inactivation of the breathing centre in the brain which takes place at relatively low concentrations. This gas is heavier than air and when unconsciousness occurs and a colleague attempts to help, the exertion and associated deep breathing will soon result in the rescuer becoming unconscious also. In high concentrations of hydrogen sulphide, it is virtually impossible to rescue the casualty to clean air unless the rescuer wears a breathing set. When the victim of hydrogen sulphide poisoning is taken into a clean area he will usually recover spontaneously if he is still breathing. If not, mouth-to-mouth breathing will be required. It is worth noting that there is no risk to the first-aider in providing mouth-to-mouth breathing in hydrogen sulphide poisoning. The important thing to remember at this point however, is to wash out the eyes.

The administration of oxygen in hydrogen sulphide poisoning may help but it is not of great importance. It is however, vitally important in the management of carbon monoxide poisoning since it will hasten the removal of carbon monoxide from the blocked haemoglobin mechanism thus restoring the oxygen supply to the tissues. In an industrial situation where there is a pressure chamber supporting a diving operation, the administration of oxygen at 2 atmospheres pressure for 30 minutes will eliminate the carbon monoxide and restore the oxygen transport mechanism (Smith *et al.*, 1962).

Injected poisons

Injected poisons usually result from a snake bite or an injection of the wrong drug by syringe. In either case there is no point in employing the method advocated in John Wayne movies — cutting the area with a knife and attempting to suck out the injected poison. A poison once injected is fixed to tissues and will not come out by sucking. This is only likely to waste time and introduce a complicating infection.

The purpose of snake venom is to paralyse the snake's prey. Man is not prey and snakes are timid and unlikely to attack unless harmed or frightened in which case they may lash out and penetrate the skin. That does not mean that venom has been injected or indeed that the full dose has been injected. It has been clearly shown that in 40% of snake bites no venom is in fact injected. All that may be necessary is to put a dressing on the wound. On the other hand, in dealing with dangerous, venomous snakes the first-aider will not know whether venom has been injected and it may be necessary to administer an anti-venom. In this case speed is of the essence and urgent transportation to a source of anti-venom is required, which is usually a hospital preferably with an intensive care unit. The casualty may deteriorate during transport and require mouth-to-mouth breathing or even full cardiovascular resuscitation but keep moving.

Shock

Shock has been left till last in this chapter since it is probably the most important aspect of emergency care and embraces all the conditions discussed before. It must not be confused with fright, emotional shock or the response to bad news. That type of shock does not end in death, the type of shock we are discussing does. It is a precise medical state which was probably best described in 1896 by an American physician, John Collins Warren. When he was rushing around a battlefield trying to determine which of the casualties required his attention most urgently, he learned to recognise a serious of signs which he described as the casualty having a "pause in the act of dying".

That very descriptive phrase indicates what shock is all about. The cells have become short of oxygen and are sick; if they are deprived of oxygen for much longer they will die. Shock is thus the clinical manifestation of that interval of time between normal and deficient oxygenation when cells are sick and having a pause in the act of dying. The body is on the countdown towards death.

Recognition of the fact that the casualty has developed shock indicates a state of emergency and establishes priority. Functioning in a remote place, the ability to recognise shock and follow its course will be of much value in the care of a seriously ill or badly injured casualty over an extended period of time. This will allow the determination of whether the casualty is deteriorating, holding his own, or even improving.

Causes of shock

The cause of this pause in the act of dying is an inadequate supply of oxygen to the tissues and there are three main groups of causes:

- Failure of oxygen to reach the tissues from the lungs and blood. This could result from exposure to a toxic atmosphere or one short of oxygen (e.g. altitude). It could also result from blockage of the windpipe in choking, a lung problem as in drowning or a problem with the mechanics of breathing as in crush injury of the chest.

- Problem with the pump (heart). Here oxygen enters the body freely but the heart is unable to deliver oxygen to the cells in the quantities they require; they become sick and after a pause, die.
- Loss of blood is the most widely recognised cause of shock. If there is insufficient blood the heart will beat faster to maintain adequate delivery of oxygen to the cells and breathing will become deeper and faster as the breathing centre notes a falling level of oxygen. This type of shock can also result from loss of fluid through damaged skin in burns, or in food poisoning from continuing diarrhoea and vomiting. It can also occur in heat stroke when as much water has been withdrawn from the cells and the blood as possible.

The above list of causes of shock include all the emergency conditions discussed thus far — gassing, choking, drowning, chest injury, heart attack, bleeding, burns, heat and poisoning. In other words, shock is the endpoint reached when things go wrong in all emergency circumstances. It is a state which leads to death from lack of oxygen.

Diagnosis of shock

The body takes automatic action to deviate the available blood containing oxygen towards the vital centres — the brain, the heart and the kidneys. This results in the surface becoming cold and pale. Adrenaline is automatically released in times of emergency and this results in sweating but the sweat is cold as distinct from that produced following exposure to heat. Skin is thus cold, pale and clammy. This is the first sign of shock.

The second sign is a rising pulse rate. Since the resting pulse rate is not known the pulse must be counted and charted from the outset so that the rise can be detected. The same is true of the breathing rate. In a serious accident as soon as the immediate first-aid has been completed, it is important to count the pulse and write it down against time every 15 minutes thereafter. It is most important that the casualty should be monitored closely until he can be handed over to receive further medical attention and any change in the situation written down and recorded against time. These recordings should be presented to the doctors on admission who will find them of value in determining the present position since only knowledge of the casualty's condition before he left and during transport can give the hospital doctors the type of information they need immediately.

The remote healthcare practitioner will of course also monitor the blood pressure and note that it falls as the pulse rate rises. It is unlikely that the lay first-aider will be in a position to monitor the blood pressure.

A final important point is the question of whether the casualty in shock should be given a drink or not. He will certainly be thirsty. Protocol first-aid teaching states that if a casualty is in shock or badly injured he should only have his lips moistened. This is true in most urban situations since ingestion of fluid may interfere with or delay the giving of an anaesthetic. There are, however, certain exceptions which must be borne in mind in remote situations and in hot climates. The fluid losses which take place in extensive burns have already been pointed out. It is thus essential that the extensively burned casualty is encouraged to drink from the outset. It is extremely important that he is allowed to drink as much as he wants during the transportation if he is to survive a long journey and a hot climate. If intravenous fluids cannot be provided by the first-aider they will be provided when he reaches hospital.

The question of time and distance also needs to be taken into account. If the casualty has a broken leg, he will need an anaesthetic when he reaches hospital, but if the journey takes several hours because the accident took place in a desert area during summer, he is unlikely to reach hospital alive unless he is rehydrated before being transferred. In summary the situations where water should be given to the casualty are:

- Burns
- Time and distance
- Heat

At the beginning of this chapter on the management of emergencies in remote places it was pointed out that panic was likely to take place in the early stages of management of an accident and for that reason it was necessary to develop a drill of priorities and actions to take.

When that initial part has been undertaken the next stage is to think through the various eventualities and to carry out the necessary first-aid treatment with an understanding of the reason for taking the various actions and modifying them in certain situations. Finally, the time arrives when judgement and thoughtfulness must be displayed — as in the question of the administration of fluids and where the action will be different in different circumstances. Provided there is a good reason for taking an action that is not normally taken, it is justified. This is the phase when thought and intelligence come into play and make the difference between routine casualty handling and inspired first-aid.

The best chance of achieving that is not only by learning and thinking about the process of first-aid but by continuing to practise it with colleagues and undertaking group exercises. As mentioned before there is no place for poor practical technique and the best way to achieve a high standard is by attending professional first-aid courses and refresher courses.

References

Norman JN, Al-Masabi SH and El-Sadig MHA. 2004. *Emergency First-Aid for Industrial and Remote Settings*. Victoria, Canada: Trafford.

Oliver E, Miller JDB and Norman JN. 1978. Steroids in secondary drowning. *Lancet* **1**: 105–106.

Smith G, Ledingham IMcA, Norman JN, Sharp GR and Bates EH. 1962. Treatment of coal as poisoning with oxygen at two atmospheres pressure. *Lancet* **279**: 816–819.

Teasdale G and Jennett B. 1974. Assessment of coma and impaired consciousness. A practical scale. *Lancet* **2**: 81–84.

Bibliography

Norman JN and Brebner JA. 1985. *The Offshore Health Handbook*. London: Martin Dinitz.

Norman JN and El-Sadig MHA. 2006. *Emergency First-Aid* (Arabic version). Cairo: Silver Information Service, ISBN 977-5709-05-9.

Resuscitation Council UK Guidelines. 2015. Available at http//www.resus.org.uk/resus-guidelines.

Roylance P and Preston F. 1983. *Travellers First-aid Handbook*. London: The Reader's Digest Association Ltd.

© 2020 World Scientific Publishing Company
https://doi.org/10.1142/9781786347510_0003

Chapter 3

Preparation for Disasters in Remote Places

J Nelson Norman and Graham Page

Introduction

The difference between an incident, a major incident and a disaster is only size because the result is equally catastrophic for the individual casualty whether he was struck by lightning while walking alone on a golf course or involved in an earthquake in a major city. The term disaster is usually only applied to a major incident, however, when the loss affects the community or society to an extent which exceeds its ability to cope using its own resources. Equally, the outcome depends on the fundamental consideration of time and distance which is the basic problem of remote healthcare in any situation. Time refers to the time taken to provide the casualty with the facilities needed for his care or survival. This can be critical even in a major urban conurbation as when a butcher's knife slips and opens his femoral artery. There are only a few moments available for someone to put a finger over the bleeding point before he loses all his blood. This stresses once again the need for universal first-aid which is just as important in a city as in a remote location. Distance in a disaster depends on the locus of the disaster. In the earthquake and tsunami in remote Indonesia in September 2018, more than a week passed before vital external help reached the disaster area. Thus, when a disaster occurs in a remote situation it raises special challenges and it has to be accepted that the chances of survival in a very remote area are less than when such an incident takes place with major hospitals or medical facilities within reasonable traveling distance. Although disasters usually occur suddenly and unexpectedly, this emphasises the need for special preparations to be made in remote areas where there is a recognised danger of a major incident taking place. Such a situation is major heavy industry such as oil exploration and production in both onshore and offshore locations. These preparations can take a considerable time to complete since they are likely to involve several responsible authorities. In the absence of detailed and tested preparations to deal with disasters, however, there is much confusion and this often results in much unnecessary morbidity and mortality.

In a dangerous place (war and terrorism) or hostile environment (flood and landslide etc.) where the possibility of a disaster can be anticipated it is possible to make preparations for management in advance. It was fortunate that the possibility of disaster was recognised by the offshore oil industry in the North Sea and detailed preparations were discussed and practised over several years before the Piper alpha disaster took place in the 1980s. This preparatory planning proved to be very important when the disaster took place. Detailed follow up by local authorities and subsequent national enquiry of the event by Lord Cullen generated a list of considerations to take into account when making plans to deal with a possible disaster and its management (Cullen, 1990).

The Major Incident Plan

It is usual for a major incident plan to be in existence in large population conurbations and this is normally the primary responsibility of the Police Directorate in towns and the Coastguard at sea. In the Middle East and many other countries, it may however be a military responsibility. If you are working for any of the emergency services it is essential for you to know which service has primary responsibility in the area, to know the detail of the local plan, how and when a major incident is declared together with what particular action you need to take whatever your position. If you are a doctor, nurse or a member of any of the response authorities which may be involved and hear an announcement of the disaster on the radio for example, you should not wait to be summonsed but repair immediately to the local assembly area of your discipline.

In Aberdeen before the Piper Alpha disaster, the authorities responsible for preliminary arrangements headed by the Chief Constable worked closely together although the medical authorities — the Grampian Health Board and the major oil companies had their own plans which they practiced individually from time to time. Once a year the three authorities held an exercise involving police, hospital and the major oil companies based on a different scenario each time.

Communications between the police, hospital and industry groups are essential and must be established immediately if the possibility of an industrial disaster is seen. Frequent practice exercises are necessary if the three groups are to act in unison and seamlessly. The problems which inevitably arise and appear during practice exercises can be minimised but not entirely prevented by further training and modification of the plan until an event occurs –even then new problems are likely inevitably to emerge. After each trial exercise it is essential to review what took place fully and in detail to learn from these problems and if necessary, to modify the plan.

Case Study 1

Some years ago a major civil air crash took place in a remote Scottish Island. There was a large number of casualties and they were taken to the local hospital which did not have the necessary resources to provide the urgent care required. The disaster was reported in the news media and attempts to mobilise medical help and advice from distant medical authorities were frustrated by the blockade of the local telephone exchange and hospital switchboard by anxious relatives and news media so that it was virtually impossible for the medical authorities to call for the support which they urgently needed.

A major incident plan should always include action to be taken to ensure communications e.g. ex-directory secure telephone lines controlled by the police.

Training

During the discussions which took place on the major incident plan before the Piper Alpha disaster, it was recognized that although the whole population at risk was trained in basic first aid there may only be one remote medical practitioner on such an installation, and he may be a nurse, a military medic or an ambulance paramedic. Arrangements were thus made to organise special training for them in the management of large numbers of casualties. This included triage, special communication skills, technology and detailed knowledge and practice of the local major disaster plan.

In addition to the general first aid training of the population at risk, additional groups were given advanced training so that casualty handling teams became available to assist the medic during a major incident until external help was available. It was recognized that this would only function effectively if the teams practiced regularly and this was achieved by constructing a series of scenarios and practice exercises which were carried out regularly and at least on a monthly basis. Eventually the teams became fully involved and motivated and were considered to function effectively. This took time and patience and much depended on the charisma of the medic training them and the commitment of the management of the installation. This system was also practiced in the Middle East oil fields and was specially advanced and regularly practiced in ADCO and ADMA of the ADNOC group of companies in Abu Dhabi, both of which were well prepared to cope with a disaster which mercifully has not occurred.

The same system was also used in the very different situation of the scientific stations of the British Antarctic Survey where there is also only one doctor. The population at risk is of course very much smaller but the same problem exists if the single doctor is not functional or is overwhelmed and could be even more serious. The main casualty could even be the only doctor! This arrangement worked well in the Antarctic and should be introduced worldwide in remote and dangerous locations where medical resources are scarce or there is only a single medic or doctor.

Casualty Clearing Area

It is necessary to create a clear space where casualties can be assembled, immediate care provided and triage carried out before transport of the casualties to hospital. This is a fairly straightforward manoeuvre when the disaster takes place within reasonable reach of a hospital but it can provide major problems when it occurs in remote places and with complicating factors such as war and terrorist activities. It may take a day or so before the casualties can be evacuated and if this takes place the consensus of opinion is in favour of the establishment of a casualty clearing station at the airport designated for evacuation and the provision there of basic resuscitation and immediate accident and emergency care facilities followed by evacuation as soon as possible. While this is generally agreed problems can arise

Case Study 2

During the war in Iraq the problem of management of casualties in the oil industry arose when the American army withdrew since the American army and its medics had undertaken responsibility for the safe evacuation of the civilian oil workers who became ill or had an accident and needed transfer through the war zone before evacuation. Since many oil companies were involved there was initial confusion on the means and extent of the preparations and facilities needed. Following a study based in Aberdeen it was finally agreed by the responsible oil companies that a casualty clearing area should be established at the airport in Basra. There had been controversy about the extent of the facilities to be provided which varied from basic resuscitation and first aid to a tertiary hospital! In the event a basic accident and emergency unit was provided at the airport which could provide immediate medical care with x-rays, immobilisation of fractures, care of wounds and intravenous fluid infusion, including blood. There were no advanced diagnostic facilities nor was there specialist medical provision. Communications with specialists at a distance were, however, provided and the staffing was by general physicians and nurses. Careful and detailed consideration was given to the extent of drug, fluid and basic equipment provision and the casualties were evacuated as soon as possible.

In the event, this system worked well but it took much time for agreement to be reached among the responsible agencies and this was only ultimately achieved when the consortium of responsible oil companies sought and took advice form an external and credible academic authority. This emphasises once again the need for prior preparation and planning when such a situation is envisaged on the horizon and well before the event takes place.

during discussion on the extent of the care provision to be provided at the clearing station and the disagreements among the responsible authorities can lead to serious delays unless the discussion takes place in advance of a possible incident.

Provision of External Medical support

External medical support will nearly always be required in any disaster situation but the nature of the support needed will vary widely. In the UK, basics have in place the support needed for major disasters on the roads while Medicine sans Fronteirs have very different but effective provision available for widely different disasters in various areas of the world varying from epidemics of serious infection, earthquakes and even terrorism and war. It can take considerable time for the necessary resources to be deployed in remote places and it took a week before help arrived following the tsunami in Borneo.

When it came to the question of the possible requirement for external medical specialist help in the event of an offshore disaster in the North Sea, the directors of the major oil companies came up against a political problem. The UK Government had decided that the management of offshore medical problems was entirely the responsibility of the industry and only became a responsibility of the National Health Service when casualties were delivered beyond the high-water mark of the UK Coastline. The available specialist anaesthetists and surgeons and the necessary equipment were, however, contained entirely within the National Health Service.

Recognising the urgency and vulnerability of the situation, a dedicated group of volunteer specialist registrars and consultants formed themselves into a team with equipment acquired from various sources and stood by in case of a sudden disaster. This was difficult for them because they were still responsible for their NHS duty rosters and now had on call commitments in addition and without mobile phones and electronic call devices which were not available at that time. Matters came to a head when it was realised that since they were not acting within their NHS contract, they had no insurance cover for loss of life or injury in a dangerous situation nor litigation cover and could be called upon to deal with a wide variety of medical problems in less than ideal professional circumstances. It seemed that they could now be called upon to manage incidents which required the professional organisation and training that they did not have. The oil companies were thus persuaded to develop and fund a professional group of specialist teams on stand by and they did this. Medics acting on humanitarian grounds can be very vulnerable and need to consider their position when industry and Government, which is ultimately responsible, is slow to act.

The team eventually deployed during the Piper alpha disaster functioned well because it was well equipped and regularly exercised and trained to work in unison. Training in medicine was not necessary for this group but familiarisation with the environment and the offshore facilities available together with the elements of the disaster plan were of much importance. It is, however, interesting to note that the specialist team was not as essential as might be expected in this case because the well trained offshore medics and their casualty handling teams functioned so well, had the burns dressed and the intravenous infusions established by the time they arrived that they had little more to do than determine the order of evacuation.

The hospital disaster plan functioned effectively and smoothly also, especially since there was time before the casualties started to arrive and beds had been cleared and additional staff called in. The medical preparations for the disaster were thus effective and not criticised in the subsequent enquiry but the situation would have been very different if the Piper alpha had exploded ten years earlier! As the British army constantly affirms, 'Prior preparation and planning prevents piss poor performance.'

Case Study 3

Some years ago, an aircraft overshot the runway at Lerwick in the Shetland Islands and landed in the sea. All the passengers were able to exit the plane before it sank but many ended up in the water. A major incident was declared and the medical staff rushed to the scene from the supporting hospital. The Shetland Islands are cold and unfortunately many of the nurses rushed enthusiastically to the scene forgetting to bring their coats. It soon became clear that they were not able to function efficiently because they were too cold! The lesson to take from this is the value of careful preparation and frequent exercise of the disaster plan.

The finesse in minimising the effects of a disaster seem to be based in careful preparation and frequent training exercises together with careful evaluation of an incident when it occurs so that the training exercises can be modified with new information and the plan modified as each new problem arises and is noted. This probably applies even more to minor problems which can achieve major significance if ignored or forgotten.

It is important that major disasters are carefully analysed after the event so that lessons can be learned and recommendations made -both major and minor- to improve the efficiency of management of future events. The oil field major disaster was examined most carefully when the Piper alpha structure in the North Sea exploded. The event was most meticulously enquired into by Lord Cullen (Cullen, 1990). It is important for those responsible for planning a major incident plan for disaster to consult as many reports of enquiries following a major incident as possible since each incident throws up new and unexpected problems which need to be taken into account. Nevertheless, disasters are so different that there will always be new and unexpected problems. It is only possible to minimise their effect by frequent revision of the major incident plan and by the institution of frequent training and exercise of the available resources.

It is also of importance to prepare for the medical and psychological responses following a disaster since these can be equally wide ranging and also require careful preparation and planning.

Reference

Lord Cullen. 1990. *The Public Inquiry into the Piper Alpha Disaster*. London: HMSO.

Bibliography

Canada-Newfoundland and Labrador Offshore Petroleum Board. 1982. Enquiry into loss of the Ocean Ranger off Newfoundland, C-NLOPB.

Cox RAF and Norman JN. 1987. Provision of back-up services. In: *Offshore Medicine* London: Springer-Verlag, Chap. 4, pp. 51–60.

Klein S and Mohamed H. 2016. Reaching a consensus on the competency and training for healthcare practitioners working in remote oil and gas operations. *J IRHC* **7(1)**: 8–12.

Norwegian Public Commission. 1981. The Alexander L. Kielland Disaster Accident Report, ISBN 80000ED27N.

Chapter 4
The Psychological Response to Major Trauma in Remote Locations

David A Alexander

Introduction

What is "trauma"?

A "trauma" is an event or circumstance which overwhelms or threatens to overwhelm a person's or a community's ability to cope. A common distinction is between "natural" disasters and "man-made" ones (including armed conflict), but it does not always stand up to scrutiny. Earthquakes are natural events but they themselves do not kill in huge numbers: poorly constructed buildings and other constructions do.

"War", strictly speaking, is armed conflict between sovereign states: other armed confrontations are "military conflicts". (I doubt if victims of these events care too much about semantic niceties.)

The impact of a major disaster should not be measured just in terms of the toll of death and injuries (as awful as they are), but also in terms of damage to the environment and the infrastructure. This was illustrated very starkly by the 2005 Pakistan earthquake. The figures and images emerging were close to overwhelming. (Certainly, to me as their Advisor.) At least 80,000 died; at least 124,000 were injured; mountains literally collapsed; bridges, roads, schools, homes, hospitals and other institutions were demolished; livestock and local industries were no more, and about 4 million people were displaced. All of this occurred over an area the size of Belgium. An excellent read is Professor Niaz's book: *The Day the Mountains Moved* (Niaz, 2006).

As an Advisor in Sri Lanka, after the 2004 tsunami, I was confronted with a new risk factor for children after major trauma. It was reported that several vehicles had been in the area of the disaster, the occupants of which were attracting the attention of many children (whose parents were either known to be dead or at least "missing") by means of various inducements including toys, food, shelter and clothing. Was this the effort of a humanitarian corps? No, it was the work of some exploitative human traffickers seeking fodder for the European sex trade.

Another risk for children is their possible recruitment as "child soldiers" (the term used to be "boy soldiers", but, unfortunately, young girls are increasingly deployed as combatants). The motive of such young persons is as varied as it is complex. However, it would be simplistic to assume that they are hapless "victims". Ominously, there is evidence that some such children, compared to adults, are: less fearful, have less respect for life, and less respect for the "rules" of military combat (NATO, 2008).

"We must do something"

Our natural concerns for others sire this attitude. However, doing "something" does not mean "anything". Enthusiasm and altruism must always be tempered by realism and careful assessment. The 19th century medical ethicist, Chomel, delivered a cautionary principle originally for doctors, but it is relevant to all "helpers": "Primum non nocere" (Above all, do no harm").

This reminds us that all interventions and decisions, however well-intended, carry the potential to cause harm. One way in which the principle is breached is by certain volunteers who parachute themselves uninvited into tragedies in foreign lands, usually the under-resourced countries. For example, after the 2004 Sri Lankan tsunami, I witnessed many "counsellors", "de-briefers" and other helpers arriving at the scene. Most had no verifiable credentials; most displayed no knowledge of the national or regional religio-cultural mores, and political influences (terrorism was rampant in the northern area), and very few had any command of the local languages. Most had no clear intervention strategy, and many were equipped with Western standardised mental health measures. (Many Sinhala in Sri Lanka use the concept of "depression" quite differently from Westerners.) It was clear some persons were genuinely motivated to help, despite their naivety and lack of preparation. However, it was equally clear that for some the disaster offered an opportunity to carry out some "research" for some degree or qualification. Many had not sought legitimate permission to carry out their work. Two personnel "just asked a local police officer" before they set up camp.

Apart from the genuine risk that some such persons may cause harm, they also consume valuable resources. They need food, drink, accommodation and transportation. Some even expected security cover. Not surprisingly, those who descend during the "convergence" phenomenon, witnessed so often after major incidents, tended to stay only briefly, rarely to return to re-stimulate the disaster response or to evaluate their earlier efforts.

There may also be something paternalistic or patronising about inviting oneself to a 3rd World or under-resourced country. Would a 'plane-load of Sri Lankan "helpers" have been welcomed after the recent terrorist incidents in Europe?

Over the years, I have developed two checklists for those going out to disasters and military conflict zones. The first addresses personal welfare issues, and the second deals with administrative ones. Respectively, these are represented in Boxes 1 and 2. Addressing these issues before departure will make life easier after arrival, and will increase your credibility.

Box 1: Welfare Matters

- Are you in a suitable physical and emotional state?
- Are your medical prophylaxis up to date, and appropriate? *(Remember the value of different anti-malarials can vary across regions even within the same country.)*
- Have you sufficient adequate clothing and footwear? *(Remember the "4 seasons in a day" phenomenon.)*
- Have you an up-to-date and relevant first aid kit?
- Do you have available and easily accessible details of your blood group and essential medical history *(e.g., allergic reactions to anaesthetic agents)*?

Box 2: Administrative Matters

- Is your passport up to date *(you commonly require 6 "extra" months after intended departure)*?
- Have you an up-to-date and accurate visa *(dates of arrival and departure can be crucial)*?
- Have you a letter of invitation from an authorised person?
- Have you suitable and up-to-date health insurance? *(Read all the small print!)*
- Have you completed a "hostage profile" *(This may be optional depending on what country is to be visited. I nearly always complete one, and leave it with a trusted and reliable person. It contains many detailed personal data about, e.g., domestic, health, social and educational/professional matters. In addition, you should record about 10 "Proof of Life" questions, the answers to which could be answered only by yourself or by a select number of persons very close to you. These are invaluable if you are taken hostage, particularly to the Foreign and Commonwealth Office and the Metropolitan Police who deal with the UK nationals abducted abroad.)*

- In the disaster zone, have you a confirmed liaison person and a base?
- Can you provide evidence of suitable training and experience?
- Do you have an adequate level of knowledge about local political, socio-cultural and religious matters?
- Have you a working knowledge and understanding of socio-cultural, political and religious factors which prevail in your area of deployment? *(You could try to identify a "cultural adviser" in that area.)*
- Have you a realistic view of what you hope to do, where, when and with what outcome?
- Is there a person in the country of the disaster area to whom you will be responsible?
- Can you provide a clear idea of what resources will be available to you that you might require?
- Have you prepared a full CV and a brief biography?

Myths about Disasters

Particularly before one's first invitation as an Adviser, it is worth checking one's beliefs and expectations. My namesake, Professor David E Alexander, University College, London (2007), has identified 56 so-called "myths" about disasters. Here are four examples.

(i) **Looting is common**

It does occur but not commonly. I admit that after the Hurricane Katrina (2005) individuals were seen to be removing unpaid goods from local shops. However, what do survivors do? There were no shop staff; there was no electricity to power ATMs or checkouts, and families were desperate for essentials, e.g., water, food and warm clothing (Gheytanchi *et al.*, 2007).

(ii) **The effects of disasters are indiscriminate**

They certainly are not. The poor and the disadvantaged suffer most as do the children, women, the elderly and the sick.

(iii) **All aid is valuable**

It is not. Many tents sent after the Pakistan earthquake disaster were totally inappropriate to the climate and terrain. Sometimes inappropriate foods are sent to Muslim and Hindu survivors, and drugs are often sent but prove to be well past their "use by dates".

(iv) Panic is common

It is relatively uncommon and is largely confined to events in which there is a lack of leadership; where there seems to be no escape, and in which help seems to be available on a "first come, first served basis" (Drury, 2012).

This seems to have been true historically. When the troopship HMS Birkenhead began to sink after being holed on rocks in 1852, there were, as usual in those days, insufficient lifeboats for all on board. Two British officers ordered most of their troops to deal with various urgent matters; the rest were assembled military style in silence whilst the women and children boarded the lifeboats. The priority accorded women and children, whilst not enshrined in maritime law, became known as the "Birkenhead Drill".

Self-care in the Trauma Zone

Those at risk?

Despite their natural resilience, high motivation for this kind of work, and effective training, it is known that "responders" of various backgrounds have an increased risk of adverse reactions attributable to the extraordinary demands of this kind of work (Alexander and Klein, 2009). Some of these reactions are captured in terms such as "secondary traumatisation" and "burnout". These are not formal diagnoses but they are useful descriptions to represent the same kind of reactions seen in casualties of disaster and conflict.

We should not be misled by "tunnel vision" and/or focus exclusively on psychological reactions. Responders may also report physical reactions, such as muscular pains, headaches, fatigue and abdominal, dermatological and cardio-vascular problems. This may be because some persons and cultures tend to "somatise" their emotional distress.

I noted what I described as the "Double Jeopardy" for police officers and military personnel who worked tirelessly after the 2004 Sri Lankan tsunami and the 2005 Pakistan earthquake. Not only were these individuals exposed to horrific and distressing scenes and events during their rescue and body retrieval work, many of them had also personally lost loved ones, homes and property. In a sense, they were, therefore, "primary" and "secondary" victims.

It should be noted that volunteer helpers, compared to professional ones, seem to be more susceptible to these problems above.

What steps can we take to help ourselves?

- We must address as best we can our basic needs such as eating, hydration, sleep, rest and exercise. (Sometimes advice in the field seems counterintuitive.) However, if Army medics tell you to drink between 8–10 litres of water in a foreign land, do not argue; they are right (as I found out in Iraq)!
- Keep one foot in reality. Your trauma work must not overwhelm everything. Check on, *e.g.*, sports scores in your country; the weather; the outcome of elections, and cultural events. This helps to remind you there is a parallel universe, and that you still belong to it. It also maintains a sense of perspective.
- Keep in touch with family and friends (ensuring there is no security risk). For some, this can be a mixed blessing. One soldier reported to me in Iraq that he did want to speak to his wife and children, but doing so left him frustrated because he could do nothing to help them with any domestic problems which surfaced. However, it is still an important option to be considered.
- "Black humour" (or "Gallows humour") has long been recognised as a way of laughing at awful events to relieve tension and to distract oneself from a disturbing experience. It rarely seems effective when dealing with dead or injured children, and females tend to use it less often than males (Alexander and Klein, 2009). What is unacceptable is cracking "black jokes" outside the original group and setting in which this humour first emerged. Such cheap humour can be offensive and hurtful to others.
- Identify before you depart, friends or colleagues who would be pleased to hear from you if you wanted "a chat", formal or informal.
- Maintain a sense of order and control over your own affairs. Disasters and military combat conspire to create disorder, indecision and uncertainty.

Personally, I find it helpful to keep daily notes on work completed; challenges met and not met, and a work plan for the following day. This is similar to Pennebaker's (1999) advice to trauma patients to write down their experiences.

How Communities and Individuals Cope with Major Adversity

Military conflict

Much has been written about the impact of military conflict. Indeed, much more was initially learned from military than from civilian tragedy. WWI and earlier wars generated a lexicon of diagnostic terms, including "nostalgia" (reported among 17th century Swiss troops) and with its counterparts "esta roto", "Heimweh" and "maladie du pays" in Spanish, German and French troops respectively. Other conditions included "disordered action of the heart", "neurasthenia", "effort syndrome", "irritable heart", and "shell shock". These differing titles confirm that the nature and aetiology of the effect of combat was not understood. Of that early list, "shell shock" stands out as the most familiar, but the diagnosis was contentious. Was it a physical or a psychological disorder? Was it even a *bona fide* disorder or was it a label of convenience for cowards and those who lacked sufficient "moral fibre"?

More recently, following its inclusion in the psychiatric taxonomy, (The Diagnostic and Statistical Manual [American Psychiatric Association, 1980]), Post-Traumatic Stress Disorder (PTSD) has become the most investigated and discussed post-traumatic condition. This will be discussed below.

As stated above, perhaps the most disturbing fact about armed conflict is the extensive and enduring impact on the civilian communities, not only in terms of a very high death toll (especially among women and children) but due to the massive destruction wrought on the infrastructure—roads, schools, hospitals, workplaces, bridges, the public utilities, and the displacement of families from their home areas.

The increasing adverse impact on civilians in a war zone is deeply worrying. In WWI, of all the casualties, 5% were civilians. Since the Vietnam War, civilians have constituted about 90% of all casualties. "Soldiers fight, civilians suffer", seems to be the hallmark of contemporary conflict.

Women and children have emerged as the most common casualties. Rape is an offensive but widely used weapon of war. Children, in huge numbers, are the victims of landmines and unexploded ordnance because of their frequent presence in the fields and open areas, where the children work and/or play. Sadly, children are attracted to weaponry and explosives as they view them innocently as toys.

Disasters

The study of the effects of civilian disasters has a much shorter history than that describing the effects of military combat. Since the 19th century, the UK has suffered many disasters of different kinds, e.g., fires, mining accidents, famines, floods and storms, transportation accidents and maritime disasters. However, very little useful information regarding their specific effects (short term and long term) on persons and communities emerged.

It was mainly since the 1980s (often referred to as the "decade of disaster" in the UK) that clinicians and academics have made systematic attempts to research the full impact of major tragedies. The global literature is now enormous, although predictably it is of variable quality. In this section, I will provide some robust findings. In the "Further Reading" list you will find more detailed descriptions of the effects of civilian disasters on communities and individuals.

Community reactions

These tend to be fairly consistent across cultures and disasters. Tyhurst (1951) has outlined three typical phases. These are displayed in Box 3.

Another community reaction is the "Ripple Effect". A disaster immediately creates "primary victims (i.e., those at its epicentre), but others may also be badly affected, e.g., families, colleagues and friends and those who just missed being at the site of the disaster.

Advisers and other helpers must be proactive to identify not only the primary victims but those who may have been more indirectly affected by the "Ripple Effect".

Generally, I have been very impressed with the resilience and resourcefulness of affected communities. That is why professionals should not attempt to take over or dominate the disaster response. We must not impede the natural healing potential of the community; we should help to develop its natural coping abilities and resources.

Box 3: Typical Community Reactions to Disaster

  (i) Impact phase
       o the community is stunned and shocked
       o the main needs are for essentials, e.g., *nourishment, safety and shelter*
 (ii) Recoil phase
       o as the tragedy unfolds, the community begins to recognise what has happened and what is needed
       o the community begins to rally, often through *ad hoc* groups, to address community needs
(iii) Recovery phase
       o this usually involves a succession of "high" and "low spells"
       o initially, there is often a "honeymoon" spell during which survivors experience much goodwill, favourable publicity and a spirit of optimism *(honeymoons do not last forever)*
       o later, harsher realities surface—accusations of culpability, legal issues, intrusive media and group conflicts

Individual reactions

There are multiple short-term reactions, but there are four main groups, as I have shown below. It must be emphasized that these are "normal" reactions. The great majority of persons display such reactions: very few persons develop frank psychopathology in the immediate aftermath of a disaster.

Emotional
- shock, denial
- fear, anxiety
- helplessness, hopelessness
- "survivor guilt" (*"Why did I survive the fire whilst my wife was killed?"*)
- "performance guilt" (*"If only I had known how to do CPR!"*)
- grief (*nearly all trauma entails some loss*)

Cognitive
- impaired memory/concentration
- confusion/disorientation
- intrusive thoughts, memories, images
- dissociation (*a sense of being "switched off"*)
- impaired decision making
- hyper-vigilance (*overly aware of risk*)

Social
- withdrawal (*survivors do not always welcome closeness; sometimes they want their own "space"*)
- irritability
- interpersonal conflict (*often over trivia*)
- avoidance (*e.g., of any reminders of the tragedy*)

Physical
- insomnia (*especially due to nightmares*)
- headaches
- gastro-intestinal complaints
- reduced appetite
- reduced energy
- hyper-arousal (*a constant state of being "on edge"*)

Responders must remain mindful of the fact that these reactions are normal in the short term. We must not "medicalise" them. Distress is not an illness nor is grief.

Grief

Some practitioners are so dedicated to identifying post-traumatic reactions, they may fail to recognise that the survivor's primary problem may be grief, through the loss of a loved one (but can also be due to the loss of a home, possessions and livestock).

A constellation of reactions to loss

Emotional
- low mood
- anxiety
- guilt ("If only I hadn't persuaded him to take that flight" (after a fatal air crash.)
- envy (because other families have not lost a loved one—hard to express as a survivor)
- loneliness (not the same as being alone)
- anger (many may become the target, e.g., even those who broke the bad news of the death; those who may be deemed [often falsely] to be responsible for the death of the deceased)

Behavioural
- searching/pining (for the deceased)
- avoidance of reminders (e.g., photographs of the deceased are put away in drawers and cupboards)
- apathy ("I've no point in living now.")
- crying (the evidence suggests that crying is universal—even among the "stiff upper-lipped")

Physical
- insomnia
- loss of appetite ("I don't deserve to enjoy my food.")
- loss of energy
- cardio-vascular problems (it seems we can die of a "broken heart")

Cognitive
- impaired concentration/memory
- changed beliefs and attitudes (e.g., to God or to an employer)
- confusion

Perception
- misperceptions (e.g., "seeing" the deceased in a crowd scene or on TV or going up in an elevator in the opposite direction to the bereaved)

- "hallucinations"/"illusions" (This is complex. What do we make of seeing "ghosts" or being aware of a "presence" [common in Scotland]? The experiences are "real" to the bereaved; regard them that way—there is no point in debating what was the cause of the experience.)

Adjustment to loss

Most persons adjust to a loss without professional help. It is impossible to be precise but generally most adjustment takes place within about 6 months after "natural" deaths (e.g., the death of an elderly relative who had not been in good health).

However, following "traumatic" deaths, adjustment may take up to 4 years, with a fluctuating pattern. That adjustment is made harder if the death were sudden and unexpected; were that of a child; if it involved violence, suffering and mutilation; where there is no body available, or when the death was due to negligence.

Other factors which may lead to a poorer prognosis are: (i) features of the bereaved (e.g., poor self-esteem, anxious and previous psychiatric history, especially anger, guilt or unresolved suffering from earlier losses; and current problems of living with no or little support), and (ii) features of the relationship (e.g., a volatile "love/hate" one or one in which there had been a high level of mutual dependence).

Pathological grief reactions

Distinguishing between "normal" and "pathological" grief reactions is not always easy as they are not discrete categories; they are on the same continuum. However, these are the four criteria to achieve a distinction.

- The extreme intensity of the reactions
- The uncommonly prolonged nature of the reactions
- A delayed onset of reactions
- The extent to which the reactions compromise the patient's ability to function (perhaps the most important single criterion)

Cultural influences

How individuals express and cope with their grief is influenced by personal, cultural and religious factors. Helpers (lay and professional) must recognise these influences. Failure to do so may cause harm and offence, and reduce their credibility.

Management

Pathological grief reactions are probably best left to the skills of specialists, usually mental health professionals. This is particularly true with regard to children and adolescents (Yule *et al.*, 2010; Dyregrov and Dyregrov, 2013).

However, the other bereaved can be helped in various ways.

- Provide comfort
- Enable the bereaved to express their feelings (but they should not be forced to do so)
- Emphasise the normality and legitimacy of their reactions
- Identify what is required for readjustment
- Facilitate their mourning practices

Most importantly, **LISTEN** and, at all costs, avoid clichés such as:

- o "don't worry you still have one son at home" (said to a grieving mother after she lost her young son at sea)
- o "I know just how you feel" (we can never fully know how another feels)
- o "we all have to go sometime"

- Do not be judgemental or defensive even if the bereaved direct their anger at you.
- Do not be afraid to use frank words, (e.g., "death" and the name of the deceased—but get it correct!)

"Ambiguous loss"

Disasters and military action quite often lead to missing bodies, mutilated bodies and just body parts. Such ambiguous loss (Boss, 2000) raises several important issues.

Bodies serve two purposes. First, they confirm the reality of the death (countering denial). Second, they provide an opportunity for the bereaved to say "Goodbye" and "I love you" etc. (Some loved ones like to put a small memento into the hand of the deceased.) Apart from important forensic investigatory reasons, the authorities should be encouraged to retrieve missing bodies if at all possible. Unfortunately, human flesh and bone can be atomised in extreme heat or blast. The military found a good solution to this by building a "Tomb of the Unknown Soldier".

With regard to viewing mutilated bodies or body parts, there are no unqualified recommendations. However, personally, I believe families should be given the choice to view but with four preconditions. First, they should be briefed accurately but sensitively about what they will see, feel and perhaps smell. Second, they should be offered to be accompanied by somebody who is familiar with post-mortem signs such as lividity and resuscitation marks. Third, they should have the opportunity for a "debrief" after the viewing. Finally, a check should be made that they are fit to travel home and have support once there, after the viewing.

The best evidence currently available indicates those who view are generally pleased to have done so, and those who did not sometimes regret it (Chapple and Ziebland, 2010).

Post-Traumatic Psychopathology

At risk factors

Not all those exposed even to severe trauma develop a psychiatric condition, and prevalence rates vary. One has to be wary about our own expectations. Some years ago, I had to deal with two pilots in the same aircraft who survived the same very disturbing "near death experience". One pilot was a quiet, introverted character and the other was an extroverted, "macho-looking", extremely confident former military helicopter pilot who had seen "action" in the Falklands. Several of us thought the latter would be the more resilient, and able to adjust more quickly. The opposite proved to be the case!

Predictors

(i) *Pre-disaster*
- Female gender (are females more frank in self reporting?)
- Extremes of age
- Sexual abuse in childhood
- Previous psychiatric history
- Disadvantaged (e.g., socially and educationally)
- Concurrent life stressors
- Unresolved matters pertaining to earlier trauma, including loss

(ii) *Peri-traumatic*
- Being trapped at the scene of a trauma
- Man-made event (e.g., due to acts of violence such as terrorism)
- Sudden and unexpected
- Extended exposure to gruesome scenes
- Proximity (there seems to be a dose-response relationship)
- Physical injury
- (Perceived) threat to life of self or other (the threat is legitimately "in the eye of the beholder")

(iii) *Post-traumatic*

- Lack of supports
- Displacement
- Financial, social or relationship problems
- Adverse reactions from others (e.g., blame and criticism)

Resilience

The pendulum has swung from a pathology-based model (which emphasizes the adverse effects of trauma) to a "resilience" one which focuses on how well survivors cope with adversity and on their reports of positive growth and change thereafter (Southwick and Bonanno, 2014).

Resilience may be underpinned by a sense of "hardiness" which is reflected in those who view potentially adverse events as "challenges" rather than as "threats" or "impedimenta". Similarly, those who regard themselves to be in control of their own destiny are more likely to display resilience compared to those who view themselves as vulnerable and hapless victims of circumstance.

Others (e.g., Joseph, 2011) emphasize the positive effects of being exposed to tragedy and risk. An early example of what is sometimes called the "salutogenic effect" was provided by my team after the 1988 Piper Alpha disaster. A large number of local police officers were deployed to remove the human remains from the wreckage of the Piper Alpha oil platform. The work was very unpleasant because of the state of the bodies, and at times dangerous. The bodies and remains were subject to post-mortem examination with the help of these officers.

The officers were assessed in terms of their mental health at three months and three years. None showed any signs of post-traumatic psychopathology. Their results, compared with those of a matched control group (not involved in the Piper Alpha disaster), showed *higher* levels of mental health, and, moreover, the officers reported feeling more confident in themselves and "stronger" than before their body handling duties.

Two officers reported spells of low mood and alcohol misuse, but these they had suffered before the disaster in an occupational health survey we had carried out by chance prior to the tragedy. They confirmed that what had helped them were such factors as good leadership, a clear definition of duties, feeling appreciated, and viewing their duties as purposeful and valuable (Alexander and Wells, 1991; Alexander, 1993).

Post-traumatic stress disorder (PTSD)

Features

This rather controversial diagnostic label entered the 3rd edition of the Diagnostic and Statistical Manual of the American Psychiatric Association (DSM – 3rd Edition,

APA, 1980). Its presence owed much to the unflagging efforts of individuals with more of a political motive than a clinical or scientific one. It has undergone several revisions (the 5th Edition is the most current), but the essential three features of the condition are still:

- the involuntary re-experiencing of the person's traumatic experience through the medium of thoughts about, memories of and vivid sensory images ("flashbacks") of the index trauma;
- the avoidance of reminders of the event (these are legion but include: places, reports, persons' clothing, noises and smells reminiscent of the original event. Even talking about it may prove to be too aversive);
- feeling hyper-aroused (due to an over-stimulated autonomic nervous system) and hyper-vigilant (over-reactive to perceived threat and risk).

The system of classification used in the UK is the International Classification of Mental and Behavioural Disorders (ICD-10) formulated by the WHO (1992). It offers a rather more flexible diagnostic criteria but they also contain those key ones represented in the DSM one. (ICD-11 is being prepared.)

Both systems insist that these symptoms should have existed for about a month. (That is why some of them were described as "normal" if they emerged only during the acute phase of the trauma.)

Prevalence

Prevalence rates vary, as is confirmed in Box 4.

Box 4: Prevalence of PTSD across Trauma

• female rape	–50%
• vehicular incidents	–15%
• non-sexual assault	
male	–12%
female	–31%
• burns patients	–45%
• childhood sexual abuse	–50%
• major disasters	–25%
• victims of terrorist attacks	–30%
• UK Gulf war veterans	–4%

In comparing prevalence rates across studies, several factors must be considered, including whether the data derived from self-report as opposed to clinical interview (the former produces higher rates); the diagnostic measures used; when the assessment was made; any specific features of the samples (e.g., whether they were litigation cases).

Although it is not an obvious factor, I found out that even political influences may play a significant role in determining prevalence rates of psychopathology. In the early 1990s I was asked to go to the Russian city of Chelyabinsk (a "closed city" in central Russia: "closed" because one has to get permission from the KGB to visit) to examine several young survivors of a horrific train crash at the foot of the Ural Mountains in which just under 2000 persons (mainly children and adolescents) had died in horrific circumstances. The young persons whom I was asked to examine had all suffered disfiguring burns, mainly to the hands and face. They had had to bear personal witness to the horrific unfolding disaster including massive damage to two trains, the deaths and serious injuries of their friends and, sometimes, siblings. There was extended exposure to the disaster scene as there was no vehicular access to the isolated site: emergency roads had to be built.

In front of an array of senior Russian paediatricians and consultant psychiatrists, I interviewed a badly burned 15-year-old girl. She displayed the archetypical psychiatric signs of a badly traumatized survivor, in addition to serious behavioural problems (violence, swearing, theft, and alcohol misuse).

I presented my carefully justified findings. Immediately, I was told by the senior Professor, chairing the meeting, that I was "wrong" because: "Russian children do **not** get PTSD". (English translation, but accurate.)

Additional pathologies

Other relevant post-traumatic conditions, as defined in the ICD-10, include in particular:

- acute stress reaction
- adjustment disorders
- dissociative disorders
- enduring personality change after catastrophic experience

What is important to remember is that PTSD is not the most common single diagnosis after trauma: in most cases, it appears in the context of co-morbidity (especially anxiety, depression and substance misuse).

Children and adolescents and trauma

Whatever are current Russian views, young persons are vulnerable to the adverse impact of trauma, lay and military (Williams, 2007).

In addition to the normal reactions, described earlier, because children and adolescents tend to act out their distress and other emotions, rather than articulate them verbally, they may display:

- regressed behaviour
- lack of trust
- inability to tolerate separation
- increased need for security
- misuse of alcohol and drugs (in the case of adolescents)

Interventions

Over many years, a number of post-incident interventions has been developed for those exposed to catastrophic events, including military conflict. Too many are based on flimsy, often just anecdotal evidence.

There is now available a number of reviews and reports which reflect informed light on the potential value of different interventions (even those which could not be subject to randomised controlled trials for ethical and practical reasons). I have set out my views largely in accordance with the NATO Guidance (2008) to which all NATO countries have signed up. I do so not just because my team contributed to its production but because it was the first effort to cull the world literature for evidence-based or eminence-based principles of practice. "Eminence-based" refers to a consensual opinion held by recognised experts in the field.

Aims

The aims of care need to be identified. Below, in Box 5, I have set out five which should be considered by those setting off to help casualties of some major trauma.

A stepped model of care

Disasters are not single unitary events: they unfold over time—sometimes over an unwelcomed long period. Thus, the needs of those affected emerge serially and pose different challenges to those who help them. Unfortunately, most attention is focused on the acute phase: help is often scant as longer term and more chronic needs emerge. The NATO Guidance recognises this in the model it has proposed (NATO, 2008).

> **Box 5: Aims of Preparing a Programme of Post-Incident Care**
>
> - Prepare individuals and communities to reduce the level of disruption in the community
> - Devise a realistic response programme which is proportionate to the disaster and which can be delivered in a flexible and phased fashion
> - Define a continuum of integrated care recognising short, intermediate and long-term needs
> - Recognise the needs of first responders, welfare providers and other helpers

We must accept that what is helpful and welcomed at one stage, may not be at another. Why do I keep reading in the immediate aftermath: "A team of trained counsellors is standing by"? What are they going to do (even if they are [mercifully] "trained")? I have never met a survivor who wants to be counselled at that early stage. Shortly after the 2005 London bombings, very few survivors wanted help from professionals to deal with their emotional needs (Rubin *et al.*, 2005).

Survivors' basic needs must be addressed first. This was brought home to me when working with a local counsellor (yes, "trained") after the Nairobi terrorist bombing. A survivor had walked two days through the bush to reach the counsellor's base (a hut!). The first thing the counsellor asked was: "When did you last eat?" Impressive!

These are recommended levels of care corresponding to the phases at which the needs of those affected by major trauma emerge.

Level 1

Provision of services aimed to meet basic needs such as safety, food and clean water, shelter and clothing.

Level 2

Provision of psychosocial services and assistance. At this stage many lay and non-specialists can be deployed under the supervision of specialists.

Level 3

Provision of screening, assessment and intervention for those who have recovered insufficiently from their immediate and short-term distress.

Level 4

Provision of primary and secondary mental health services for the minority who require them.

Psychosocial interventions

Specific steps such as the following provide support, facilities and encouragement for those affected by major adversity.

- Restore normal social activities
- Restore normal community activities
- Institute religious events (e.g., services and memorials)
- Restart schooling (In Sri Lanka I saw the value of this, particularly because the local authorities had equipped the children with lovely new uniforms, and re-opened the schools quickly.)
- Establishment of outreach programmes, walk-in centres and helplines. (You need to consider for how long these provisions should be available.)

Psychological First Aid [PFA]

Raphael's (1986) innovative programme of provisions has undergone various revisions but they all reflect her fundamental model.

It is not a "treatment": it involves a collection of provisions and services (including some of those psychosocial ones listed above) aiming to meet very basic needs which commonly challenge survivors and their families. These can generally

---

Box 6: Essentials of Psychological First Aid

- Normalise reactions
- Address basic needs (e.g., shelter, safety, food and fluids, clothing, sanitation)
- Provide *accurate* information
- Allow the **voluntary** expression of feelings
- Provide support
- Provide "psycho-education" (i.e., what are short-term and longer term reactions, when and where to get help, and how to help oneself)
- Encourage resilience, independence, coping and adjustment
- Initiate a period of "watchful waiting" (This term derives from guidelines produced by the National Institute of Clinical Excellence [NICE], 2005). It advocates allowing about a month to lapse to allow the remission of normal reactions before considering specialist mental health intervention.)
- Re-establish links with family, friends or colleagues
- Initiate a system of triage (using the "at risk" factors described above to identify those who are likely to require different levels of care)

be delivered by lay persons who are sensitive to local socio-cultural and other moves. (In Pakistan, my team successfully trained senior medical students, social workers, imams, health visitors and other interested persons who had no specific professional background.) Orner and Schnyder (2003) provide a detailed list of items which are subsumed under the title of PFA. There is also a PFA manual for children (Yule *et al.*, 2013).

Peer support

Numerous studies of lay, emergency and military personnel have confirmed the value of the support provided by their peers. Creamer *et al.* (2012), using the Delphi method, defined a set of guidelines for how to facilitate this kind of support which is favoured by so many (because peers have "credibility" as they share the same values, code of conduct, and language as those needing help, and they understand the demands of their jobs).

Of course, consideration must always be given to the need for confidentiality and for the need to assure that seeking support does not compromise professional standing and career aspirations (Alexander and Klein, 2009).

Critical Incident Stress Debriefing [CISD] (Everly and Mitchell, 1997)

This post-incident intervention has become a contentious one. It was first developed for emergency service personnel, and became very popular in the 1990s. Its popularity led it to being used by inappropriately trained personnel, at inappropriate times, for inappropriate samples of participants, and for inappropriate reasons. Subsequently, its critics challenged its claim to prevent PTSD. Further, they emphasized its potential to cause harm (Alexander and Klein, 2009). A review of post-traumatic interventions proposed that CISD should not be used as a mandatory one-off intervention (NICE, 2005).

More recently, Hawker and Hawker (2015) have offered an excellent balanced review of CISD arguing against extreme over-generalisation for and against it as a method of reducing distress, which is generally seen favourably by emergency service, military and humanitarian aid personnel.

Trauma Risk Management [TRiM] (Greenberg et al., 2011)

This non-specialist peer support and assessment programme was first developed by the UK Royal Marines. It has face validity, and is now well-received by other military units, emergency service personnel and by the UK Foreign and Commonwealth Office. Its longer term value awaits rigorous assessment.

The TRiM protocol requires those persons exposed to a particularly disturbing event to be offered the opportunity to be seen by a trained peer at about 3 and

28 days thereafter. Participants are assessed as to their likely need to be seen by a mental health professional, on a list of 10 "at risk" factors.

It must be noted that this is not a treatment for post-traumatic pathology.

Specialist services after disasters

Throughout the UK there are now a number of trauma clinics providing specialist care, involving the use of psychological and psychopharmacological methods.

The two psychological methods recommended in the NICE (2005) Guidelines are: trauma-focused cognitive behavioural therapy, and eye movement desensitizing and reprocessing therapy (EMDR). Psychological therapies are recommended as the first line treatments.

Sometimes medication may be required, e.g., when there are no trained staff to deliver the above treatments; when the patient cannot or refuses to undergo these treatments; when these treatments have failed to achieve relief, or when symptoms are particularly severe and overwhelming (Alexander, 2005).

The NICE (2005) Guidelines advocated the use of four pharmacological agents:

- Paroxetine and mirtazapine for use by non-mental health professionals
- Amitriptyline and phenelzine for use by mental health professionals

These guidelines do not imply that other interventions might not be effective; it is just that at this stage there is insufficient evidence to support their use, particularly for PTSD.

Conclusion

Disasters and other major trauma are numerous, and we now hear more of their effects because of the rapid global network of communication. Their effects commonly cannot be calculated with great accuracy, and even the best estimates cannot reflect the intensity and scale of human suffering. It is even a challenge to estimate the breadth of the "Ripple Effect", which extends well beyond (in time and place to) the epicentre of the event, to implicate many persons. Responding to such events cannot be fuelled exclusively by good intentions. They may even cause more harm through helpers disrupting the natural healing resourcefulness of individuals, families and communities. Alternatively, some helpers who migrate uninvited from outside local communities may cause difficulties through their ignorance of socio-cultural, political, and religious sensitivities.

There is now an extensive research base relating to how catastrophe affects victims and others, how they cope, and how they can best be helped. Thus, whenever possible, assistance should reflect evidence-based or eminence-informed principles of practice which acknowledge the natural resilience of the human spirit.

References

Alexander DA. 1993. Stress among police body-handlers. A long term follow up. *Br J Psychiatry* **163**: 806–808.

Alexander DA. 2005. Early mental health intervention after disasters. *Adv Psychiatr Treat* **1**: 12–18.

Alexander DA and Klein S. 2009. First responders after disasters: a review of stress reactions, at-risk, vulnerability, and resilience. *Prehosp Disaster Med* **24**: 87–94.

Alexander DA and Wells A. 1991. Reactions of police officers to body-handling: a before-and-after comparison. *Br J Psychiatry* **159**: 547–555.

Alexander E. 2007. Misconception as a barrier to teaching about disaster. *Prehosp Disaster Med* **22**: 95–103.

American Psychiatric Association (APA). 1980. *Diagnostic and Statistical Manual of Mental Disorders*, 3rd Ed. Washington DC: APA.

Boss P. 2000. *Ambiguous Loss: Learning to Live with Unresolved Grief*. Cambridge, Mass: Harvard University Press.

Chapple A and Ziebland S. 2010. Viewing the body after bereavement due to traumatic death: qualitative study in the UK. *Br Med J* **340**: doi:http://dx.doi.org/10.1136/bmj.c2032

Creamer MC, Varker T, Bisson J *et al.* 2012. Guidelines for peer support in high-risk organisations: an international consensus study using the Delphi method. *J Trauma Stress* **25**: 134–141.

Drury J. 2012. Collective resilience in mass emergencies and disasters: a social identity model. In: *The Social Curve: Identity, Health and Well-being*. (eds.) Jetten J, Haslam C and Haslam SA. Hove: Psychological Press.

Dyregrov A and Dyregrov K. 2013. Complicated grief in children—the perspectives of experienced professionals. *OMEGA* **67**: 291–303.

Everly G and Mitchell JT. 1997. *Critical Incident Stress Management: A New Era and Standard of Care in Crisis Intervention*. Ellicott City, MD: Chevron.

Gheytanchi A, Joseph L, Gierlach E *et al.* 2007. The dirty dozen. Twelve failures of the Hurricane Katrina response and how psychology can help. *Am Psychol* **62**: 118–130.

Greenberg N, Langston V, Iversen AC *et al.* 2011. The acceptability of "trauma risk management within the UK armed forces. *Occup Med*: doi:10. 1093/occmed/kqr022.

Hawker D and Hawker D. 2015. What can be learnt from the debriefing controversy? In: *Early Interventions for Trauma* (eds) Yule W, Hawker D, Hawker D *et al.* Leicester: British Psychological Society.

Joseph L. 2011. *What Doesn't Kill Us? The New Psychology of Post-Traumatic Growth.* New York: Basic Books.

National Institute for Clinical Excellence (NICE). 2005. Post-traumatic stress disorder (PTSD): the management of PTSD in children and adults in primary and secondary care. London: National Collaborating Centre for Mental Health.

Niaz U. 2006. *The Day the Mountains Moved.* Canada: Sama Books.

North Atlantic Treaty Organization (NATO). 2008. Psychosocial care for persons affected by disasters and major accidents.

Orner R and Schnyder U. 2003. Progress made towards early interventions after trauma: principles of evidence-based practice. In: *Reconstructing Early Interventions After Trauma.* (eds.) Orner R and Schnyder U. Oxford: Oxford University.

Pennebaker JW. 1999. The effects of traumatic disclosure on physical and mental health; the value of writing and talking about upsetting events. *Int J Emerg Med Svcs* **13**: 9–18.

Raphael B. 1986. *When Disaster Strikes. How Individuals and Communities Cope with Catastrophe.* New York: Basic Books.

Rubin JG, Brewin CR, Greenberg N *et al.* 2005. Psychological and behavioural reactions to the bombings in London on 7 July 2005: cross sectional survey of a representative sample of Londoners. *Br Med J*: doi10.1136/bmj.38583.728484.3A

Southwick SM and Bonanno GA. 2014. Resilience definitions, theory, and challenges: interdisciplinary perspectives. *Eur J Psychotraumatol* **5**: 25338-http://dx.doi.org/10.3402/ejpt.v5.25338

Tyhurst JS. 1951. Individuals' reactions to community disaster: the natural history of psychiatric phenomena. *Am J Psychiatry* **107**: 764–769.

Williams RJ. 2007. The psychosocial consequences for children of mass violence, terrorism and disasters. *Int Rev Psychiatry* **19**: 263–277.

World Health Organization (WHO). 1992. International Classification of Mental and Behavioural Disorders. Geneva: WHO.

Yule W, Dyregrov A, Raundalen M *et al.* 2013. Children and war: the work of the children and war foundation. *Eur J Traumatol* **4**: 1–8.

Bibliography

Blythe BT. 2006. *Blindsided.* New York: Penguin Putnam.

Bourne I. 2013. *Facing Danger in the Helping Professions.* Berkshire, UK: Open University.

Jones E and Wessely S. 2003. *Shell Shock to PTSD.* East Sussex: Psychology Press.

Law Commission. 1998. Liability and psychiatric illness. Law Commission No. 249. London: The Stationary Office.

Neria Y, Galea S and Norris FH. 2009. *Mental Health and Disasters*. Cambridge: Cambridge University Press.

Ursano RJ, Fullerton CS, Weisaeth L *et al.* 2007. *Textbook of Disaster Psychiatry*. Cambridge: Cambridge University Press.

Chapter 5

Communications and Telemedicine

J Nelson Norman

Historical Development

Communications form the basic requirement of any system of remote healthcare. Medical communications with extremely remote communities often had to rely on radio, and sometimes even Morse code, until relatively recent times. This was certainly the case for groups of explorers, ships at sea or even early oil related offshore workers in the North Sea in the 1970s. The urgent requirements of larger occupational groups such as the rapidly expanding Offshore Oil Industry in the North Sea or the strategic and academic importance of the Antarctic following the Falklands war caused rapid advances in communication technology. Fax machines, tropospheric scatter and radio telephones were introduced by the North Sea industry in the 1980s as a means of speeding up communications and ensuring accuracy in medical diagnosis and the provision of advice and management. This made a huge difference in offshore healthcare provision at that time (Norman and Brebner, 1987; Brebner, 1990).

The breakthrough in medical communications had come earlier, however, when NASA was preparing to explore the moon and developed technology for the medical support of the astronauts during the flight. There had been extensive research and technological development in preparation, and following the lunar landing, several very sophisticated communications equipment was now available for other functions. This was initially mounted on a mobile caravan and used to explore its use in healthcare provision for remote communities in the USA — particularly isolated areas of Arizona (Bashshur and Lovett, 1977). The concept was then picked up by Memorial University in Newfoundland where Max House used it to review and read all the EEGs for the vast remote areas of Newfoundland and Labrador. This worked well and it was followed by the establishment of a remote nursing programme in Memorial University, St Johns, with a view to establishing its graduates in a series of remote clinics throughout the extensive remote provinces of Newfoundland and Labrador. They were communicated by voice via the new satellite communications once per day from Memorial by a panel of doctors and were able to discuss their clinical problems and the progress of their patients. The system worked very well and provided a good start to the development of healthcare for remote communities.

When offshore oil exploration was initiated off Nova Scotia, Memorial University of St Johns in Newfoundland sought advice from Aberdeen University on the medical care which could be required for the expanding offshore workforce, working in a similar hostile environment as the North Sea. The two Universities collaborated for some years thereafter researching and developing remote healthcare for the oil industry.

Memorial had picked up the NASA technology as had the medical directors of the oil industry in the Grand banks but when telemedicine was introduced to Aberdeen and the North Sea it was initially received with reserve. The problem was that the technology had advanced only to the level of slow-scan television and the still images were considered of only limited diagnostic value and accuracy. Nevertheless, an experiment was established between the Robert Gordon University in Aberdeen and Memorial University where a series of X-rays was transmitted across the Atlantic and the correct diagnosis was obtained in all cases — albeit considering the images were read by the chief radiologist at each end!

The breakthrough undoubtedly came when digital technology was finally introduced and it was found that the transmitted X-ray images were now of equal quality to the originals — and could even be enhanced to improve quality! The quality of X-ray transmission was regarded as the gold standard of visual image quality (Dunn *et al.*, 1980; House and Roberts, 1977).

Development of Medical Communications and Telemedicine in Aberdeen

A further series of experiments was then established in Aberdeen where two rooms were connected electronically and simulated patients were managed by telemedical means. This established many important basic points such as the importance of a preceding precise communication between the distant practitioner and the base doctor before the telecommunication was established. For this a special form was developed. A second point was on the positioning of the camera so that important parts of the patient could be observed by the base doctor and his body language observed during both the history taking and the examination by the remote practitioner. During the examination it was also seen to be important for the base doctor to be able to position the remote examining practitioner so that he could observe the position of his hands during, say, abdominal examination and to advise on the pressure applied while also observing the body language of the patient — specially his facial expressions. These practical points were seen to be of much importance when the action moved to the true clinical situation offshore and in support of the healthcare of the explorers for the British Antarctic Survey which was the next step.

A concern raised early in the investigation of telemedicine was that of medical confidentiality. This was largely solved by extending existing communication privacy requirements among medical and support personnel originally but is now taken care of by advanced new technology. Advanced new technology has indeed provided much improvement in the healthcare which can be provided for those who live in remote areas and considerable benefit for the doctors responsible for their care. An example is in ante-natal care. Either the pregnant women need to travel long distances to an ante-natal clinic in a main hospital or the obstetrician needs to travel long distances to hold clinics in remote peripheral hospitals. This problem was alleviated when the remote mid-wives were trained in the operation of ultrasonic equipment and transmitted the images electronically, together with the results of their consultation, to the obstetrician at the hospital base.

Another example is in orthopaedics when a patient treated in hospital for a fracture requires follow up visits to an out-patient clinic during recovery and rehabilitation. This was studied in Aberdeen and telemedical equipment was set up in the A&E department at Aberdeen Royal Infirmary to communicate with the nurse-led departments at the cottage hospitals in the region. This experiment successfully demonstrated that follow up could be successfully achieved from a central A&E department led by doctors and consultants and nurse-led peripheral units. This is now routinely provided there and in certain Accident and Emergency Departments in the main regional hospitals via telecommunication by a consultant there with the A&E Department of a remote peripheral hospital. The consultant is able either to communicate with a remote GP or nurse or directly with the patient. This has provided considerable advantages for both patients and consultants in hospitals serving wide peripheral areas such as in Aberdeen and Inverness.

A further area considered was whether a patient would be concerned about discussion of his problem over a telemedical link with a distant doctor. This proved not to be a problem and indeed it was found that in psychiatric practice the patient often felt more at ease discussing his problems from a closed studio and much less threatened than attending a clinic at a hospital.

The direction of developments in travel now suggests that advancing technology will now result in more and more routine consultations in urban medical practice. Hospital follow-up consultations may eventually take place routinely also by electronic means aside from the use of telemedicine in remote healthcare.

There are two aspects in determining the quality of audio-visual communication — the quality of the image and the quality of the sound. Of these it has been found by experience that sound is the more important for minor faults in imagery can be forgiven if the sound is of good quality. In international telemedicine, sound can have its own problems due to language difficulties and regional or international accents. Difficulties with sound in such situations as the helium speech of saturation divers has been overcome by the introduction of scramblers and the technological revolution has taken care of the international language problems by the development of automatic translation initially during writing and now while speaking in one language. This has some way further to go in development but undoubtedly such technical progress is being made rapidly enough that interpreters will eventually become outmoded. This will of course not only result in great progress in medical communication but also in the whole area of international understanding and debate.

In visual communication the quality of colour has importance in certain areas of clinical diagnosis, such as in skin conditions but also in the diagnosis of pathological specimens and histological slides. Second opinions are frequently requested in difficult histological diagnosis where colour plays a part but a problem of greater importance arose when it was pointed out that in such cases it was necessary for the pathologist to be able to move the slide around the microscope so that several fields could be viewed. This problem was solved by advancing technology which made it possible for the slide to be moved freely from a distance.

Development of Medical Communications and Telemedicine in the Middle East

The action next moved East from the North Sea to the UAE and collaborative research was initiated between the Aberdeen Universities and the Faculty of Medicine and Clinical Sciences at the UAE University in Abu Dhabi. While the basic aim of this research was to determine whether telemedicine would be of value in improving healthcare for remote communities of the UAE, it was soon realised that though telemedicine had been established for clinical purposes, it was equally important and useful in teaching. Discussion in this area was initiated during a conference of medical deans on undergraduate medical education held in Abu Dhabi, which had the advantage at that time of having the only digital telephone exchange in the Middle East. This was required since international telemedical exchange was by ISDN telephone at that time.

A demonstration was established where the Dean of the medical faculty at Aberdeen University simultaneously taught a class of students in Aberdeen and one in Abu Dhabi on a case of renal failure. The teaching was interactive with questions and answers being exchanged easily between Aberdeen and Abu Dhabi. Thereafter the Aberdeen Dean presented a case of ambulatory peritoneal dialysis, which was a new technique developed in Aberdeen and not yet practised in the Emirates. While the Deans were impressed by the feasibility now available in international educational collaboration, many of those present were even more impressed when the UAE students were invited to describe their Community Medicine projects to the Aberdeen students and the Aberdeen students reciprocated by describing their elective projects to the UAE students. Both groups of students plunged into easy animated discussion including such detail as which faculty provided funding for the travel involved, completely oblivious to the very prestigious, international audience in attendance.

This demonstration heralded the development of international, collaborative medical education. Like many initiatives, however, it requires a committed and enthusiastic leader or driver for success for there is much preparation and continuing communication to be undertaken. Experience has shown that transcontinental or even collaborative telemedical education will not function successfully and be sustained unless there is an equally committed driver at both ends. This is, of course, often the case in many other aspects of remote healthcare or collaborative research (Norman et al., 1995).

This first demonstration of transcontinental education was a major step forward and it was followed by consideration of how the new technology could be used to advantage in educational areas which were difficult to provide in the Middle East. Post-mortem pathology was particularly difficult to provide for students in the Middle East because at that time the local culture required bodies to be buried as soon after death as possible. In Scotland, post- mortem demonstrations were regarded as a key element of undergraduate medical education and were often carried out on a daily basis during the appropriate part of the curriculum. A video link was used between the autopsy room and the lecture theatre in Aberdeen University and consideration was given as to whether this link could be extended to the lecture theatre in Abu Dhabi. This was found to be technically feasibly using ISDN telephone lines.

The lecturer in Aberdeen was provided with the names of the UAE students and a plan of where they would be seated. Once again the teaching was entirely interactive and after the lecturer had announced the case they would be considering (of a seventy year old man who had presented with severe chest pain and had suddenly died), it was interesting to note the reaction of the student who was asked the first question, "Ahmed, what is the first possible cause which comes into your mind?" Ahmed rose about a foot from his seat at being imperiously selected for questioning by a lecturer four thousand or so miles away! Thereafter the students were at attention and the teaching progressed well, with much satisfaction from both students and staff in attendance (Brebner et al., 1997).

A research project was established to determine whether the UAE examination results were improved in the classes taught by telemedical means and the classes where this technology was not used. The result showed clearly that the telemedical teaching produced significantly better examination results. This initial experiment was followed by other areas. An advantage which emerged was that the teaching was of a consistently good quality since it required careful preparation by the lecturers. A further advantage was that the lecture could be videoed and the recording served as lecture notes so that the students could concentrate on the teaching rather than scribbling down often inadequate notes and missing out on vital points in understanding.

ISDN telephone communication was however expensive and that was a limiting factor even for wealthy areas such as the Emirates. Advances in communication technology have however solved that problem and video-conferencing now provides international, collaborative education at a reasonable cost. This is vital to allow education to penetrate into poorer and less privileged areas in the world. Further advances in technology have also allowed lectures to be delivered into several sites simultaneously by bridges and this has allowed individual study in remote places such as oil rigs and isolated communities. It can even apply to other aspects of education where lectures are given simultaneously to different schools. Interaction between teacher and pupils is, of course, an essential aspect of successful remote teaching (Brebner, 1997).

The next logical step was the determination of whether telemedical communications could be extended to the facilitation of major international medical conferences and discussions. This was initiated when a research paper submitted by a faculty member of the UAE University was accepted by the organisers of a major international conference on general medical practice to be held in Glasgow. Following a further feasibility study the paper was duly presented from Al-Ain using basic Picturetel equipment and a document camera. The presentation was very successful and was followed by an equally successful interactive period of questions and answers.

This rapidly led to a second session where three complex surgical problems were presented to a meeting of the Association of Surgeons of Great Britain and Ireland once again in Glasgow. The cases were presented by consultant surgeons from the municipal hospital in Al-Ain. In this case, however, more sophisticated equipment was used and it was possible to accompany the consultants' oral presentations with investigations including x-rays, histology, biochemistry and in one case a colonoscopy. Thereafter surgeons in Glasgow were able to question the patients in the UAE directly, in addition to their consultants, and the attendees of the meeting in both Glasgow and Al-Ain entered into an interactive discussion on management of these complex and difficult problems. This was technically highly successful but it required much careful preparation and the attendance of a technical member of the UAE group in Glasgow — emphasising once again the importance of a driver at both ends. It also pointed out the considerable economy possible in conference attendance both in terms of funding and time. It was also possible for a large number of personnel in Al-Ain to attend the conference by video link or even just the occasional paper which was of interest to them without organising international travel. The use of sophisticated video-conferencing techniques can now be practised with some ease but, though full of obvious advantages, is far from routine as yet. This is unlikely to be due to technical problems which have all now been solved but by human factors in the need for enthusiastic involvement at the various local sites and their relationship with the conference organiser (Norman *et al.*, 1997).

The original concepts of remote medicine established in the North Sea oilfields had already extended into the oilfields of the Middle East with particular reference to training, but clinical aspects of telemedicine were slow to develop in the UAE oil industry. This was due to local legal constraints and medical uncertainty as had been experienced initially in the North Sea oil industry. The university sector, however, pushed ahead in other community areas and the UAE had the advantage of its digital telephone exchange.

Road traffic accidents, including the management of the resultant casualties, was under the control of the Ministry of the Interior and thus the police directorate. Road traffic accident victims were thus not well managed medically since most attention was directed towards the cause of the accident and the collection of evidence leading to possible prosecution. Negotiation with the police directors in Al-Ain and Abu Dhabi, however, led to the establishment of training courses in first-aid for traffic policemen along the lines of those used for laymen in the offshore oil industries in the North Sea and Abu Dhabi. This rapidly greatly improved the mortality and morbidity of the casualties.

The rapport and collaboration which developed between the police directorate and the University not only resulted in continuing first-aid training for traffic policemen but established joint research into prevention and management of road traffic accidents. It also allowed for the development of communication with overseas police forces by the use of telemedical technology. In particular, this was established during the annual conferences held by the Abu Dhabi Police directorate which now included participation from overseas forces using the new technology available. One joint conference was with Grampian Police in Aberdeen on prevention of road traffic accidents and another was with the international agency in London responsible for the control and management of illegal drugs. Telemedical technology had thus spread outside medicine and eventually provided considerable benefit to the UAE in the prevention and management of road traffic accidents.

As was emphasised at the beginning of this book and in many sections, the start point in any successful innovation must be the process of research. That is if the project is to be achieved in a reasonable timescale. This was clearly recognised by the emerging Middle East Universities but it takes many years for a useful research culture to develop in a University. It was thus necessary for UAE personnel to visit Europe or America to receive research training and qualifications. A start was made towards research self-sufficiency by the University of Kuwait which invited Aberdeen University to establish an MSc course by research for a group of its medical graduates which was responsible for improving the quality of local healthcare. The course was to be held in Kuwait so that the students could remain at home and study local issues rather than those prescribed by foreign countries. This was agreed and 12 students were enrolled as part time MSc students at Aberdeen University.

This was a two-year experimental course and it was commenced by attendance at Aberdeen University during the long summer vacation which then existed at Aberdeen when the lecture and computing facilities were available. Each student selected a subject for study from a problem identified in the area with which he was involved in Kuwait. Students were given instruction in the basic elements of research methodology such as protocol design, statistics, epidemiology, literature review etc. After agreement on their experimental protocol they returned to Kuwait to collect data in line with their protocol. They were supervised from Aberdeen by e-mail and visited in Kuwait once each term by the Aberdeen supervisors. After the first year they returned to Aberdeen, once again during the long vacation, where they were instructed in data analysis and statistics and were supervised in the analysis of their own data. They were also given instruction in scientific writing and thesis presentation and returned home to complete their analysis and write the dissertation. Once again, they were assisted by e-mail and visited once per term during the second year. The dissertations were presented to an experienced external and an equally experienced internal examiner both of whom then visited Kuwait and conducted a careful and very full viva. All the students passed the examination and were awarded the Aberdeen degree, one with distinction.

This episode represented a further step forward in the development of international educational and research collaboration but it was difficult to administer and provide good supervision. It was noted by many who were involved that the course would be greatly improved if telemedicine had been available. This was in terms of administration, supervision and economy both for the students and their supervisors. This led logically to the next step which was the involvement of the UAE University which had led development in medical telecommunication technology. This was of course largely by virtue of the digital telephone exchange in Abu Dhabi and the various medical communication initiatives developed by means of ISDN telephone lines.

Appropriate administrative arrangements were thus made with Aberdeen University to accept UAE students to study part-time for higher degrees at Aberdeen University with supervision by telemedicine using a supervisor in Aberdeen and a second supervisor at the UAE University. Basic Picturetel equipment was used once again for communication and it was supplemented by the use of a document camera for the transmission of graphs and tables. Depending on the requirement of the research projects, communication was conducted by these means between the Aberdeen supervisor and students in the UAE on a weekly or monthly basis. This was a collaborative experiment between the two universities and it was agreed that the UAE student should spend at least 6 months of his registered studentship in Aberdeen.

A main advantage of this process was that it allowed the UAE student to remain at home and in his own environment rather than moving himself and his family to a foreign culture and way of life. In addition, it could also allow him to continue his employment at home on a part-time basis rather than requiring him to resign and start again. It also provided considerable economic advantages in both travel and subsistence. This allowed many to achieve a higher degree which would not otherwise have been possible and it allowed research and academic understanding to develop further between the universities.

Once again two examiners were appointed and the theses were examined in Aberdeen by the normal system of that University. The viva was, however, conducted in Abu Dhabi by telemedical means with one examiner in Aberdeen and the other in Abu Dhabi. By these means, 10 PhD studies and 5 MSc studies were taken to satisfactory completion in a six-year period with only two failing to complete for one reason or another. Considerable enthusiastic administrative support was provided by both Aberdeen and the UAE Universities. With the passage of time, however, and personnel changes in both Universities, this programme has not been sustained, once again emphasising the point made several times already on the vital support required at both ends by a key leader or driver. Now that Western universities and governments are recognizing both the academic and economic importance of such collaborative academic activity, support may improve — it may be a bit late however for UK involvement since many former third world universities are now actively developing their own research culture and higher degrees!

The largely historical approach taken in this chapter has preceded the rapid and amazing technological advances in communications technology which have been required by the energy and other major industries. In a relatively short time, medical communications for the support of those living in remote areas have advanced from Morse code and flag signals to a degree of sophistication which could not have been envisaged as little as twenty or thirty years ago. Technology is no longer a problem but a basic understanding of what is possible and how to use the new and at times complex equipment available is important for the emerging remote healthcare practitioner.

References

Bashshur RL and Lovett J. 1977. Assessments of telemedicine: results of the initial experience. *Aviat Space Environ Med* **48**: 65–70.

Brebner EM. 1997. Telemedicine and medical education. University of Aberdeen, UK: MSc thesis.

Brebner EM, Brebner JA, Norman JN, Brown PAJ, Ruddick-Bracken H and Lanphear JH. 1997. Intercontinental post mortem studies using interactive video. *J Telemed Telecare* **3:** 48–52.

Brebner JA. 1990. The provision of healthcare in remote and hostile environments. Robert Gordon University, Aberdeen: PhD thesis.

Dunn E, Acton H, Higgins C and Bain H. 1980. Telemedicine links patients in Sioux lookout with doctors in Toronto. *Can Med Assoc J* **122:** 484–487.

House AM and Roberts JM. 1977. Telemedicine in Canada. *Can Med Assoc J* **117:** 386–388.

Norman JN and Brebner JA. 1987. *The Offshore Health Handbook.* London: Martin Dinitz.

Norman JN, Brebner JA, Brebner EM, Lloyd OL, Ruddick-Bracken H, El-Sadig M, Catto GRD and Ledingham IMcA. 1995. Telematics in undergraduate teaching. *Med Educ* **29:** 403–406.

Norman JN, Brebner JA, Brebner EM, Ruddick-Bracken H, McIlvenny S and Sim AJW. 1997. International telemedicine. *J Telemed Telecare* **3:** 1–2.

Chapter

6 Acute Surgical Problems

J Nelson Norman

The Acute Abdomen

Abdominal pain can cause much concern even to an experienced surgeon. This is probably because a situation which seems relatively innocuous can deteriorate or develop with alarming suddenness into a serious life-threatening situation which requires immediate action. Immediate surgery is often not possible however, in remote and isolated situations and the remote healthcare practitioner may not have much or any surgical experience. Even if he does, the patient's chances of survival could be greater if management was by a more conservative regime. It is worth remembering the time-tried approaches to conservative therapy which were used with good effect in the pre-antibiotic, pre-sophisticated anaesthetic era.

The remote healthcare practitioner needs to have a means of determining what is likely to be wrong in the abdomen, to have a means of communicating to a source of specialist advice and he also needs to have a knowledge of how to manage an acute abdomen, even though he does not have a precise diagnosis, nor is equipped to undertake surgical treatment.

Abdominal pain

In surgical diagnosis the characteristics of abdominal pain are the key factors in determining action, and this is why surgeons become irritated when patients admitted to the wards are given powerful analgesics before they have had the opportunity to see them. In general terms there are three types of pain which are of importance:

- colic
- peritoneal pain
- referred pain

Colic

The abdomen consists of a number of organs, many of which are hollow and connected by a series of tubes which transmit material from one part to another. The tubes and organs are supplied with muscles so that they can undergo movements designed to propel their contents onwards. The walls of these organs are poorly innervated and one is not normally conscious of their actions because they do not intrude upon consciousness. If one of these structures becomes inflamed or the lumen becomes blocked, the muscular efforts often become exaggerated and the movements then reach conscious appreciation. This is interpreted as abdominal pain and the type of pain is known as colic. Colicky abdominal pain is a poorly localised discomfort, of which the pain site is indicated by the patient with the palm of his hand and movement over a fairly large part of the abdomen. It is useful to distinguish between three types of abdominal colic:

1. Fore gut colic
2. Mid gut colic
3. Hind gut colic

1. Fore gut colic
Where the patient complains of fore-gut colic he complains of a spasmodic, ill-defined pain, and the hand passes across the upper abdomen above the umbilicus. When you see that, you can say that it is likely that the problem lies anatomically somewhere from the lower end of the oesophagus to the second part of the duodenum. In common disease terms that means hiatus hernia, peptic ulcer, gastric neoplasm, cholecystitis or pancreatitis. As soon as you see the flat of the hand passing across the abdomen above the umbilicus you have begun to hone down on the diagnosis.

2. Mid gut colic
When a patient complains of mid gut colic he complains of spasmodic abdominal pain and his hand passes across the umbilicus. He is therefore complaining of some kind of problem from the second part of the duodenum to the hepatic flexure of the colon. Once again, in disease terms, he could be complaining of — a small bowel obstruction which is most likely to be caused by the bowel becoming caught up in an external or an internal hernia. The internal hernia may be an adhesion so you should look for a previous abdominal scar, or it may be a congenital band or a recess of the peritoneum. It can of course also be caused by something blocking the lumen of that part of the bowel known as the mid gut. The most common part of the lumen that becomes blocked to produce that symptom is the appendix. In food poisoning the gut reacts fiercely to rid itself of the noxious substance and that produces the same type of griping and spasmodic abdominal discomfort, but it is of course associated with diarrhoea and vomiting.

3. Hind gut colic

When the patient complains of hind gut colic he is complaining of ill-defined, spasmodic pain, and the hand passes across the abdomen below the umbilicus. He is thus referring to a colonic problem from the hepatic flexure of the colon to its termination. This is where any discomfort associated with constipation is likely to be felt, but probably the most common disease is either a neoplasm of the sigmoid colon or diverticular disease. These problems are of course less likely to occur in the younger age groups. It is thus obvious that just listening to the patient and observing him closely can take you quite a long way in abdominal diagnosis.

When the disease process proceeds and extends outwards to involve the whole thickness of the tube or organ and its peritoneal covering becomes involved, the character of the pain changes, since, unlike the walls of the organs and tubes, the peritoneal lining is richly supplied with pain nerve endings. Thus, when the disease process reaches that point, the patient complains of a different type of pain — peritoneal pain.

Peritoneal pain

When peritoneal pain takes place, it is a sharp, shooting, intense pain which is precisely localised and therefore pointed out by the patient with a finger, rather than the palm of the hand. Thus, in the early stages of cholecystitis when the outlet of the gallbladder may be blocked by a stone and its contents become infected the patient will complain of pain of the fore-gut colic variety. If the diseased gallbladder wall becomes so involved that the overlying peritoneum is affected, the patient will then say that he now has a sharp, lancing, excruciating pain and point with his index finger to the region of the ninth costal cartilage. The emergence of peritoneal pain suggests that the process has progressed to one of greater urgency than that manifested by colicky pain alone.

Referred pain

Referred pain is pain which indicates a disease process in an organ referred to where the organ develops. It can thus be of help in determining where the seat of a problem is if one remembers where certain key organs develop. For example, if a peptic ulcer leaks or a gallbladder becomes inflamed and either process causes peritoneal irritation on the under-surface of the diaphragm, the pain may be felt at the shoulder tip. This is because the diaphragm developed in the neck and took its nerve supply with it. This comes from the third and fourth cervical segments of the cord. Equally, the testis develops alongside the kidneys and testicular pain is sometimes felt in the loin, rather than the scrotal region. A frequently serious mistake made in examining the abdomen is not to inspect or palpate the scrotum and its contents. Loin pain could mistakenly be associated with a minor renal problem when the real answer to the problem is a tumour of the testis or an early torsion.

Before you begin to treat the acute abdomen it is essential that you learn as much about the problem as possible. Thus, always stick to the tried and tested routines of the old physicians:

1. Take the history
2. Conduct the abdominal examination
3. Carry out such investigations as are necessary or possible
4. Consider the diagnosis at this point or establish a working diagnosis with a view to determining management

1. Take the history

This is the most important part of the diagnostic process; it will take you time and you need to get it right. First of all, you need to establish the central complaint and its timing and duration. The timing and the order of appearance of the various signs and symptoms in abdominal disease is probably more critical in achieving a diagnosis than anything else. It is thus essential to stick rigidly to the rules of history taking if you hope to get a clear picture of the developing disease process. The most useful first question in establishing the timing sequence could be "When did you last feel entirely well?" When that point has been established the next thing to ask is "What happened next, and when was that, what happened after that and when did that take place?"

Remember, where possible, never to ask direct questions, always show patience and listen to the patient talking, guiding him only slightly to keep him on the rails. Eventually you will need to ask direct questions in order to define points precisely, but that should be right at the end of the interview. If, for example, you wish to determine whether the patient was jaundiced, you must think of several ways of asking the same question before you can be sure he has completely understood you. The first question can be something like, "Have you noticed any change in the colour of your skin at all?" If that answer is in the negative you can pursue it by saying, "Not even in the whites of your eyes?" Alternatively, "Have you noticed any change in the colour of your urine or of your bowel motions?" as compared to "Have you noticed dark urine or pale stools?" It takes time and patience to determine each point with certainty.

You can build up the sequence of events and the order in which they took place, and having defined the central complaint and the timing and order of appearance of the various events, it is now time to begin the examination. No attempt should be made to touch the patient in any way until a clear and precise history has been obtained. Experienced clinicians will tell you that if they have little idea of the diagnosis by the time the history has been taken it would be unusual for them to be further advanced in the diagnosis after the examination. The examination confirms and substantiates suspicions and facts that have already emerged in the history.

2. Conduct the abdominal examination

You will only get one chance to examine the abdomen properly and if you make a mistake early in the examination you may fail to elicit relevant information to your satisfaction. The biggest mistake you can make is to be in too much of a hurry. You must gain the patient's confidence for him to allow you to poke around amongst his inflamed and tender viscera.

The first thing to do is to look at the abdomen. To look at it you must expose it. Remember that the abdomen begins at the lower end of the chest and includes the hernia orifices and scrotum, while the digestive tract begins at the mouth and ends at the anus. The first thing to look at is the patient's attitude in bed. If he is complaining of severe pain and is writhing about trying to find a comfortable position it is likely that he is suffering from some type of colic. If, on the other hand, he is complaining of severe pain and is lying very still it is more likely that the pain is of the peritoneal type. In this case, movement will cause an exacerbation of the pain as the inflamed layers of the peritoneum rub against each other.

Equally, breathing is restricted in the face of peritoneal pain for the same reason. If the abdomen is distended with gas this may be due to a fairly low intestinal obstruction and you may be able to suspect or detect that by looking at the at abdomen. In a small bowel obstruction, you may even see bowel movements through the abdominal wall if they are sufficiently exaggerated.

Elicit all the information you can by looking at the abdomen. Having gained the confidence of the patient by talking to him quietly, you should next get into a comfortable position so that the palm of your hand is able to rest very gently on the abdomen as far away as possible from the area which he has indicated to be painful. Pass the flat of your hand gently over the four quadrants. You are not trying to achieve anything at this time other than to gain the patient's confidence and to make him feel that you are not going to hurt him. Continue with this sort of movement and now try to determine whether there is any difference in the consistency or feel of the abdominal wall in each of the four quadrants. This will be indicated by involuntary guarding which is caused by muscle spasm with a view to preventing too much movement of the underlying peritoneal lining or inflamed organ wall. If there is some abnormal constituent or hard lump you will probably feel this at the same time but that is about all you can achieve. In fact, if you are able to localise the area of pathology by this means, you will in fact have achieved quite a lot.

When you have completed this stage of the examination, and say for example that you have located an area of tenderness in the right lower quadrant, you may wish to determine whether there is a precise area of tenderness which could be caused by the tip of an inflamed appendix touching the peritoneal lining of the abdominal wall. You are now in a position to use the tips of your fingers to determine whether there is a precisely localised area of tenderness. Gradually push your fingers deeper into the abdomen, separating the layers of the peritoneum slowly. When you suddenly withdraw your fingers, the inflamed surfaces rub over each other rapidly producing an excruciating stab of pain. This is diagnostic of peritoneal irritation. Usually you only get one chance to elicit this.

When you have examined the main area of the abdomen, turn your attention next to the hernia — orifices, both inguinal and their femoral. At least once each year in most surgical wards, a patient is admitted having vomited for three or four days and in a serious state of dehydration, because the hernia orifices were not properly examined and a small femoral hernia had gone undetected.

Finally, the scrotum must be inspected and examined. The cause of the pain may be torsion of a testicle and if that is the case you do not have long to take corrective action before the testicle is lost. Remember also the congenital abnormality which allows this to happen is often bilateral. Equally, in a young man a testicular tumour may present as a painless, slightly enlarged testicle on one side. Survival depends upon early diagnosis and thus in all routine examinations of the abdomen, the scrotum should always be carefully examined even if it is only to exclude this possibility.

Having completed the examination, the findings must now be carefully recorded. This is for two purposes. In the first instance it allows the formulation of the message you will pass to the clinician at a distance who will advise on management and secondly it will allow you to recall additional features with timing as they occur if you are in clinical charge for a prolonged period.

3. Carry out such investigations as are necessary or possible

You may not be in a position to undertake any special investigations but it is always worthwhile to examine the urine particularly for the presence of blood. This could suggest a stone somewhere in the urinary tract. The estimation of the haemoglobin might suggest slow and chronic bleeding of an ulcer while a high ESR could indicate the possibility of neoplasia or inflammation. A white blood count greater than 10,000 cells per cubic millimetre may provide evidence of acute appendicitis if the other signs and symptoms are present.

4. Consider the diagnosis

If the various signs and symptoms elicited are to be of value to you in making a diagnosis, it is useful to have a knowledge of the classical presentation of the common abdominal complaints so that you are in a position to determine how closely the clinical picture elicited from your patient relates to the classical features of the common conditions. A series of thumbnail sketches is thus given below of the prominent features of the most common conditions you will meet.

We will consider:

1. Peptic ulcer
2. Cholecystitis
3. Pancreatitis
4. Intestinal obstruction
5. Appendicitis

1. Peptic ulcer

A peptic ulcer may occur in either the stomach or the duodenum. What happens is that for one reason or another, part of the lining of the organ is destroyed, leaving a shallow ulcer crater in which there are exposed nerve endings. When the acid level rises to a critical value, the nerve endings are stimulated and pain occurs. Pain is of course, of the fore-gut colic variety, and it is relieved when the acid level falls again. This is achieved either by taking food or alkali mixtures.

Pain associated with eating is known as dyspepsia and the dyspepsia associated with peptic ulcer is periodic in nature. That means that there are periods of time when the patient has a great deal of trouble with his stomach and periods of time when he is free of pain. This is presumably due to the partial healing of the lesion and the covering of the exposed nerve endings.

The characteristic features of a peptic ulcer are thus periodicity, characterised by periods of trouble which may last for a few weeks, and then periods of freedom which may last for a few weeks or even months.

The second feature is that the pain comes on when the stomach is empty. The patient will often say that it is related to meals and that it comes on after a meal. You have to dig quite deeply to determine that when he says after a meal, he in fact may mean two or three hours after a meal or in other words just before the next meal.

The classic presentation of peptic ulceration is thus of a periodic dyspepsia which comes on when the stomach is empty and is relieved by both food and alkalis.

It is often worthwhile to seek possible complications in trying to confirm a diagnosis. The main complications of a peptic ulcer which one might find is bleeding and that is usually made manifest by the appearance of coffee ground particles in the occasional vomit or by dark or even tarry stools. Vomiting is, however, not a common feature of early peptic ulcer.

2. Cholecystitis and gallstones

Cholecystitis results in a dyspepsia which is different from that caused by an ulcer, although the site of the pathology may be very close anatomically. When the gallbladder becomes inflamed the presenting symptom is the same as that shown by peptic ulcer — fore-gut colic, the palm of the hand passing across the abdomen above the umbilicus. The dyspepsia is, however, not periodic. It can occur in attacks at any time, and since it is an infective condition caused by blockage of the gallbladder by a gallstone in the cystic duct it may be associated with some fever. In this case the dyspepsia is certainly associated with food and is caused directly by it, and is not relieved by alkali mixtures. When food passes into the duodenum a hormone is released which causes the gallbladder to contract releasing bile into the upper gut to assist in the process of digestion. If the gallbladder is inflamed, pain will result when its wall is squeezed in much the same way as pain will result if you squeeze an inflamed finger.

Since bile is particularly important for the digestion of fat discomfort will be most marked when fatty foods impinge upon the duodenum and that is why the gallbladder patient is often intolerant of fat.

There is thus no periodicity in gallbladder dyspepsia, pain is caused directly by food, particularly fatty foods, and it is not relieved by alkali mixtures. Associated complicating features relate to the presence of gallstones and the possible obstruction of the common bile duct by a stone or merely the swelling of the gallbladder. Thus, we are looking for the possibility of mild fever on the one hand and mild jaundice on the other. This can either manifest itself by a yellowish discolouration of the sclera or by associated dark urine or pale bowel motions.

In general terms, peptic ulcer usually occurs in the 20s and affects ambitious, active young people, with a predominance in males. Gallbladder problems usually manifest themselves a bit later, in the mid-30s or early 40s. There is a tendency to mild obesity in sufferers from this condition and there is a predominance in females.

3. Pancreatitis

Occasionally the pancreas undergoes an acute aseptic inflammatory reaction for reasons which are not always clear, but are often associated with alcohol in some cases and with gallstones in others. When acute pancreatitis strikes, it usually does so with dramatic suddenness and a condition is produced which is indistinguishable from a perforated peptic ulcer or gallbladder. In other words, there is generalised abdominal pain with a rigid, hard abdominal wall. The diagnosis can often only be confirmed in hospital by blood tests such as the level of serum — amylase. In a remote situation the accurate diagnosis of acute pancreatitis may not be possible but its management would be the same as the management of a perforated ulcer and this will be discussed below.

There is also a condition of chronic, relapsing pancreatitis and when this occurs it is difficult to distinguish from chronic peptic ulcer or even chronic cholecystitis. The manifestations are much the same in terms of pain which is, of course, of a fore-gut, colicky nature but it is difficult to relate the dyspepsia to that found typically in peptic ulcer or the gallbladder variety. The only distinguishing feature is that the pain often radiates through to the back and is felt between the shoulder blades.

4. Intestinal obstruction

There are three main features of intestinal obstruction:

1. Vomiting
2. Colicky abdominal pain
3. Distension

In general terms the site of the obstruction can be placed anatomically if it is accepted that the lower the obstruction the greater will be the distension and the lesser the vomiting. On the other hand, the higher the obstruction the greater will be the vomiting and the lesser the distension. Thus, in a high, small bowel obstruction there will be copious vomiting but little distension since the bowel beneath the obstruction will be collapsed. On the other hand, in a large bowel obstruction the gut has to fill totally with fluid and gas before it spills over and vomiting takes place. Vomiting may thus not occur for several days or even occasionally weeks after the colon has become partially obstructed. Thus, in the early stages of diagnosis vomiting may not be a feature in intestinal obstruction and it is important to remember also that absolute constipation is not an immediate feature either, particularly if the obstruction is high and the whole bowel has to empty beneath the obstruction before absolute constipation takes place.

The one common feature will be colicky abdominal pain and it will of course be either fore, mid or hind gut colic depending on the locus of the obstruction. When you are led to suspect the possibility of intestinal obstruction always examine the hernia orifices very carefully with special reference to the femoral orifices, and look for previous abdominal surgical scars which could suggest the presence of adhesions.

5. Appendicitis

Appendicitis is a condition which is sometimes very difficult to diagnose if the appendix does not lie in its usual position. You must always remember that the tip of the appendix may lie deep in the pelvis or the whole appendix may be wrapped up in coils of small bowel.

The classical features of appendicitis were originally described by an Irish surgeon named Murphy. He stated that the classical picture of acute appendicitis was present if five symptoms/signs presented in a particular order. If any symptom or sign was missing or if the order was different you could not positively diagnose appendicitis. Equally, if they were all present in the stated order the diagnosis was almost certain. Murphy's five signs of appendicitis are, in order:

1. Mid gut colic
2. Nausea or vomiting
3. Peritoneal pain in the right iliac fossa
4. Fever
5. Leucocytosis

Appendicitis is a rapidly developing condition and it is unlikely to be present if the symptoms have been around for several weeks. Right iliac fossa pain under these circumstances would be more likely to be due to something like constipation rather than appendicitis. The fever is usually modest and the temperature usually not much more than 38°C. A confusing picture is always presented if there is an absence of peritoneal pain localised to the right iliac fossa. This can occur if the appendix is wrapped up in small bowel but this is uncommon. It is much more common however, for the tip of the appendix to lie deeply in the pelvis and it is for this reason that a rectal examination as part of the examination of the abdomen is important and particularly if appendicitis is suspected.

How to conduct a rectal examination

Lay the patient on his side and ask him to pull his knees up towards his chest. Insert the index finger to its full extent into the rectum and attempt not to touch any of the surrounding rectal wall. Next, say to the patient that you appreciate that he is now suffering some discomfort. Ask him to appreciate the level of that discomfort before doing anything further. The prostate is directly in front of your finger and there is a pouch on the right side and one on the left side. If there is an inflammatory exudate or an inflamed appendix at the tip in the pelvis you then move your finger forwards to prod the pouch on the right side; it will produce severe sharp discomfort since the pouch is lined with peritoneum. It is only possible to be sure that the pouch is tender if you have first made sure that the patient appreciates the discomfort of having a finger in the rectum and is then able to say that you have greatly increased that discomfort by prodding the peritoneal pouch.

Management of the Acute Abdomen

In the management of an acute abdomen, the first thing you need to do is establish communication with a distant clinician who is preferably a surgeon. Following consultation, a diagnosis or at least a working diagnosis should be established. This may not be possible but you may be fairly certain that it is something serious. In any event something needs to be done. You can either buy time and observe carefully hoping that the picture becomes clearer with time. Alternatively, you can start treatment on the basis that it is likely that the abdominal problem is of an inflammatory order or obstructive nature.

The first thing to do is to put the gut at rest. This can be done to several degrees depending upon your feeling of how serious the condition is. The first degree is to stop the patient eating. If you think it is more serious than that, then reduce the oral intake to sips of water or bland fluids. If you think it is even more serious than that, you can stop the patient eating and drinking totally. Finally, if you wish to put the gut totally at rest you need to pass a naso-gastric tube and aspirate the contents of the alimentary tract continuously. If you do this however, for any length of time, it is necessary to establish intravenous replacement fluids and electrolyte therapy.

You have not initiated specific treatment directed towards the gut itself but at the same time it is important that precise progress notes are kept so that you are in a position to determine the development of the condition. It is also worthwhile monitoring pulse, temperature and blood pressure on a regular basis and preferably hourly if you are concerned about the patient. These measures will be sufficient to buy time in the diagnosis of most abdominal conditions and will also form the basis of conservative treatment.

All that is necessary in addition, for example, in the management of acute cholecystitis would be the addition of an antibiotic. All that you require for the conservative management of appendicitis would once again be the addition of an antibiotic and possibly small doses of morphine to reduce gut movements even further. It is even possible to treat a perforated peptic ulcer by these means, if necessary, and it has been shown in the past in high-risk cases that the survival rate is almost as good by conservative management as by operative management in these conditions. If you have been able to establish a good line of communication with a distant clinician and you have the appropriate kit you should be able, given a bit of luck, to manage an acute abdominal condition conservatively. If you have failed to establish a point of communication and are not able to evacuate your patient you need a little more knowledge in order to maintain the fluid and electrolyte replacement therapy adequately until help arrives or the condition resolves.

Fluid and Electrolyte Therapy

Fluid replacement therapy is quite easy provided you follow a few simple guidelines. If you are working in a remote or isolated place you may not have access to laboratory control so you need a system which will provide good results over a long period of time without laboratory control. Some people are quite cavalier about this form of treatment, and consider that it doesn't really matter what you put in since the kidneys will sort things out in the long run. While this may be so, but if the subject is really ill, the kidneys are probably not functioning effectively. You may get away with infusing a few bottles indiscriminately for the first day or two, since it will only be after a week or so that the real problems which are caused by this kind of therapy will emerge — and the patient will probably have moved on to another person's care by that time! Whether you are to be looking after the patient for a prolonged period of time or only until evacuation can be arranged, you should always begin intravenous therapy as though you are going to be in charge of it yourself for at least six weeks.

If 24 hours urine flow is not known, then it would be reasonable to start your prescription on the urine flow which you would like to see, and the reasonable figure would be 1.5 litres. The scheme set out below works well without laboratory control for several weeks. It is important however, that you choose a logical sequence from the outset.

Basic maintenance therapy

Here we consider what is required to maintain fluid and electrolyte balance in the subject who, for one reason or another, is just not able to take fluid by mouth. The prescription is based on a fluid balance chart, such as is shown in Figure 1, and it is prescribed for a period of 24 hours. The prescription is based on the fluid lost in the previous 24-hour period, thus as far as the prescription is concerned, we are always working 24 hours in arrears and thus we need to know how much was lost in the previous 24-hour period. If we assume that 1.5 litres of urine was passed in the previous 24 hours, we also need to know of any other sources of fluid loss. If we allow 400 ml was lost in insensible perspiration and 600 ml fluid from the respiratory tract that makes a total of 1.0 litres for insensible loss. If we add that to the urine loss, that makes a total of 2.5 litres to replace during the next day.

The way to write the prescription is to write down the number of 0.5 litre bottles required on the left-hand side, and then to write the time for the confusion of each bottle on the right. That is, of course, obtained by dividing the number of bottles into 24 so in this situation where five bottles (2.5 L) are to be infused, the first four bottles will be infused over five hours each but the final one in four. An example of such a fluid prescription may be seen in Figure 2.

Intake		Losses	
Tea	600ml	Urine	1500ml
Water	1200ml	Insensible sweat	400ml
Juice	300ml	Insensible respiratory	600ml
Soup	400ml	**Total**	**2500ml**
Total	**2500ml**		

Figure 1:   Summated fluid balance chart for 24 hours.

Fluid to be infused	Time for infusion
1..5% dextrose	5 hours
2..5% dextrose	5 hours.
3..5% dextrose	5 hours.
4.. 5% dextrose	5 hours.
5. 5% dextrose	4 hours.

Figure 2:   Example of 24 hour IV fluid prescription providing basic maintenance of water for the following 24 hours.

While we want to prescribe water, we of course require an isotonic solution and an isotonic solution which provides pure water is 5% dextrose. Thus, in order to give the patient who has passed 1.5 L of urine during the previous 24-hour his water requirements for the next 24 hours, this would require a prescription of five bottles of 5% dextrose.

Replacement of electrolytes

It must be remembered that salt is being lost constantly as is potassium, but, once again if we use rule of thumb figures, we will not go wrong. About 5 g of salt is lost by a normal subject in 24 hours and 5 g of salt is contained in one bottle of 0.9% physiological saline. Thus if one of the bottles of 5% dextrose is replaced by one of 0.9% saline we have prescribed both for the water and for the salt requirements.

The next fact we are required to know is that around 3 g of potassium is lost in 24 hours. If we add 1 g of potassium to each of three of the bottles of 5% dextrose, we will have prescribed the water, the salt and the potassium requirements for the next 24 hours. An example of the fluid prescription which provides this basic maintenance can be seen in Figure 3.

This is a very simple system to follow since all you really need to know, and thus to measure, is the urine flow over each 24-hour period. If you wonder where to start when you commence this type of therapy, particularly if you do not have measurement of the previous 24 hours of urine flow, it would be reasonable to

Fluid to be infused	Time for infusion
5% dextrose...5 hours	
5% dextrose +KCL...5 hours.	
5% dextrose+KCL..5 hours.	
5% dextrose+KCL..5 hours.	
0.9% saline...4 hours.	

Figure 3:   Example of 24 hour fluid prescription which provides basic maintenance of both water and salts.

start your prescription on the urine flow which you would like to see, and the reasonable figure would be one and a half litres.

In practice, when prescribing fluids for the subsequent 24 hours, the natural tendency is to round up the urine flow to the nearest half litre since people do not pass urine in precise half litre volumes. This minor over-prescription usually results in a slightly increased urine flow the next day, which results in a slightly increased rounding up until the patient may be passing several litres per day. When this takes place, and you notice it, you should not take sudden action, but gradually pull back on the prescription and for a day or two prescribe a bottle less until you "arrange" for the urine flow to be in the region of a litre or litre and a half. This is part of the art which accompanies the science of good healthcare! It is always worth maintaining a reasonably substantial urine flow in the face of intra abdominal pathology or in the face of injury, as you wish to — prevent toxic products of tissue breakdown from appearing in a concentration which is too high in the renal tubules. Whatever other form of fluid the patient may require intravenously you must always start by giving him his basic maintenance requirements.

Fluid requirements during illness

We now consider the prescription for the patient who has a naso-gastric tube in place and which may be producing a reasonably high aspirate and who may be losing fluid also from other sources. The prescription of fluid is worked out from the fluid balance chart and giving, once again the volume of fluid which was lost in the previous 24 hours. This is done by taking the urine flow, adding the insensible loss and writing the basic maintenance prescription as suggested above. We then add the volume of aspirate together with any other source of fluid loss and replace that volume of fluid with 0.9% physiological saline. The reason for this is that the fluids which are lost from the body will have a constitution not dissimilar to extracellular fluid and will already have a substantial quantity of salt within them. We therefore replace all the additional losses in the form of physiological saline and then add 1 g of potassium to every additional bottle added.

We may end up with a fairly substantial fluid prescription which could result in the need to infuse one half litre every two hours or so. Even so, if these rules and guidelines are followed from the word go, it is unlikely that any serious disturbance of fluid and electrolyte balance will take place — even without laboratory control.

Monitoring fluid and electrolyte therapy

If a patient is sufficiently ill to require fluid and electrolyte therapy, it is necessary to measure the pulse rate and the blood pressure at regular intervals to determine the general state of well-being. It is also essential to measure the urine flow, not only from the point of view of the fluid prescription, but also to determine whether the patient is passing sufficient urine. If the urine flow falls below 1 L in 24 hours he is likely to become dehydrated and needs rather more fluid. If the urine flow rises about 2 L or so, it is likely you are giving him too much and should cut back a little on your prescription.

Another sign worth noting is the state of skin turgor. Pinch up a little skin on the back of the hand, and if the subject is young and reasonably fit, it will spring back into place very rapidly. If he is reasonably young and fit, and it does not spring back into position but remains creased, it is likely that he is requiring more water and salts. On the other hand, if you give him too much fluid, the first place where this will leak out is into the lungs and respiratory rate will begin to rise. He may begin to cough up some clear frothy fluid and if you are able to auscultate the chest you will hear moist sounds at the lung bases.

With close attention to all these signs and an understanding of the guidelines for fluid prescription, it should be quite possible for you to maintain your patient in a reasonable state of hydration and electrolyte balance until the disease process subsides or he begins to recover or is able to be evacuated for specialist care. It is essential, however, that you have some understanding of what you are doing, because this type of therapy is equally as much an art as it is a science, and it can only be practised safely and well by those who have not only an understanding of what they are trying to achieve, but also a clinical sense for the patients' well-being.

Bibliography

McLatchie G, Borley N and Chikwe J (eds.). 2013. *Oxford Handbook of Clinical Surgery*, 4th Edn. Oxford: Oxford University Press.

Innes JA, Dover A and Karen Fairhurst K (eds.). 2018. *Macleod's Clinical Examination*, 14th Edn. Amsterdam: Elsevier.

Thomas J and Monaghan T (eds.). 2014. *Oxford Handbook of Clinical Examination and Practical Skills*, 2nd Edn. Oxford: Oxford University Press.

Ranasinghe L and Clements O. 2019. *RevMED: 300 SBAs in Medicine and Surgery*. London: World Scientific. Available at https://doi.org/10.1142/q0203.

Williams N, O'Connell PR and McCaskie A (eds). 2018. *Bailey & Love's Short Practice of Surgery*, 27th Edn. Boca Raton, Florida: CRC Press.

© 2020 World Scientific Publishing Company
https://doi.org/10.1142/9781786347510_0007

Chapter

7 Diagnosis and Management of Medical Emergencies

Thomas French

Introduction

The wide variety of acute medical complaints and the management of these can cause anxiety even in the most experienced physicians who have access to a full complement of diagnostic aids, as well as peers experienced in a wide array of sub-specialties. The remote clinician is often an independent practitioner who may be both geographically and personally isolated from easy to access resources. It is important that the remote clinician develops skills, particularly in the field of clinical diagnostics, to manage diagnostic uncertainty and sensibly manage the risk that this entails. They must be able to utilise those skills in often challenging environments with limited resources.

The remote clinician will often have access to basic investigations, be it biochemical, haematological or radiological tests. The skill lies in how they interpret these and apply the results of available investigations to the clinical problem with a realistic approach.

Acutely unwell medical patients will present in a variety of ways and this chapter will not cover all of them; but it will help the clinician to adopt a systematic approach to common medical complaints that they may be faced with. As with any medical complaint the importance of taking a clear and accurate history from the patient is paramount, this combined with examination will often lead to a clear diagnosis, that would otherwise in a non-remote setting be supported by further investigations. A working diagnosis may be just as valuable, and the ability to think critically and revisit potential diagnoses should not be undervalued.

Assessing the Acutely Unwell Medical Patient

All medical patients should have a basic set of observations taken and recorded. These include, respiratory rate, pulse rate, systolic blood pressure, oxygen saturations, conscious level, and oxygen saturations. There are various clinical early warning scores that have been developed, and in general they are useful at helping to clarify how unwell a medical patient is at a point in time. They will also allow the clinician to categorise deterioration or improvement in condition. Each parameter is assigned a score and the summation of these will give an indication of the severity of illness and clinical risk. However, they are not perfect, and if the clinician feels that a patient is more unwell than the parameters suspect, clinical suspicion should not be ignored. An experienced clinician may be more adept at picking up patient deterioration that is impending or otherwise than a set of parameters can.

An example of an early warning score system is the National Early Warning Score System as advocated by NICE. Initially borne out of need to better recognise the septic patient, they are now applied more widely in most clinical settings (RCP London, 2017).

When approaching the acutely unwell patient, the clinician should approach the clinical scenario as dictated by the most pressing problem. For example, patients who have clear hypoxia, should be given oxygen. An ABCDE approach has been advocated for many years and is well established amongst the profession in the initial assessment of acutely unwell patients (Thim et al., 2012).

A — Airway
B — Breathing
C — Circulation
D — Disability (conscious level/neurological compromise)
E — Exposure, glucose level and everything else

Variations of this approach have been adopted in many basic resuscitation courses, such as ALS, ATLS, and IMPACT. The order in which the patient is assessed as a systematic approach will help ensure that life threatening problems are managed in an appropriate way. The military, following the medical advances made in multiple combat theatres, have moved on to parallel resuscitation. This involves clearly defined roles within teams and parallel assessment of multiple problems at the same time. The management of complex trauma patients is ever evolving with the development of trauma teams and trauma centres improving patient outcomes (McCullough et al., 2014). The same system operates when a cardiac arrest team arrives to manage a patient in cardiac arrest with feedback being given to a central team leader. This may not be possible in the remote setting as the clinician will often be on their own. It is now recognised that the non-technical skills used in the management of critically unwell patients play an important role in their outcomes.

The advantages of adopting this systematic approach is that, under pressure, the clinician is less likely to miss something important and deal with this appropriately.

In patients that are more stable it is the tenets of good basic medical practice that come to the fore. Crucially the ability to take a good history and focus the examination to this. A well taken history will save time and save lives.

Common Medical Complaints and Presentations

Chest pain

Patients will present in a variety of ways with chest pain and the history is often enough to help discriminate between the various causes.

Common complaints include cardiac related chest pain, pulmonary thromboembolism (PTE) and pneumothorax. However, dyspepsia, gastroesophageal reflux disease and musculoskeletal chest pain can often mimic these presentations. This can cause anxiety amongst even the most competent medic and lead to over investigation.

When taking a history in relation to chest pain the pneumonic SOCRATES is a helpful reminder as to what to ask.

Sight
Origin
Character
Radiation
Associated Symptoms
Timing and Duration
Exacerbating/Relieving Factors
Severity

Cardiac related chest pain in males tends to present with a classical dull ache in the centre of the chest. It lasts minutes to hours. In patients who have a history suggestive of myocardial infarction there are often associated with autonomic symptoms such as nausea, flushing, vomiting. Women, often present more atypically, and this should be borne in mind. Diabetic patients may present with no pain at all, the 'silent MI' (Niakan et al., 1986).

There is likely to be a history of escalating symptoms in patients who have pre-existing coronary artery disease. These are often exertional but may not be. They will often have risk factors for the development of coronary artery disease, be it family history, high cholesterol levels, or predominantly a history of smoking.

An ECG demonstrating ST segment elevation or changes consistent with a posterior myocardial infarction are medical emergencies and they should be dealt with as such. The pain in these patients is often pathognomonic of ongoing ischaemia and myocardial damage. Reducing pain, and myocardial oxygen demand is vital. A troponin in these patients is unlikely to tell you anything different, and if possible, they should be transferred to a tertiary centre. However, if this is not possible thrombolysis should be considered to restore coronary artery perfusion. There are a few contraindications to thrombolysis that should be considered, and tertiary advice should be sought.

The initial management should be centred around stabilising the patient and providing basic cardiac care. This typically includes: Morphine, Oxygen, Nitrates and Aspirin (MONA). Reduction of pain and improving oxygen delivery to the cardiac muscle will help to reduce cardiac myocyte damage. Nevertheless, this historical practice has now progressed to include other treatments, and the pneumonic "THROMBINS2" has been proposed (Kline *et al.*, 2015).

Classical angina is a clinical diagnosis, and should be managed based on symptoms, those with a negative troponin, often now available with the advent of near patient testing, should have this diagnosis considered and managed appropriately.

Unstable angina with symptoms at rest is different and, depending on the availability of tertiary care, it may be more appropriate to transfer the patient for angiography as it could herald an impending myocardial infarction. In this scenario inpatient management until symptoms are controlled or myocardial infarction becomes apparent is preferable.

In some instances, a troponin is very useful. Particularly when the history is suggestive of an ischaemic cause and may indicate that the patient has suffered a non-ST segment elevation myocardial infarction (NSTEMI). These patients often go on to require angiography, however, it can be in the remote setting managed medically in the first instance, and this may be all that is possible.

Troponins may rise in other circumstances and this should be borne in mind, such as in the case of myocarditis, or as a secondary insult from other pathology. This is often noted to be a type 2 MI and treating the underlying cause is often the best course of action (Thygesen *et al.*, 2007). Serial troponins can help to elicit if there is a cause for concern from a cardiac perspective. The routine testing of troponins in all patients with chest pain may seem like a good idea, but it is often counterproductive and may confuse the situation. All investigations should be targeted.

Pulmonary thromboembolism

Patients presenting with pleuritic chest pain in combination with a history of breathlessness should be assessed for the possibility of a PTE. This is even more so in the presence of an otherwise unexplained tachycardia. Hypoxia may be obvious or subtle. Various clinical scores have been created and heavily researched to predict whether a patient may have a PTE. However, a low risk Wells score in combination with a negative PERC score (Pulmonary Embolism Rule-out Criteria) strongly correlates with a patient being unlikely to have a PTE and there is no need for further investigation. This negates the need for a D-Dimer. This is useful in patients who are younger, and generally fitter (Kline *et al.*, 2004).

In those patients who do not meet the criteria as detailed in a PERC score but still have a low probability Wells score for PTE, a D-Dimer may be required to exclude a PTE.

If a patient has a Wells Score likely to indicate the presence of a PTE then a D-Dimer is not useful and the patient should be commenced on low molecular weight heparin prior to CT pulmonary angiography (CTPA) if possible. Though often overlooked, a plain film chest x-ray may be helpful in patients presenting with features of PTE through the presence of the Westermark sign or even evidence suggestive of pulmonary infarction. The Westermark sign is the presence of dilated pulmonary vessels proximal to the embolism, with collapse of vessels distal to it. It is remarkable how many times this is missed on many a plain film. A plain film may also reveal a further cause for the chest pain which may have been overlooked, such as pneumonia.

Patients with PTE are often managed now in an ambulatory fashion, and those with confirmed PTE and no adverse features, or those suspected of having PTE can be risk stratified to allow this. Patients can be assigned a PESI (Pulmonary Embolism Severity Index) score. Patients with low risk PESI score can be safely managed in an ambulatory manner (Aujesky *et al.*, 2005).

PTEs are often caused by other pathology or recent insult to the body and this should be borne in mind. Where possible it is important to investigate for these. Simple general examinations of the patient including of breasts and testicles can go a long way to reassuring the clinician. Where a family history of embolism is highlighted, a thrombophilia screen is unlikely to change initial management, but may indicate the need for life long anticoagulation. Within reason it is suggested that 6 months of anticoagulation is needed in most cases. With the advent of direct oral anticoagulants (DOACS) treatment of thromboembolism is becoming easier and more patient friendly. In a small number of cases a DOAC may be unsuitable, and low molecular weight heparin (LMWH) or warfarin may be the only suitable alternatives. Equally, patients may choose these treatments in preference to a DOAC.

In the remote setting, CTPA is not likely to be available. The use of CXR, cardiac echo, and clinical skills could be enough to reach a diagnosis and manage the patient as required. The clinician should not delay treatment of PTE as it carries a significant mortality risk.

Pneumothorax

As previously highlighted, a history of sudden onset shortness of breath and pleuritic chest pain does not always mean a pulmonary embolism is the cause, but pneumothorax is common. Classically tall and thin patients will present with pneumothorax. The British Thoracic Society guidelines on the management of pneumothorax are freely available and should be considered a useful directory (Macduff *et al.*, 2010).

A good CXR will likely reveal the presence of pneumothoracies. Normally, well patients can tolerate pneumothoracies for some time before presentation but will often have worsening breathlessness or pain.

A tension pneumothorax is quite different and is a medical emergency. ALS guidelines should be followed in respect of these with immediate needle decompression in the second intercostal space on the mid clavicular line. Tracheal deviation is a late sign and may not be present, but examination may reveal profound hypoxia, in combination with a lack of chest wall movement on the affected side with or without intercostal recession. Subcutaneous emphysema may be present, and this can often be dramatic. Patients with voice changes should be monitored carefully as there is a risk to the airway. Fortunately, placement of an intercostal drain will improve this rapidly.

If aspiration fails or is as indicated by the presence of other factors an ICD may be merited. Once a chest drain is inserted the patient should be educated to look after it. They will last a lot longer, and once the drain is no longer bubbling, a repeat CXR may demonstrate resolution. Rapid decompression can lead to re-expansion pulmonary oedema and the clinician should be mindful of this. Patients who have an ICD in situ should have adequate analgesia to prevent hypostatic pneumonias forming.

The management of pneumothoracies is often simple, and in most cases, the insertion of an intercostal drain is enough. Following successful treatment of a pneumothorax the patient should be advised that travel by air carries risk of recurrence for some time, and sub aquatic activities are contraindicated unless they are cleared to do so by a cardiothoracic surgeon.

If a pneumothorax fails to respond to treatment in a remote setting, consideration should be taken as to whether transfer to a facility capable of further management is warranted, particularly if the patient is still symptomatic. This is more common in patients with pre-existing or advanced lung disease.

Musculoskeletal chest pain

Musculoskeletal chest pain is a common presentation that can cause worry, unfortunately, palpation of an injured area is not well correlated with the exclusion of more serious insults, and so the clinician should be wary. However, in essence, pain that follows injury to a muscle and is worse on movement is often reassuring.

Sometimes there may be no clear diagnosis, and this is acceptable. Good worsening advice and safety netting will allow most patients to feel reassured. They will re-present if there is a problem.

In all patients presenting with chest pain, plain film CXR may lead to a concrete diagnosis, point the clinician towards alternative diagnosis or be ultimately reassuring. Ultimately the history taken will guide the clinician as to the appropriate next step.

Palpitations and syncope

Palpitations and transient loss of consciousness are common medical complaints, and in general patients will often present with a history of such without physical findings. Often the cause is never found, and this can be disconcerting.

Most patients presenting with palpitations will have benign findings and can be reassured. Caffeine overuse is a common cause of palpitations for example and is not worrying. Whereas constitutional symptoms may point to a broader underlying problem such as thyrotoxicosis. This is rare. The clinician should be more worried in patients that present with palpitations followed by syncope. Particularly if that syncope is exertional and this should lead to further investigation.

Abnormal ECGs and syncope without obvious warning is also more worrying and these patients may require additional monitoring. Listening to the heart sounds and identifying pathological murmurs is important in these cases. Patients who have lost consciousness without the prodrome typical of vaso-vagal syncope may have something else more sinister underlying and this should be borne in mind. In some rarer cases there may be a family history of early cardiac death, or unexplained death and this should alarm the clinician as to the need for further investigation.

It is important to take a good history from these patients, eliciting what they recall, if anything, how they felt in the moments before syncope and also what medications the patient may or may not be taking.

Environmental factors such as heat may predispose people to increased vagal responses as may emotional distress. Careful history taking will elicit most of these. A collateral history from a witness may also reveal further details of vital importance that will lead to a diagnosis or exclude more serious pathology. However, collateral historians will often recount visualising what they believe to be symptoms of a seizure and these should be teased out carefully. As previously alluded to, a family history of early cardiac death should not be overlooked.

When managing patients who have had a syncopal event, it is important to consider what the underlying cause might be and whether this is going to have an impact on their current lifestyle or ability to carry out specific occupational roles. Injuries from syncope to themselves or others can therefore be avoided. Many organisations, such as the oil industry, will have strict policies in place to safeguard staff and by and large they are there to protect the individual. Nonetheless, patients in this context may be resistant to acknowledging their symptoms and this should be considered.

Respiratory problems

By and large, asthma, Chronic Obstructive Airways Disease (COAD), and pneumonias will form the largest group of presenting complaints. The approach to these patients is no different than to any other group, thorough history combined with examination will elicit most diagnoses.

Asthma

Asthma is a condition that can worry the most experienced clinician. There are numerous stories of patients being discharged early coming into difficulty. In remote settings this can be particularly challenging. The management of a sick asthma patient requires the clinician to identify the severity of the asthma exacerbation and respond appropriately to what is in front of them (SIGN, 2016).

The severity of the initial asthma exacerbation will indicate the possibility of the patient's likelihood to deteriorate, but also allow recognition of improvement. The initial management of all patients has two steps in common, the use of nebulised salbutamol and ipratropium and the commencement of steroid therapy. Not all exacerbations require antibiotics, and some may benefit from antiviral medications. If flu is suspected as a cause of the exacerbation, then they should definitely be considered as it has been demonstrated that commencement of antiviral therapy such as Tamiflu is associated with a reduction in mortality in patients with asthma.

In those who have an oxygen saturation of less than 94% or when consolidation is suspected, a plain CXR is useful to look for other causes of hypoxia, such as a secondary pneumonia.

Features of acute severe asthma include:
Peak expiratory flow (PEF) 33–50% of best known or predicted peak flow
Unable to complete sentences in one breath
Respiration rate of ≥ 25 breathes per minute
Pulse rate ≥ 110 beats/min

Life threatening features include:
PEF < 33%
SpO_2 <92%
Silent chest, cyanosis or feeble respiratory effort
Arrythmia or hypotension
Exhaustion or altered consciousness

In patients who present with any life-threatening conditions, it is optimal to undertake blood gas analysis. The presence of acidosis, severe hypoxia or a 'normal' PaCO2 is concerning. Unless already given, IV magnesium should be considered in these patients. In some circumstances it may be necessary for IV theophylline to be considered to alleviate the bronchospasm and this is another treatment option that should be available in remote settings. IV salbutamol is usually only the preserve of intensive care physicians but may be life sustaining.

The monitoring of these patients is vital to allow the clinician to pick up on both improvement and deterioration. Patients should be monitored in the following ways:

SpO_2 oximetry achieving > 94–98%

Repeat blood gas analysis if initially required 1 hour after commencing management

Repeat PEF every 15–30 minutes after commencement of therapy

Once the patient is stable, PEF monitoring should be taken at least 4 times a day whilst the patient remains under the care of the clinician. Fortunately, most patients will respond well to initial therapy. Prior to discharge from the care of the clinician a review of inhaler technique and worsening advice should be given. Virtual follow up with dedicated asthma services should also be considered.

In those patients who have COAD as an underlying diagnosis, the treatment is much the same, however, there is less reversibility and they often tolerate lower SpO2 ranges. In an effort not to drive hypercapnic respiratory failure it is prudent to maintain oxygen saturations at 88–92%.

The use of non-invasive ventilation (NIV) is usually preserved for those patients with hypercapnia and respiratory acidosis, however, it can be used as a temporising measure in asthma patients. Nonetheless, it should be used with extreme caution in those with asthma, as the possibility of air trapping and stacking in these patients can lead to worse outcomes. In some asthma patients with poor chest movement, manual chest decompression may be required. This is often carried out better when the patient is formally mechanically ventilated. They will often have significantly raised pressures when ventilated and can be tricky to manage.

If formal mechanical ventilation is unavailable, then NIV can be used as a bridging technique to give other therapies time to work. This tactic is not generally advocated, but in the remote environment with no prospect of critical care intervention it may be useful. The use of NIV in patients with asthma exacerbations is not considered to be standard practice in the UK. There are few indications for using NIV in severe asthma and should the clinician choose to do this they must be aware of the signs of NIV therapy failure (Gianfranco et al., 1996).

Near fatal asthma is heralded by the presence of a raised PaCO2 or in those who have higher pressures when mechanically ventilated. Patients who have evidence of near fatal asthma on initial presentation in the remote setting should be aggressively managed, and tertiary advice be sought early on. It is appropriate to transfer these patients to a facility that is more equipped to manage them.

Upper GI bleed, inflammatory bowel and liver disease

Upper GI bleed

Upper Gastrointestinal Haemorrhage presents with a spectrum of disease and these might not be immediately apparent. In the absence of endoscopy services, it may be prudent to attempt to stop haemorrhage by whatever means is medically necessary.

Most patients presenting with upper GI haemorrhage in the absence of underlying liver disease will likely have gastritis, gastric or duodenal ulcers. General examination and the presence of adverse features will dictate the management of these patients.

A useful scoring system, the Glasgow-Blatchford Bleeding score allows pre-endoscopy management to be carried out in most patients safely (Chen et al., 2007). This scoring system picks up on most adverse features and those with a score of 1 or more have a 50% chance of requiring endoscopy or transfusion of blood products to manage the underlying haemorrhage. In those presenting with a score of 0, the chances of requiring further intervention is low and they can be managed effectively as an outpatient, such as with oral proton pump inhibiters (PPI). Helicobacter stool samples can be taken prior to commencement of PPIs and should they prove positive, eradication therapy will reduce the chances of further instances of UGI complications.

In the remote setting, where endoscopy may not be available, resuscitation should be aimed at maintaining the circulatory volume, and strategies developed to treat the most likely underlying cause. The Hong Kong protocol is traditionally used as a post endoscopy therapy; however, in the remote setting it may be more appropriate to commence this. IV PPI, with or without tranexamic acid may help to safely manage patients who are bleeding. Bowel rest and careful monitoring would be prudent in the scenario.

If blood transfusion is available, then it is important that this scarce resource is managed appropriately. Patients should not be transfused above a haemoglobin target of 7g/dL. Patients who have been transfused to a higher level have not been shown to have any mortality benefit, and may have worse outcomes. The debate over tranexamic acid is ongoing, however, there is evidence that it is of benefit currently, and therefore it is worth considering (Bennett et al., 2014).

In some patients who are on antiplatelets, for example clopidogrel, other blood products such as platelet transfusion should be considered if available and when all other options have been exhausted. Often a pool of platelets is enough to counteract the effects of antiplatelets in the short term. Patients who are taking a DOAC should have consideration for the intravenous use of prothrombin complex if they are shocked as well as IV Vitamin K if there is concern regarding deficiency. This may be dietary or otherwise. In general, this should be a rare occurrence and supportive resuscitation with a balanced crystalloid may be enough to tide them through the initial period of haemorrhage. In patients who take warfarin and require prothrombin complex it is vital that vitamin K is co-administered to avoid rebound anticoagulation.

In variceal haemorrhage, chiefly present in those with pre-recognised cirrhosis and portal hypertension, resuscitation in the remote setting can prove challenging. Recognition of severity of the bleeding, followed by appropriate resuscitation is key. A Sengstacken tube with a correctly inflated gastric balloon, though unpleasant for the patient, may be life saving. Inflation of the oesophageal balloon is not always required and may cause oesophageal wall necrosis and subsequent perforation. This in itself can prove fatal.

With variceal bleeding the same principles of treatment still apply, restoration of blood circulating volume and the supplementation of coagulation factors.

It is good practice that all patients who present with upper GI bleeding and require admission have at least two large bore cannulae sited so that prompt resuscitation can take place if required. In the remote setting, permissive hypotension may be helpful as over-resuscitation may encourage further bleeding. This technique has been widely used in the context of trauma.

Inflammatory bowel disease

Exacerbations from inflammatory bowel disease are common and can be extremely debilitating. Patients will often present with abdominal pain, colic, and rectal blood loss with or without mucous. This subgroup of patients also has a higher incidence of infection. In order to gain control of the exacerbation, where infection is not suspected, IV methyl prednisolone at a dose of 30mg BD is now a recognised initial therapy. If infection is suspected or confirmed IV steroids are not routinely advocated, and if the clinician decides to do this, careful consideration and monitoring is required.

In patients who are of concern, transfer to a facility that has both medical and surgical centres may be required. This is more often the case in those with advanced disease, or significant signs of abdominal concern, such as peritonism or guarding. Supportive management with careful fluids, bowel rest and IV antibiotics may be all that can be achieved in the remote setting prior to evacuation.

Most patients who have inflammatory bowel disease will have been educated as to the signs and symptoms to look out for, and in the remote setting they may become particularly adept at self management. They will often know more about their condition than the treating clinician and they should be listened to. Treatment of inflammatory bowel disease is highly specialist, and advice from gastroenterologists should be sought at the earliest convenience. Basic investigations and plain abdominal films can go a long way in providing the advising clinician enough to provide realistic advice.

Alcohol related hepatitis

Alcohol related hepatitis is an autoimmune condition arising from ingestion of alcohol with a characteristic pattern of liver function testing abnormalities. In general, it is not usually fatal. However, a subgroup of patients will go on to develop fulminant hepatic failure. A Glasgow Alcohol Hepatitis Score ≥9 conveys a higher mortality, and these patients should be given IV steroid therapy (Forrest *et al.*, 2005). Ultimately the management is supportive, but good supportive care can reduce the mortality associated with the condition.

There are multiple other causes of hepatitis and a detailed history will point the clinician in the right direction as to the underlying cause. If available, a liver screen should be taken and sent for further analysis. Viral hepatitis is common, and in particular Hepatitis C is now a curable disease. Supportive treatment may be all that is available remotely and the patient should be encouraged to seek help where needed from tertiary centres.

Patients with decompensated hepatic disease are also often nutritionally deplete and have lower nutritional reserves to call upon. Providing additional nutritional support may be required to improve the patient's chances of survival. In those presenting with ascites, and fever or peritonism, always consider spontaneous bacterial peritonitis as a source of infection and treat this accordingly. Supportive management on top of this may be all that can be achieved, but good supportive management will prevent unnecessary death.

Diabetes, DKA, and HHS

Hyperglycaemia will present in many patients and comes with significant morbidity if left unregulated. Not all patients require insulin but being aware of which patients do will lead to a reduction in poor outcomes and unnecessary hospital admissions. In general patients who are thin, losing weight, polyuric and thirsty are type 1 diabetics. Patients who are obese will likely have insulin resistance and are therefore more likely to benefit from non-insulin treatments. This pathological process is often found in patients with type 2 diabetes.

In patients who present with hyperglycaemia and are more likely to have type 1 diabetes it is important to establish whether they have the presence of ketones and acidaemia. Those who have both are in diabetic ketoacidosis which should be considered a medical emergency. In those without ketosis and acidaemia they can usually be managed with SC insulin and occasionally IV rehydration. Ketone production can only be stopped with the introduction of carbohydrates. Eating food containing carbohydrates is usually enough to achieve this.

Diabetic Ketoacidosis (DKA) management has gradually become increasingly prescriptive within hospital settings with the development of DKA pathways. DKA can present with varying severity, from patients who are relatively well, to those with evidence of critical illness. Severe DKA with profound acidosis can present with reduced conscious level, and multi organ dysfunction. There is often a triggering illness, though in some cases no cause is identified. In assessing patients who present with DKA it is important to elicit any underlying cause and treat this appropriately. Infection is one of the most common causes, as normal glycaemic control becomes impossible.

The mainstay management of DKA pathways involve the use of intravenous insulin, IV fluid replacement, monitoring of electrolytes and the introduction of carbohydrates. Once the bicarbonate level is above 22, re-commencement of the patient's normal insulin regime can begin. If a patient is already taking a long acting insulin it is important not to withhold this. Various intravenous insulin regimes are available and should be followed. If a patient is not able to eat and drink as they normally would, it is prudent to continue an insulin sliding scale. Most patients with DKA will improve over the course of 24–48 hours. It is prudent that the remote clinician has an available pathway to follow in the advent of presentation of this group of patients. Following management, it is also vital to understand how the patient came to be in this situation and take steps to address this. Re-education of the patient, potentially with the help of virtual diabetic clinic appointments may be required.

Hyperosmolar hyperglycaemic state

This is a life-threatening condition that occurs mainly in patients who have type 2 diabetes. Formerly known as HONK (Hyperglycaemic hyperosmolar non ketotic coma). Its onset is often more insidious and there is usually no evidence of ketosis. Serum glucose levels are often much higher than those associated with DKA and there is often no metabolic acidosis. Patients will often present with delirium and can have altered conscious levels.

A serum osmolality greater than 320 has to be demonstrated, with hyperglycaemia usually greater than 30 mmol/L and the patient must be severely dehydrated or unwell for the diagnosis to be reached. They will often have marked biochemical abnormalities and acute kidney injury. Patients are usually older, between 50–70 years old, and as with DKA there is often an underlying triggering pathology.

Similar to DKA the mainstay of treatment is fluid replacement and glycaemic control (Joint British Diabetes Societies, 2012). However, rapid resolution should be avoided. The blood glucose level should fall at rate of 4 — mmol/hour and fluid replacement should be guided by firstly calculating the estimated fluid deficit. This is usually in the range of 100–220 ml/kg. Thorough assessment of the fluid status of the patient should be undertaken, eliciting both clinical and biochemical signs.

Crystalloid replacement in the initial phase will result in a fall in serum glucose levels, and this may in turn cause the serum sodium level to rise. This should not be of concern if the calculated osmolality is falling. Intravenous insulin should not be commenced as it may result in precipitous falling of the serum glucose level in patients that are not insulin deficient and may herald cardiovascular collapse. Only in patients with significant ketonemia should insulin be considered, and this at a rate of 0.05 units/Kg/h, reducing blood glucose levels at 5 mmols per hour.

After the initial phase of fluid replacement, and once the glucose level is no longer falling, intravenous insulin can then be safely commenced. Potassium replacement is also likely to be needed in these patients, and this should be done in light of their current potassium levels. Those with a K+ of >5.5 do not need K+ replacement, whereas those with a potassium level of 3.5–5.5 will need 40 mmol/L replacement. Those with levels lower than 3.5 will likely require more. It is therefore important to repeat available blood tests as required, and hourly in the first few hours to ensure correction of the condition is at an appropriate rate.

These patients are at particular risk of developing thrombosis and embolic events, ranging from PTE to ischaemic gut, and therefore, LMWH should be given subcutaneously at a prophylactic dose.

Given that these patients, particularly those with severe hyperosmolar hyper-glycaemic state (HHS), are likely to need significant monitoring for a prolonged period of time, it may be prudent to transfer them to a tertiary facility for further management once the initial phase of treatment has begun.

All diabetic patients are at risk of developing foot ulcers, and examination of the feet should not be missed. Diabetic foot ulcers herald the development of morbidity, and an infective ulcer may be the predisposing condition to both DKA and HHS.

Common Neurological Presentations

Headaches

Headaches are a common presentation to any acute medical setting, and the remote setting will be no different. Being able to recognise the difference from a likely primary headache to that of a secondary headache will stand the clinician in good stead when facing these occasionally challenging diagnostic conundrums. As with any medical complaint a thorough history and examination of the patient can point towards a diagnosis.

Primary headaches are benign, often recurrent and are not caused by underlying pathology or structural problems, nonetheless they can cause particular angst amongst patients and re-assurance is often required. The majority of all headaches will fall into the primary category.

All patients presenting with a headache should have a detailed history taken and a full neurological examination. Any positive findings indicate a need for further assessment. Examination in all cases should include fundoscopy, looking for papilledema, pupillary reactivity, and new pupillary asymmetry.

Examples of primary headache disorders include migraine with or without aura, medication over-use headaches, tension headaches, and cluster headaches. Each of which has specific criteria which must be met as set out in the ICD-10 classification.

Red flags suggestive of secondary causes include:

Sudden onset severity, reaching maximal intensity within 5 minutes

Change in neurological status, personality, or a new focal neurological deficit

Aura lasting over 1 hour that is atypical for the patient in conjunction with combined oral contraceptive use

Dizziness suggestive of ischaemic event

Fever

Vomiting

Trauma or head injury within the last 3 months

Patients with these features are more likely to have a secondary cause for the headache such as subarachnoid haemorrhage, venous sinus thrombosis or meningitis (Beithon *et al.*, 2013). There are many other signs which can be elicited in this cohort of patients and the reviewing clinician should have an awareness of these. In those with focal neurology, particularly of sudden onset, evacuation for secondary consideration and imaging is often necessary.

If meningitis is suspected IV antibiotics should be administered as soon as is feasibly possible. Not all patients with meningitis will require transfer, and this should only be considered if deemed necessary. Viral meningitis may be indistinguishable from bacterial in the remote setting, and whilst the management of viral meningitis is supportive, it is a diagnosis that should be made with caution. Patients with headache, fever, photophobia and a rash should be treated as if they have bacterial meningitis without exception. Patients presenting with a headache and altered mental status or who go on to have seizures should have encephalitis considered as an underlying cause. Focal neurology in this group of patients is worrying and evacuation should be considered.

Seizures

Epilepsy is a common medical condition in the general population that conveys higher risks to the individual and or others in remote settings. Employment in remote settings for sufferers of epilepsy may be prohibited by the employing organisation with occupational health departments strictly controlling deployment of such individuals. The remote clinician may encounter patients who have new onset seizures, and this may therefore have implications for employment.

The management of seizures and the seizing patient is supportive in the first instance, with protection of the airway and safety provision in the environment. The treatment of convulsions with rectal or intravenous benzodiazepines is often enough to raise the seizure threshold and prevent further seizures.

In some cases, the seizures may continue. In patients who have seizures without spontaneous cessation or those that continue in spite of benzodiazepines in the remote setting, IV Levetiracetam (Keppra) should be considered. There is increasing evidence that IV Levetiracetam is just as efficacious in the management of status epilepticus as IV phenytoin and has fewer side effects (Dalziel *et al.*, 2019). Patients should be considered to be in status epilepticus if they have a seizure lasting more than 5 minutes, or two or more seizures without the person returning to normal between them within a 5-minute time period.

All patients presenting with seizures should have basic electrolytes checked, including a magnesium level check. A small subgroup of patients will require anaesthesia to achieve status resolution though the burden of this to the individual should be taken into account and it may not be possible to offer this to all in the remote setting.

It is good practice that patients presenting with seizures as a first presentation should be offered at the least CT brain imaging. This need not be done immediately if the patient is well, and may not anyway be possible in the remote setting. Normally the commencement of oral antiepileptics is reserved for secondary specialists, in the remote setting it may be more prudent to establish the patient on antiepileptics prior to secondary review later. This is particularly the case in patients who have had a witnessed seizure requiring intervention.

Stroke and transient ischaemic attack

Stroke is a medical emergency that can lead to significant morbidity and mortality. It is characterised by sudden onset neurological deficit in the context of pre-existing vascular disease. Though this is not always apparent. A careful history is vital in picking up both strokes, transient ischaemic attacks (TIA), and stroke mimics.

In the remote setting the clinician will come into contact with two subgroups of patients, those that present within a time frame suitable for intervention and those that do not. The vast majority of patients who present with stroke will have had an ischaemic event. The clinical judgement of the reviewing clinician is paramount in discerning which patients are at risk of deterioration or subsequent events and which are not. Remote clinicians should have specific training in the recognition and management of stroke.

Access to immediate brain imaging may not be possible in the remote setting. Patients presenting with a TIA can be risk stratified as having low, moderate, or high risk of recurrence through clinical scoring systems. The ABCD2 score is one such classification (Johnston *et al.*, 2007). Those with a score ≥4 are at more risk of having a completed stroke within 2 days and should be considered for transfer to a facility more equipped at managing stroke patients.

In the absence of ongoing symptoms or signs of focal neurology it is prudent to start high dose aspirin in the remote setting prior to CT imaging. Typically,

300 mg aspirin once a day. In the presence of atrial fibrillation these patients will have a higher risk and should be transferred to a facility capable of imaging the brain so that a DOAC can be safely commenced.

Stroke classification

Classification of stroke is less important in the remote setting, as opposed to recognising the presence of a likely stroke in the patient and the severity of the stroke. Nevertheless, being able to classify the stroke territorially based on the symptoms is a useful skill to have when determining the potential outcome and possible treatments. The Oxford Classification of Stroke allows for this.

The four main classifications as outlined are:

Lacunar Circulation Stroke (LACS)

Posterior Circulation Stroke (POCS)

Partial Anterior Circulation Stroke (PACS)

Total Anterior Circulation Stroke (TACS)

Posterior circulation strokes are hard to clinically delineate from many stroke mimics and can be easily missed. Brainstem strokes are rare and even harder to clinically detect as they often present with odd symptoms that wax and wane over time, even months.

In patients who have had a treatable stroke, they should be transferred to an appropriate facility capable of CT brain imaging, and the swiftness of transfer is critical. In the developed world, mechanical thrombectomy has been shown to improve the outcome in some patients up to 24 hours after the index event. However, in general patients who have suffered a stroke and are beyond 7.5 hours from this, intervention will not be considered. Where thrombolysis is the intervention available, patients will not benefit from this after 4.5 hours from the index event. In deciding which patients will benefit from intervention it is important to quantify the severity of the stroke by examining the patient thoroughly. The National Institute of Health Stroke Scale (NIHSS) score will provide the clinician with enough information to justify any decisions made and is a well recognised tool to help determine the severity of a patient's stroke (Johnston et al., 2003). There are inherent risks in thrombolysis, and without CT brain imaging confirming the absence of haemorrhage or significant areas of ischaemia it is not recommended.

As previously stated, patients who have suffered a significant stroke should be transferred to a specialist facility with dedicated stroke services for further investigation and subsequent multidisciplinary management. In deciding this the patient and their family should be consulted. It may not be appropriate to transfer patients who have suffered a TACS for example as it may be more appropriate to consider this a terminal event, particularly in the elderly. Death may not be imminent, and the dying phase can last for some time. The families should be counselled as to this. In patients who have suffered a middle cerebral artery event this can lead to MCA infarct syndrome and in the absence of cranial decompression can be fatal. It will present with worsening conscious level and features of raised intracranial hypertension. Surgical decompression does not reduce the burden of morbidity in these patients but can preserve life.

In the remote setting the clinician may only be able to administer antiplatelets and manage secondary pathologies, however, agreed pathways should be in place to help the clinician manage these patients safely and effectively. Early engagement with secondary care and stroke specialists is advisable. The advent of telehealth medicine has improved access to stroke specialist care in the remote setting and contact with secondary services should be made as soon as is reasonably practical. If there is any doubt, evacuation is warranted. A missed stroke and untreated stroke convey higher morbidity and mortality.

Poisonings and Toxidromes

The poisoned patient is an increasingly common medical complaint and in the remote setting can present in many ways. The approach to managing these patients will fall broadly into two groups. Those with ingestion or exposure to a known poison and a proven remedy, and those who present without the poison being known.

Access to regulated databases such as 'Toxbase' will provide the clinician with helpful advice on the management of specific poisons and antidotes should the need arise. However, often, and increasingly with the advent of new psychoactive substances, the poison or toxin may not be immediately identifiable. In these circumstances the ability to recognise typical clinical symptoms and constellation of signs will point towards the type of poison or at least its likely consequences. As with any patient, basic history taking, clinical examination, basic biochemistry and an ECG are important paths to a working diagnosis.

In poisoned patients of unknown substance, the presence of a group of symptoms and clinical signs can suggest a specific toxidrome which aids initial management. An ABCDE approach to these patients will highlight these and inform the clinician of any life-threatening problems that need to be addressed.

The main toxidromes are:

Anticholinergic

Tachycardia, hypertension, hyperthermia, hypervigilance or agitation, dilated pupils, reduced or absent bowel sounds and decreased diaphoresis, urinary retention. (Hot as hades, mad as a hatter, blind as a bat, dry as a bone, and red as a beet.)

Cholinergic

Bradycardia or tachycardia, confused or comatose, pinpoint pupils, bradypnea, hyperactive bowel sounds, and increased diaphoresis. (Salivation, lacrimation, urinary and bowel incontinence, emesis.)

Opioid

Bradycardia, hypotension, hypothermia, CNS depression or coma, pin point pupils, hyporeflexia, reduced or absent bowel sounds, reduced diaphoresis. Occasionally pulmonary oedema.

Hallucinogenic

Tachycardia, hypertension, hyperthermia, hallucinations or agitation, dilated pupils, nystagmus.

Sympathomimetic

Tachycardia, hypertension, hyperthermia, dilated pupils, hyperreflexia, rigidity, seizures, hyperactive bowel sounds and increased diaphoresis.

Sedative-Hypnotic

Bradycardia, hypotension, bradypnea, CNS depression or coma, dilated pupils, hyporeflexia.

Serotonergic

Tachycardia, hypertension, hyperthermia, dilated pupils, hyperreflexia or clonus, tremor or myoclonus. These patients may also seize.

Armed with an awareness of the constellation of signs and symptoms elicited through basic examination and a history, collateral or otherwise, the clinician should be able to identify the possible or probable toxin type. This will inform early management and establish a working diagnosis. The monitoring of these patients will be dictated by the severity of their presentation.

The toxidrome and the trajectory of the patient's condition should be considered and in the remote setting it is advisable to seek tertiary centre advice as the risk of deterioration is high. Maintenance of normal physiological parameters and biochemistry may be all that is possible. In most cases, particularly in those who present without adverse features a period of observation may be all that is required. Whether an antidote is recommended will depend on situation and should be done with caution. Rapid reversal of toxins can have unintended consequences, such as acute opioid withdrawal, or seizures with the use of flumazenil. Unless there are significant adverse features, the presence of a toxidrome for example, reversal or antidote use should be guarded.

Different populations will have different risk factors for poisons dependent upon wildlife in the immediate environment and the existence of industrial chemicals that may in other countries be prohibited. There may also be differing societal pressures. When operating in remote settings it is advisable that the clinician has a working knowledge of potential toxin sources for the geographical area they operate in.

In industrial situations it is imperative not only to consider the presenting patient, but to consider wider affected individuals and to activate alert systems in place. If there are significant casualties or poisoned patients, understanding the predicted trajectory of patient outcomes will allow the clinician to both plan for and request immediate support.

Sepsis

The timely recognition of the septic patient can be lifesaving, particularly in the remote setting, and if in doubt it is always advisable to consider this in the differential of any patient presenting with the constellation of signs and symptoms that could either be precursors to sepsis or sepsis itself.

The recognition of the systemic inflammatory response syndrome (SIRS), with the addition of a suspected source of infection in the remote setting should be considered as a medical emergency and requires the clinician to act promptly. Every hour of delay in the treatment of severe sepsis will result in higher mortality. Although there are now pressures to move to different scoring systems, in the remote setting the recognition of the SIRS response in a sick patient is readily achievable and therefore valuable (Simpson, 2018).

The SIRS criteria are:

Temperature <36°C or >38°C

Heart Rate >90 beats per minute

Respiratory Rate >22 breaths per minute

Neutrophil count of <4 or >12

In the remote setting the neutrophil count may not be immediately available and if the clinician suspects sepsis then treatment should not be delayed. If no immediate source is identifiable then the clinician should manage the patients with broad spectrum antibiotics until a source is identifiable and a more targeted approach becomes achievable.

The management of sepsis has changed significantly over the years, but treatment of severe sepsis defined as those who have sepsis with evidence of end organ dysfunction has broadly followed the same principles. Resuscitation with a balanced crystalloid solution and prompt initiation of IV antibiotics will go some way to stabilising most patients (Rhodes et al., 2016).

Should the patient have developed septic shock, as defined by a lack of response to fluid resuscitation manifesting itself as refractory hypotension, then vasopressors are usually indicated. Multiple trials have also failed to suggest if steroids are of benefit. They may be, and in the remote setting with limited resources, the supplementation of IV steroids may be helpful in the management of septic shock. Ultimately, patients with septic shock, or those who are unstable will likely require evacuation to a facility capable of delivering critical care. Specialist retrieval teams will often be able to initiate critical care management, including the use of vasopressors and if a patient is presenting with signs of shock early discussion is vital.

Ambulatory Care Systems, Pathways and In-Home Management Services

The development of acute medicine as a specialty, and the ever-rising pressures on hospital systems to cope with rising demand and patient expectation has led to the development of ambulatory care pathways designed to deliver safe and effective hospital standard care to the patient in an outpatient setting. The same strategies can be utilised to deliver care in the remote setting where resources will be finite and time more precious. Successful pathways have patient centered care and realistic medicine as overarching principles.

Examples of ambulatory care are numerous, from management of atrial fibrillation, to management of cellulitis. However, all pathways have a few basic tenets for the safe delivery of care and the management of specific conditions.

1) Criteria of inclusion for management of a defined condition or illness
2) Criteria of exclusion for management of a defined condition or illness

> 3) Ability of the patient to be ambulant
> 4) Good safety netting and worsening advice
> 5) Subsequent admission criteria if ambulatory care fails

These pathways are adaptable and have a strong grounding in clinical governance. If any pathway covers the core outlined areas above, it has every chance of being successful.

In the remote setting the management of cellulitis and infection in an ambulatory fashion may be even more preferable, as it allows the remote clinician to safely treat patients who would traditionally require hospital admission with brief encounters. The once daily administration of a 3rd generation cephalosporin as opposed to four times daily administration of a penicillin is much less time consuming for an individual clinician. Patients with simple cellulitis can be managed safely and effectively in this manner.

In increasing numbers, patients are being managed in their own homes with the clinician and clinical teams coming to them. This may be face-to-face clinician patient interactions, virtual interactions, or a combination of both. Although not without risks, with improving technology it is now possible to remotely monitor patients and this capability will only increase demand for delivery of realistic, cost effective care in the patient's home. This form of care will require the remote clinician to be highly mobile but will often improve patient outcomes. Keeping patients at home and supported with ancillary services is preferable to both patient and clinician. If domiciliary care is provided in a structured manner it will also reduce the burden on healthcare provision for the area and therefore the clinician. Empowering patients to be part of their healthcare and the practice of patient centred realistic medicine is crucial to sustainability of remote clinical services. It is also crucial to the sustainability of the remote clinicians themselves.

Telehealth and Communication Strategies

Effective communication between remote clinicians and clinicians in secondary or tertiary centres is vital to ensure that accurate information is conveyed in a timely manner. Failure to communicate effectively can have disastrous consequences for the patient and the clinician.

Many communication strategies have been developed in multiple fields from the airline industry to medicine, from the battlefield to ambulance control rooms. A useful and simple tool in providing communication is the SBAR communication tool (Müller *et al.*, 2018).

Situation — Description of current clinical problem

Background — Relevant past medical history

Assessment — Detailed findings and observations

Recommendation — Request for response required

The initiator then asks the receiving team to repeat back to them the information they have understood.

This template has been advocated by NHS improvement to allow clinicians to readily communicate clinical problems in a concise and focussed manner allowing appropriate management of patients. In the remote setting the ability to concisely refer patients or seek additional recommendations will help reduce time on the phone. Focusing the communication between teams as to what is medically relevant and required is essential for good outcomes.

An example of this would be:

Situation: This is Dr X, in X location. I have a 45-year-old male, called Y who has chest pain, it started 30 minutes ago.

Background: Y has type 1 diabetes and hypertension

Assessment: He has ST elevation on the ECG consistent with an acute myocardial infarction. I have given him aspirin, GTN, and morphine. The observations are RR, 20, BP 160/80, HR 100, and temperature 37 degrees celsius. I am concerned that the pain is ongoing.

Recommendation: I believe he needs primary coronary intervention, and needs to be evacuated to X to have this.

By using this tool, the receiving team will be left with no doubt as to the urgency of the situation and will be able to act accordingly. The above example, though simple, is concise, accurate, and detailed enough to get the result required for effective patient care.

In some circumstances, the recommendation may be for further advice, and this can then be documented and carried out. It enables shared care of critically unwell patients, and therefore shared responsibility.

As previously alluded to, with the advent of telehealth communication it may be possible to get specialist advice in remote locations. This is particularly useful when the diagnosis is as yet unknown or in doubt. In patients who have strokes, for example, telehealth medicine has been used to remotely manage patients who are suitable for thrombolytic therapy, enabling patients to be visualised and directly counselled by physicians who would otherwise not be able to attend to them. Thrombolysis is then carried out remotely. Telehealth medicine is an invaluable resource and is covered by other chapters in this book.

Transfer Decisions

In deciding when to transfer patients who are medically unwell, it is important to consider the risk to the patients and the patients' wishes. Although the need for evacuation or transfer rises with severity of illness, it may not be in the patient's best interests or wishes. Prior to transfer, all that can be done to stabilise a patient should be undertaken. Transfer medicine is its own discipline and the risks involved with transferring patients, particularly by air are considerable.

Decisions to transfer patients should be made in conjunction with specialist retrieval teams and secondary facilities. In most of the cases, early evacuation is better than late once a patient has been stabilised to the best of the clinician's ability. In some cases, the clinician may not be able to stabilise the patient, and this is where swift evacuation is warranted. Transferring a patient requires planning for all eventualities to minimize the risk to both the patient and the clinician. Risks are either modifiable or not, and they encompass scenarios arising from situations outside the control of the referring clinician, such as the weather.

Remote Clinician Resilience

Above all, the remote clinician will be responsible for the lives and health of a population that is often outside the reach of traditional healthcare services; with this comes an element of risk that the clinician will encounter on a daily basis. In communities where they serve as the sole medic, that individual will often have an influential voice and elevated societal position. This can take its toll on even the most resilient of clinicians as it is a role that is all encompassing, with patients becoming known to them on a personal and clinical level.

The remote clinician is therefore at increased risk of burnout syndrome. The challenge of staying abreast of the latest clinical evidence and delivering healthcare with limited resources to an ever-aging population is a challenge faced by all healthcare workers, but the added occupational stress of isolation can be damaging to healthcare providers.

Recognising when one is developing burnout syndrome is an important skill to have. Remote clinicians should have specific training to cope with this, and the organisations they are working for should have policies and protocols in place to address this.

The key features of clinician burnout syndrome are measured by the Maslach Burnout Inventory, or more specifically the Maslach Burnout Inventory — Human Services Survey for Medical Personnel (MBI-HSSMP) (Maslach *et al.*, 2016).

It describes the following as key indicators of the syndrome, each rated on a scale correlating with the likelihood of diagnosis. These are: emotional exhaustion, depersonalisation, and personal accomplishment. The syndrome itself encompasses a wide range of both physical and psychological manifestations of symptoms that if left unchecked will prove costly both to the individual clinician, the employing organisation and the health of the population served as a whole. The development of clinician resilience is therefore vital in maintaining the health of the remote clinician so that they can continue to practise and deliver healthcare with a high degree of autonomy and efficacy.

Summary

In summary, the challenge of delivering acute medical care in the remote setting is all consuming. When faced with medical challenges the key skills of history taking, clinical examination, and the interpretation of basic medical tests underpinned with a good grounding in medical sciences will stand any clinician in good stead. They must always remember that communication is paramount, be it to the patient or wider clinical teams and be comfortable at recognising their own limitations. Being able to recognise one's limitations in the remote setting is not a weakness, but a vital skill and could mean the difference between life and death.

References

Aujesky D, Obrosky DS, Stone RA, Auble TE, Perrier A, Cornuz J, Roy PM and Fine MJ. 2005. Derivation and validation of a prognostic model for pulmonary embolism. *Am J Respir Crit Care Med* **172**: 1041–1046, doi:10.1164/rccm.200506-862OC.

Beithon J, Gallenberg M, Johnson K, Kildahl P, Krenik J, Liebow M, Linbo L, Myers C, Peterson S, Schmidt J and Swanson J. 2013. Institute for Clinical Systems Improvement. Diagnosis and treatment of headache. Updated January 2013.

Bennett C, Klingenberg SL, Langholz E and Gluud LL. 2014. Tranexamic acid for upper gastrointestinal bleeding. *Cochrane Database Syst Rev*, doi:10.1002/14651858.CD006640.pub3.

Chen I-C *et al.* 2007. Risk scoring systems to predict need for clinical intervention for patients with nonvariceal upper gastrointestinal tract bleeding. *Am J Emerg Med* **25**: 774–779.

Dalziel SR *et al*. 2019. Levetiracetam versus phenytoin for second-line treatment of convulsive status epilepticus in children (ConSEPT): an open-label, multicentre, randomised controlled trial. *Lancet* **393**: 2135–2145.

Forrest EH, Evans CD, Stewart S, Phillips M, Oo YH, McAvoy NC, Fisher NC, Singhal S, Brind A, Haydon G, O'Grady J, Day CP, Hayes PC, Murray LS and Morris AJ. 2005. Analysis of factors predictive of mortality in alcoholic hepatitis and derivation and validation of the Glasgow alcoholic hepatitis score. *Gut* **54**: 1174–1179, doi: 10.1136/gut.2004.050781.

Gianfranco UM, Cook TR, Turner RE, Cohen M and Leeper KV. 1996. Noninvasive positive pressure ventilation in status asthmaticus. *Chest* **110**: 767–774, ISSN 0012-3692, doi:10.1378/chest.110.3.767.

Johnston KC, Connors AF Jr, Wagner DP and Haley EC Jr. 2003. Predicting outcome in ischemic stroke: external validation of predictive risk models. *Stroke* **34**: 200–202, doi: 10.1161/01.str.0000047102.61863.e3.

Johnston SC *et al*. 2007. Validation and refinement of scores to predict very early stroke risk after transient ischaemic attack. *Lancet* **369**: 283–292.

Joint British Diabetes Societies, Inpatient Care Group. 2012. The management of the hyperosmolar hyperglycaemic state (HHS) in adults with diabetes.

Kline JA, Mitchell AM, Kabrhel C, Richman PB and Courtney DM. 2004. Clinical criteria to prevent unnecessary diagnostic testing in emergency department patients with suspected pulmonary embolism. *J Thromb Haemost* **2**: 1247–1255, doi:10.1111/j.1538-7836.2004.00790.x.

Kline KP, Conti CR and Winchester DE. 2015. Historical perspective and contemporary management of acute coronary syndromes: from MONA to THROMBINS2. *Postgrad Med* **127**: 855–862, DOI: 10.1080/00325481.2015.1092374.

MacDuff A, Arnold A, Harvey J *et al*. 2010. Management of spontaneous pneumothorax: British Thoracic Society pleural disease guideline. *Thorax* **65**: ii18-ii31.

Maslach C, Jackson SE and Leiter MP. 1996–2016. *Maslach Burnout Inventory Manual*, 4th Edn. Menlo Park, CA: Mind Garden.

McCullough L, Haycock JC, Forward DP and Moran CG. 2014. Early management of the severely injured major trauma patient. *Br J Anaesth* **113**: 234–241, ISSN 0007-0912, https://doi.org/10.1093/bja/aeu235.

Müller M, Jürgens J, Redaèlli M *et al*. 2018. Impact of the communication and patient hand-off tool SBAR on patient safety: a systematic review. *BMJ Open* 2018: e022202, doi: 10.1136/bmjopen-2018-022202.

Niakan E, Harati Y, Rolak LA, Comstock JP and Rokey R. 1986. Silent myocardial infarction and diabetic cardiovascular autonomic neuropathy. *Arch Intern Med* **146**: 2229–2230, doi:10.1001/archinte.1986.00360230169023.

Rhodes A, Evans LE, Alhazzani W *et al*. 2016. Surviving sepsis campaign: international guidelines for management of sepsis and septic shock. *Intensive Care Med* **43**: 304, https://doi.org/10.1007/s00134-017-4683-6.

Royal College of Physicians (RCP). 2017. National Early Warning Score (NEWS) 2: Standardising the assessment of acute-illness severity in the NHS. Updated report of a working party. London: RCP.

SIGN 153. 2016. British guideline on the management of asthma. ISBN 978 1 905813 47 4.

Simpson SQ. 2018. SIRS in the time of sepsis-3, *Chest* **153**: 34–38, ISSN 0012-3692, https://doi.org/10.1016/j.chest.2017.10.006.

Thim T, Krarup NHV, Grove EL, Rohde CV and Løfgren B *et al.* 2012. Initial assessment and treatment with the Airway, Breathing, Circulation, Disability, Exposure (ABCDE) approach. *Int J Gen Med* **5**: 117–121, doi: 10.2147/IJGM.S28478.

Thygesen K, Alpert JS and White HD. 2007. Joint ESC/ACCF/AHA/WHF Universal Definition of Myocardial Infarction, Task Force for the Redefinition of Myocardial Infarction. *J Am Coll Cardiol* **50**: 2173–2195; doi: 10.1016/j.jacc.2007.09.011.

Chapter 8

Remote Healthcare and Psychiatric Emergencies

Alison Carroll

Introduction

Remote sites vary widely. Geography, climate, distance to definitive care, number of personnel, medical resources and culture all have an influence on how cases should be managed; dealing with a psychiatric emergency in a remote location can be one of the most challenging situations for the practitioner.

Often, he/she has little experience of psychiatric illness, it is also unlikely that anyone else will be experienced in such a situation to give help, and transport to definitive care can be problematic.

Adding to this is the risk the disturbed patient can present in a very dangerous worksite which presents many opportunities to cause damage to themselves and others.

This chapter is not intended to be an introduction to psychiatric illness, diagnosis or management but is rather a collection of handy hints to assist practitioners who may find themselves faced with this problem.

More than any other medical condition, the presentation of psychiatric illness is significantly affected by cultural background.

To give some examples of this:

(a) Delusions of persecution and auditory hallucinations are not necessarily signs of schizophrenia. Some countries have culturally validated beliefs in sorcery and witchcraft.
(b) In some cultures, depression presents with predominantly physical symptoms.
(c) Some psychiatric illnesses tend to occur only in very specific areas such as Multiple Personality Disorder which is seen only in North America.

Remote worksites are usually multi-cultural so it can be helpful to discuss what is seen as normal or abnormal with workers from the same background as this may significantly alter your assessment.

There are also many factors in the remote worksite that may trigger psychiatric illness or induce a relapse in those who have a previous psychiatric illness. People are separated from family and support structures and, in addition, language difficulties can lead to a sense of isolation.

Pre-mobilisation medicals do not address this in any great depth so it is not unusual for vulnerable employees to be assigned to unsuitable posts.

Differential Diagnosis — Is this Actually a Psychiatric Illness?

The first and most important step to take in reaching a diagnosis is to consider whether the patient has an acute medical condition with symptoms which could be mistaken for psychiatric illness or whether this is, indeed, a psychiatric condition.

There are a great number of physical illnesses which can present with symptoms which may superficially suggest psychiatric disorder and mistaking them for a psychiatric illness results in a delay in managing the underlying condition which may prove fatal. Some examples of those which may present in the typical remote site population are:

(a) Drug or alcohol withdrawal
(b) Hypo or hyper-glycaemia
(c) Head injury
(d) Encephalitis
(e) Hepatic encephalopathy

There are some simple "rules of thumb" to differentiate between the two.

1. In physical illness, acute confusion is predominant. The patient is disorientated to some degree — usually time and place rather than person. A psychiatric illness presents in clear consciousness so any drop in Glasgow Coma Scale should be presumed to have a physical cause.
2. As a rule of thumb, auditory hallucinations are psychiatric in origin while physical illness may have visual hallucinations. We can all recall the pink elephants meant to be associated with alcohol withdrawal!
3. Symptoms come on more rapidly in a physical condition compared to a psychiatric illness.

4. There will be signs of the underlying illness — pyrexia, abnormal pupil size or reaction, low blood sugar for example.

The American Psychiatric Association recommends that any one of the following should make you think of an organic cause:

(a) A patient over 40 years old with no psychiatric history
(b) Disorientation, lethargy, stupor
(c) Abnormal vital signs
(d) Visual hallucinations

Case Study 1

A young Nigerian gentleman arrived for his second trip on a production platform in the offshore UK sector. He was based there temporarily to do some specialised work. He was fit and healthy and on no medication.

He had been noted to not be coping well with the work on this trip although there were no reported problems from his first trip.

One day, he failed to attend to start his 12-hour shift and he was found still asleep in his cabin.

The medic was called to assess him and found him denying any symptoms other than sleepiness. He was described as confused, unsteady with signs of dehydration. After giving him fluids, the medic spoke to the project manager and the supervisor who said he was not coping with the work, had become very stressed and they had made arrangement for him to go home the next day without finishing his tour of duty.

The onshore doctor was called for further advice and his notes follow:

"Colleagues have noted that he has a stressful job and not coping.

Patient orientated in person but not in place otherwise observations normal. Blood Sugar 7.9. Has passed urine. No hallucinations or delusions. Admit to sick bay and observe overnight. Will come onshore tomorrow and be reviewed."

Over the next 12 hours the patient's condition was closely monitored as he steadily deteriorated. He became increasingly confused and lethargic; he was described as "withdrawing" from people as he didn't respond to questions. His speech was unintelligible.

BP steadily fell as pulse rate and respiratory rate rose. The glucometer reading was reported as "lo" which was interpreted as meaning "low".

Eventually at 7 am next morning his BP was 92/63, pulse 101, blood sugar still "lo" and he was responding only to pain so a rescue helicopter was called to transfer him to the nearest hospital. Here his blood sugar was found to be 72 and it became apparent he was a new onset insulin dependent diabetic in a hyperglycaemic coma.

Clearly this patient did not have a psychiatric illness but rather was suffering from an acute medical condition.

What should have indicated this was a physical and not a psychiatric disorder?

(a) He was disorientated. His GCS was initially 15 then 14 then dropped even further.
(b) He had clear signs of physical illness — tachycardia even when asleep in bed, increased respiratory rate, falling blood pressure.

Two main errors led to his near fatal deterioration. The first was deciding early on that he was psychiatrically unwell which resulted in clear signs of physical illness being ignored. The second was a faulty glucometer which the medic did not know how to use.

This case highlights the dangers of leaping to an assumption about the diagnosis.

Acute Confusional States

An acute confusional state (sometimes called delirium) is an acute, transient and reversible state of confusion, usually the result of other organic processes (infection, drugs, dehydration etc.). The onset is acute and the mental state of the patient can be highly fluctuant over a short period of time.

There are two main types — hyperactive and hypoactive — and fluctuation between the two is common.

Hyperactive is the most common picture:

- Agitation
- Delusions
- Hallucinations
- Wandering
- Aggression

Hypoactive — more difficult to spot:

- Lethargy
- Excessive sleeping
- Inattention

History and examination

It may not be possible to get a coherent history from the patient but try to establish if they are orientated in time and place and ask specifically about hallucinations — ask the patient what they are seeing/hearing or experiencing. Get any history possible from those who have been closest to the patient — for example, when did they start noticing symptoms?

Possible causes:

- Hypoxia
- Infection
- Metabolic disturbance
- Hepatic or renal dysfunction
- Drugs
- Alcohol withdrawal

Do whatever examination and investigation is possible, given your circumstances:

- Temperature, respiratory rate, oxygen saturation
- Pulse, blood pressure
- Urinalysis
- Blood sugar
- Look for signs of hepatic dysfunction — for example, yellow sclera

Management

There are too many possible causes to consider each one in depth. What follows is a description of how to manage alcohol withdrawal, chosen since this remains one of the more common causes for acute confusion in the remote site population.

Alcohol withdrawal symptoms classically begin 48–72 hours after cessation of drinking. Many men drink heavily whilst at home, stopping abruptly just before they return to work. These people often have a history of always being "under par" for the first few days of a tour of duty, many complaining of nausea, loss of appetite, headaches and tremor. This usually resolves without any intervention and the patient goes on to work normally.

In some cases, however, possibly related to a heavier than normal alcohol intake on his time off or a gradual worsening of his alcohol dependence, the symptoms continue to worsen after day three.

The patient begins to show signs of restlessness and fear with confusion, hallucinations and delusions. His tremor is uncontrollable, he cannot eat or drink and he may have ataxia. He will have a marked tachycardia and pyrexia. In some patients they progress to seizures.

This acute condition is known as delirium tremens or DTs and has a 20% mortality rate if untreated. Death is usually caused by status epilepticus or hypoglycaemia.

- Treatment is to nurse the patient in a quiet but well-lit room — dim light casts shadows which may add to the patient's hallucinations.
- A reducing regime of benzodiazepines should be given, probably intra-muscularly as, at this stage, the patient usually cannot take anything orally because of nausea and/or vomiting. Which benzodiazepine to choose is dependent on local protocols or which one is stocked on site. Diazepam or chlordiazepoxide are among the most commonly used. The severity of the patient's dependence needs to be determined before starting the regimen using the Severity of Alcohol Dependence Questionnaire (SADQ, see Figure 1). Both the SADQ and table of daily dosage are given at the end of this section, however bear in mind the dosage may need to be increased or decreased depending on the patient's reaction. If it is not possible to get the patient to complete the questionnaire then start at the second highest level and monitor the patient carefully.
- Fluids — the patient will be very dehydrated but unable to keep down anything given orally, so IV access should be gained and fluids given. Alternating bags of saline and dextrose may be given until blood sugar is stable. The confused patient will often try to remove the IV line so ensure it is well protected.
- Blood sugar must be checked regularly. The patient is at risk of hypoglycaemia.
- The patient needs urgent transfer to hospital. There is a risk of Wernike's Encephalopathy and subsequent Korsakoff's Psychosis developing so IM Vit B1 (thiamine) injections are necessary to prevent this. This is seldom available in remote locations.

1. The day after drinking alcohol, do you wake up feeling sweaty? *
   ○ Almost never ○ Sometimes ○ Often ○ Nearly always

2. The day after drinking alcohol, do your hands shake first thing in the morning? *
   ○ Almost never ○ Sometimes ○ Often ○ Nearly always

3. The day after drinking alcohol, does your body shake violently first thing in the morning if you don't have a drink? *
   ○ Almost never ○ Sometimes ○ Often ○ Nearly always

4. The day after drinking alcohol, do you wake up drenched in sweat? *
   ○ Almost never ○ Sometimes ○ Often ○ Nearly always

5. The day after drinking alcohol, do you dread waking up? *
   ○ Almost never ○ Sometimes ○ Often ○ Nearly always

6. The day after drinking alcohol, are you frightened of meeting people first thing in the morning? *
   ○ Almost never ○ Sometimes ○ Often ○ Nearly always

7. The day after drinking alcohol, do you feel at the edge of despair when you wake up? *
   ○ Almost never ○ Sometimes ○ Often ○ Nearly always

8. The day after drinking alcohol, do you feel frightened when you wake up? *
   ○ Almost never ○ Sometimes ○ Often ○ Nearly always

9. The day after drinking alcohol, do you like a drink in the morning? *
   ○ Almost never ○ Sometimes ○ Often ○ Nearly always

10. The day after drinking alcohol, do you gulp your first few drinks down as fast as possible? *
    ○ Almost never ○ Sometimes ○ Often ○ Nearly always

11. The day after drinking alcohol, do you drink to get rid of the shakes? *
    ○ Almost never ○ Sometimes ○ Often ○ Nearly always

12. The day after drinking alcohol, do you have a strong craving for drink when you wake up? *
    ○ Almost never ○ Sometimes ○ Often ○ Nearly always

13. During a heavy drinking period, do you drink more than 1/4 bottle of spirits (or 1 bottle of wine, or 4 pints of beer) each day? *
    ○ Almost never ○ Sometimes ○ Often ○ Nearly always

14. During a heavy drinking period, do you drink more than half a bottle of spirits per day (8 pints of beer, 2 bottles of wine)? *
    ○ Almost never ○ Sometimes ○ Often ○ Nearly always

Figure 1:   Severity of Alcohol Dependence Questionnaire (SADQ)

15. During a heavy drinking period, do you drink more than a bottle of spirits per day (3 bottles of wine, 5 litres of cider or 10 pints of lager) *
○ Almost never ○ Sometimes ○ Often ○ Nearly always

16. During a heavy drinking period, do you drink more than 2 bottles of spirits per day (7 bottles of wine, 9 litres of cider, 20 pints of beer). *
○ Almost never ○ Sometimes ○ Often ○ Nearly always

17. Imagine you have been abstinent for a few weeks, then drink heavily for a couple of days. The morning after would you start to sweat? *
○ Not at all ○ Slightly ○ Moderately ○ Quite a lot

18. Imagine the same scenario again, would your hands shake? *
○ Not at all ○ Slightly ○ Moderately ○ Quite a lot

19. Imagine the same scenario again, would your body shake? *
○ Not at all ○ Slightly ○ Moderately ○ Quite a lot

20. Imagine the same scenario for the last time, would you be craving for a drink? *
○ Not at all ○ Slightly ○ Moderately ○ Quite a lot

Figure 1:   (*Continued*)

- If the patient has an epileptic seizure, the only management necessary is to ensure that they do not harm themselves during the tonic/clonic contractions. The use of oxygen is rarely successful because of patient movement.
- If seizures continue without the patient fully recovering between each fit this is termed Status Epilepticus. This is defined by UK NICE Guidelines as a life-threatening neurological condition of five or more minutes of either continuous seizure activity or repetitive seizures without regaining consciousness. It should be treated as an emergency and the most important aspect of treatment is to try to stop the seizure.
- Treatment options in the remote location are limited by the drugs available and many drugs seen as first line in the hospital setting are not commonly stocked. The two drugs most commonly available are buccal midazolam and rectal diazepam.
- Buccal Midazolam dose is 10 mg, then 10 mg after 10 minutes if required.
- Rectal diazepam dose is 10 mg, then 10 mg after 10 minutes if required, administered at a rate of 1 mL (5 mg) per minute.
- The greatest risk associated with these is depression of respiration so ensure respiratory rate is monitored and be prepared to assist with a bag and valve mask if necessary.

Once the convulsions have ceased, the patient should be given oxygen and closely monitored.

Scoring answers to each question are rated on a four-point scale:

- Almost never 0
- Sometimes 1
- Often 2
- Nearly always 3

→ A score of 31 or higher indicates "severe alcohol dependence".

→ A score of 16–30 indicates "moderate dependence".

→ A score of below 16 usually indicates only a mild physical dependency.

→ A chlordiazepoxide detoxification regime is usually indicated for someone who scores 16 or over.

Chlordiazepoxide Regime:

https://www.nice.org.uk/guidance/cg115/resources/sample-chlordiazepoxide-dosing-regimens-for-use-in-managing-alcohol-withdrawal-pdf-4489950493

Ultimately, he tested positively for amphetamines and benzodiazepines. It is believed he regularly used amphetamines at home then, just before he was due to return to work, he stopped them and took a short course of benzodiazepines to help him return to normal. Being called back to work earlier than usual disrupted his schedule, leading to his strange behaviour.

Case Study 2

A young rope access technician was called to return offshore unexpectedly because a colleague had become ill and needed to be transferred to hospital. He arrived late at the heliport with a confused story about a car accident on the way, however, there was just time to get him aboard before take-off.

On arrival, he and the others from the same flight were given time to eat before reporting for a Safety Induction. The patient didn't turn up for this and was found asleep in his bunk. It took considerable time and effort to wake him at which stage he began to act strangely.

He was described as alert but disorientated in time and place. Speech was not slurred but jumbled and not coherent. He was trying to stand on the television and dressing/undressing repeatedly.

He had difficulty walking. He denied any history of head injury or drug taking. Although, when asked, he agreed to take a drug test; he was overheard trying to persuade another crew member to take it for him.

Psychoses

The essential features in psychoses are delusions **in clear consciousness**. The patient is not disorientated nor does he have any reduction in conscious level.

Terminology:

- A hallucination is a perception without a stimulus.
- A delusion is a fixedly held false belief that is not shared by others from the patient's community.

The two main psychotic illnesses encountered are schizophrenia and mania/hypomania.

Schizophrenia

Schizophrenia is a complex illness with many differing presentations but it has nothing to do with "split personality" which is a common misconception. The main symptoms can be classified as follows.

Positive symptoms

Lack of insight

- Failure to appreciate that symptoms are not real or caused by illness.

Hallucinations

- Hallucinations can occur in any sense — touch, smell, taste, or vision — but auditory hallucinations are the most common (usually "hearing voices").

Delusions

- Delusions often develop along personal themes; for example:
  - Persecution — patients think they are victims of some form of threat or are central to a conspiracy.
  - Passivity — patients think that their thoughts or actions are being controlled by an external force or person.
  - Other — delusions can develop along any theme; for instance, grandiose, sexual, or religious.

Thought disorder

- Manifests as distorted or illogical speech — a failure to use language in a logical and coherent way.
- Typified by "knight's move" thinking — thoughts proceed in one direction but suddenly go off at right angles, like the knight in chess, with no logical chain of thought.

Negative symptoms

- These include social withdrawal, self-neglect, loss of motivation and initiative, emotional blunting, and paucity of speech.

In practice, few schizophrenics work in remote locations. This is especially true when the "negative symptoms" predominate. Living in an isolated community in close proximity to others is likely to be particularly challenging to someone who suffers from social withdrawal and people who have significant loss of motivation and drive are unlikely to be in any demanding employment.

On occasion, first onset cases of schizophrenia have occurred or, more commonly, those without significant negative symptoms are employed during a stage when their positive symptoms are well controlled. They often stop their medication and relapse quickly once exposed to the stressors of remote life.

Case Study 3

A young medic had been recently employed on a large offshore platform in the UKCS. She had completed one trip with no concerns being raised, however it quickly became apparent early in the second trip that all was not well.

The OIM contacted the onshore doctor and described how her behaviour had become increasingly unusual. By the time of the call, she had to be restrained as she attempted to barricade herself and a group of workers in a lounge, believing that ill-defined forces were trying to take over control of the installation. She thought she was saving their lives and was increasingly distressed when they resisted her attempts. She was able to speak to the doctor on the phone and it was established that, in addition to this delusion, she was also experiencing auditory hallucinations with voices telling her what actions she should take to save her colleagues. It was difficult to decide whether she also had thought disorder as the interview was understandably brief.

Eventually she was persuaded to take some anti-psychotic drugs and was taken onshore heavily sedated and restrained in a helicopter.

Later, after she was treated and had recovered from the acute episode, she was able to describe having a history of several years of schizophrenia, usually reasonably controlled on depot anti-psychotic drugs. She had been unable to work as a nurse onshore because of this history and so decided to conceal it by applying for an OGUK medical.

Sadly, her career as a medic was brief but in such a safety critical role, the risk was unacceptably high.

Hypomania and mania

These terms are often used to indicate the severity of the symptoms. Hypomania is at the milder end; mania has lasted longer and the patient has deteriorated to the extent that they cannot be tolerated socially or in the workplace.

Hypomania

Hypomania is defined in ICD-10 as elevated or irritable mood that is abnormal for the individual and is sustained for at least 4 days. Features such as over-familiarity, increased activity or talkativeness, distractibility, or reduced sleep should also be present, but these symptoms are not present to the extent that they lead to severe social disruption of work or result in social rejection. Criteria for a manic episode should not be met, nor should hallucinations or delusions be present.

Mania

Mania is defined as elevated, expansive or irritable mood that must be sustained for at least 1 week.

Accompanying symptoms may include increased activity or talkativeness, flight of ideas, disinhibition, reduced sleep, grandiosity or reckless behaviour, which lead to severe interference with personal functioning in daily living. Mania may occur with or without psychotic symptoms, which may be mood-congruent or mood-incongruent. Typical mood-congruent hallucinations would take the form of voices telling the individual that he/she had superhuman powers. Mood-incongruent psychotic symptoms may include voices speaking about affectively neutral topics, or delusions of persecution.

Frequently the layman imagines this to be the opposite of depression and expect the main feature to be an excessively cheerful and happy mood. Except in the very mildest of cases, this is unlikely to be the case and irritability is more often the overriding mood.

It is a recurring condition which, when adequately treated, results in a complete return to normality between episodes. Drugs may be given to reduce the frequency and/or the severity of the relapses with Lithium being traditionally the mainstay. Lithium is a dangerous drug with the therapeutic dose being very close to the lethal one so it is not usually acceptable in remote work places.

Some people suffer from episodes of depression as well as hypomania/mania in which case the condition is termed bi-polar disorder. We will not consider this specifically because at any one time only one will be present and the patient is unlikely to remain long enough in the workplace for both conditions to be manifest.

Usually the onset happens over a period of time, from hypomania to mania although often this is only obvious in retrospect.

Case Study 4

A young steward worked on an offshore platform for several years. He was well known and liked and had never displayed any psychiatric symptoms in the past.

At the beginning of one trip he was noted to be sleeping very little. At night, when he would usually be sleeping, he was often to be found offering to help his night shift colleagues with their work. Initially, during the day, he was getting through his work at great speed but with a lack of attention to detail; however, as the days went on, he became increasingly unable to settle at any task for more than a few minutes, so nothing was completed. His speech became rapid and he jumped from one subject to another until it became hard to follow.

He seemed superficially elated, however, he became extremely irritable when his supervisor tried to encourage him to complete tasks properly. He felt that he was well qualified to tell others how to do their jobs no matter how little he knew about most of them. When he was teased about this by some of the drill crew, he became extremely angry, shouting and waving his fists at them.

Finally, he woke the OIM up at 4am and presented him with several dozen sheets of paper minutely covered with rambling, handwritten notes explaining where the OIM was failing in running the installation and how he could do it better.

Although there were no psychotic features — hallucinations or delusions — at this stage, his condition would now seem to have moved from hypomania to mania, based on the social and work problems it was causing.

He was persuaded to take oral anti-psychotic drugs and returned to shore with surprisingly little fuss although he was accompanied by four well built colleagues to ensure everyone's safety.

It transpired that he had several such episodes in the past but more recently, his family had learned to recognise the early symptoms and prompt treatment prevented any escalation of symptoms. On this occasion, he had been on holiday without any family members and had come straight offshore on his return from overseas. He, of course, had no insight into his developing relapse.

Depression

Depression is a commonly used term but medically, it does not apply to the low mood people feel as a reaction to life events or problems.

Here we will look only at what is classed as major depressive illness or clinical depression.

Cause

The cause of major depressive disorder is unknown however there are two main schools of thought:

- The biopsychosocial model proposes that biological, psychological, and social factors all play a role in causing depression.
- The diathesis–stress model specifies that depression results when a pre-existing vulnerability is activated by stressful life events. The pre-existing vulnerability can be either genetic or resulting from views of the world learned in childhood.

Whatever the cause, the stresses of work in a remote area and isolation from friends, family and other support systems can trigger illness in a susceptible person or cause rapid deterioration in an illness already present. Suicide happens regularly, if not frequently, so it is important to be alert for symptoms indicating someone is at risk.

Symptoms

The symptoms of depression are characterized by an overwhelming feeling of sadness, isolation, and despair that lasts two weeks or longer at a time. Depression isn't just an occasional feeling of being sad or lonely, like most people experience from time to time. Instead, a person feels like they've sunk into a deep, dark hole with no way out — and no hope for things ever changing.

- Depressed mood most of the day, nearly every day. In some, irritability may be predominant.
- Loss of interest or pleasure in most or all day to day activities, such as zero interest in hobbies, sports, or other things the person used to enjoy doing.
- Not coping at work — not managing workload or finding it difficult to make decisions.
- Significant weight loss when not dieting.
- Insomnia, particularly early morning wakening.
- Feelings of worthlessness or excessive or inappropriate guilt (e.g., ruminating over minor past failings).
- Diminished ability to think or concentrate, or indecisiveness (e.g., appears easily distracted, complains of memory difficulties).
- Recurrent thoughts of death, recurrent suicidal ideas without a specific plan, or a suicide attempt or a specific plan for committing suicide.

The use of standardised scoring systems to diagnose depressive illness is not particularly helpful. Many are designed, not for diagnosis, but to monitor progress in an already diagnosed condition. Others need training before they can be used effectively. A good history specifically covering the points mentioned above is much more likely to assist in reaching a diagnosis.

Red flags

- Physical symptoms like weight loss
- Early morning wakening. Patient awakens suddenly in the middle of the night and cannot get back to sleep.
- Diurnal variation — mood at the lowest ebb on first awakening with some slight improvement towards evening
- Failure to attend to personal hygiene, dishevelled appearance
- Inability to see a future, hopelessness, despair
- Suicidal thoughts — planning

In the presence of red flags, the patient will need to be closely supervised until they reach definitive care.

Agitated depression

This is a particular sub-set of major depression which may be driven by hypomania. Many depressed people have a degree of agitation, however, here it is the prominent symptom. It is more common in the middle aged and elderly and is associated with a higher risk of self-harm. The diagnostic criteria for an agitated depression are:

- Major Depressive Episode
- At least two of the following symptoms:
  - Motor agitation
  - Psychic agitation or intense inner tension
  - Racing or crowded thoughts

Symptoms are:

- Extreme irritability
- Outbursts of complaining or shouting
- Racing thoughts and incessant talking
- Restlessness and pacing
- Anger
- Agitation
- Hand-wringing and nail-biting
- Pulling at clothes or hair
- Picking at skin
- Fidgeting

Sedation and preventing the patient harming themselves or others is the main approach.

Suicide

This is one very important feature to address in the depressed patient since it is the leading cause of death among men under the age of 50 in the UK. Those who suffer from schizophrenia, bi-polar disorder and personality disorder are also more likely to kill themselves. Risk factors include:

- Sex — men kill themselves more often than women
- History of mental illness
- History of drug or alcohol abuse
- Marital breakdown and/or family breakdown
- History of attempted suicide
- Family history of suicide
- Social isolation
- Low intelligence
- Low socio-economic status

For many people suicide happens after a period of some months thinking about it. Over this period of time their mood and behaviour can be noted to change, for example:

- Feeling depressed, withdrawn, anxious
- Loss of interest in work, hobbies, socialisation and even appearance
- Expressing ideas of hopelessness or purposelessness
- Acting impulsively
- Giving away things, sorting out their affairs or making a will
- Talking about suicide, wanting to "end it all"

Management of suicide risk

Suicide risk should be assessed on the basis of the history and identification of red flags. The use of questionnaires such as SAD should be avoided as there is evidence these are no better than a random decision.

Some useful questions to ask:

- How does the future look to you? What are your hopes?
- Do you wish you could just not wake up in the morning?
- Have you considered doing anything to harm yourself, or to take your own life?
- Have you made actual plans to kill yourself? What are they?
- What has stopped you from doing anything so far?

Many people worry that, in asking about suicide, they may be actually planting the idea in the patient's head and making it more likely to happen. This is not the case. Often the patient feels relief that they can openly talk about these distressing thoughts.

It is easy to commit suicide in an industrial worksite with access to heights, heavy machinery and isolated areas. In offshore sites drowning is the commonest but hanging has also occurred.

Some choose to commit suicide at work to save their family from having to discover their body, others because they feel even more isolated and hopeless separated from their family.

The patient should be confined to the single cabin and have someone sitting with them at all times. The room should be cleared of anything sharp or anything that could be made into a ligature. They should be accompanied to the lavatory and not permitted to lock themselves in there under any circumstances. Similar supervision is necessary during transport.

It is a kindness to people in this state of distress to prescribe some sedative medication such as a benzodiazepine, night sedation can also be useful.

Management of a successful suicide

If a body is found and suicide is suspected, it is important to follow any local police guidelines to ensure this is managed in a way consistent with the legal requirements.

Should there be any possibility of a successful resuscitation, the usual ABC approach must be taken. If the patient is found hanging, try to cut them down without damaging the knots in case there is a subsequent investigation. In general, try to preserve evidence, but be very clear that the resuscitation has priority.

If there is no possibility of resuscitation e.g., if there is rigor mortis or decomposition then preservation of the site becomes the priority.

Later it transpired that his wife had left him because of his problem drinking and taken the children. He had sunk heavily into debt and as a result lost his house, so he could no longer have the children to stay on visits.

He had sought treatment for his depressive illness but had only just started the medication.

Case Study 5

A 50-year-old chef had been noted to gradually be acting differently. He became less sociable, spending as much time on his own as he could and he didn't communicate while working except for what was essential for the job.

He had no interest in his work and didn't seem to care about standards in the galley which was very unusual for him.

He had been found to be neglecting his personal hygiene and his eyes often looked red as if he was crying. People tried to ask him if anything was wrong but he denied this and was quite irritated at the question.

One day he failed to report for duty and he couldn't be found in his room or in any other part of the accommodation area. An extensive search was undertaken and eventually he was found in an isolated part of the worksite having hanged himself.

Management of the Acutely Disturbed Patient

It is important to remember that most mentally ill people are not violent, however most acts of violence committed by individuals with serious mental illness are carried out when they are not being treated. This means that there is an increased risk in the remote environment where patients are unlikely to be taking medication (Figure 2).

Someone who has paranoid delusions or hallucinations may be very frightened and a frightened patient, acting on his delusions, can lash out and cause harm to themselves or others.

The usual scenario is that other workers have noticed a change in behaviour in a colleague over a period of days but that senior staff and the remote practitioner have not been told of their concerns until a crisis develops.

This may not happen until the patient has started to threaten violence, so you are faced with an extreme situation from the outset.

The aims in managing the situation are:

- To make sure there is no threat to the safety of the operation
- To ensure the safety of other staff
- To move the patient to a safe area where he can be managed

The first approach should be with a view to talking to the patient. You should observe some basic rules when attempting this:

i. Approach calmly and politely
ii. Avoid prolonged eye contact as this can be seen to be threatening
iii. Keep at a safe distance
iv. Keep your exit route clear — never let the patient get between you and your escape route.

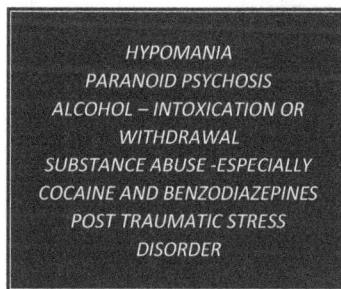

> HYPOMANIA
> PARANOID PSYCHOSIS
> ALCOHOL – INTOXICATION OR
> WITHDRAWAL
> SUBSTANCE ABUSE -ESPECIALLY
> COCAINE AND BENZODIAZEPINES
> POST TRAUMATIC STRESS
> DISORDER

Figure 2: Psychiatric Disorders Associated with Violence

Do not disagree with the patient if he discusses delusions or hallucinations. Use an empathic non-confrontational approach, but set boundaries. The aim is to persuade him that you are on his side and will work with him to keep him safe from any harm. Offer him food or drink and clothing if appropriate. Try to divert the patient from his emotions by raising neutral subjects. It is useful at this stage for the patient to see that there is a large team of people standing by to help you deal with the situation (Figure 3).

If you are successful, then the patient should be persuaded to accompany you to a room which has been prepared by removing all furniture and objects that can be lifted.

The next step is to try to persuade him to take some anti-psychotic drugs orally. It is surprising how often patients do not object to taking medication whilst simultaneously being adamant that their delusions are absolutely real.

If your attempts to persuade the patient to come with you quietly fail and he is still presenting a risk then you have no choice but to restrain and sedate him.

Planning is essential for restraint to be effective and cause as little distress as possible. If you are unsuccessful at the first attempt, a second will be much more difficult. You should identify five people whom you know are physically fit and able to take instructions in a heated situation. You will act as the leader, four of your team will be assigned a limb each with a spare person to help where necessary. Each member of the team should hold their assigned limb with one hand on the joints — wrist and elbow or knee and ankle. The fifth person assists in lowering the patient to the ground.

Be clear exactly what you want them to do and practise it beforehand.

Restraint in the face up position is safer for the patient but more difficult than the face down position. The face down position restricts the leg movements and prevents the patient biting. It is probably best therefore to use the face down position but make sure that you do not compromise the patient's breathing in any way. Ensure no pressure is put on the patient's back which would restrict breathing or even result in asphyxia.

Your role is to act as team leader, administer the medication once the patient is restrained and continually monitor the patient's breathing. The medication should be drawn up and ready to administer.

Anger
Demanding attention
Loud voice
Excitement
Staring eyes, flared nostrils
Flushed face
Hands clenched
Pacing and rapid movements

Figure 3:   Signs of Impending Violence

Guidelines differ on which drugs to use, and the evidence is limited and unconvincing. The choice ultimately comes down to what is available on site.

Suitable medication falls into two categories — benzodiazepines and anti-psychotics. Benzodiazepines are usually used as an adjunct to anti-psychotics in the inpatient situation and seldom on their own. All should be used intra-muscularly.

The most commonly available drugs at the remote site are haloperidol and chlorpromazine. The effective dose is extremely variable but 2.5–10mg of haloperidol or 50–100mg of chlorpromazine give some indication of a starting point.

The risks of sedation are considerable and include respiratory depression and pulmonary aspiration, sudden cardiac death, dystonic reactions and hypotension.

Once you choose to start chemical sedation, you have full responsibility to maintain the patient's airway, breathing, circulation, provide bladder care, hydration, and general nursing care to that patient.

Ideally you are looking to have the patient at 0 or minus one of the Sedation Assessment Tool (SAT, see Figure 4).

Transfer of the patient to definitive care is likely to be challenging because of the need to achieve a balance between over-sedation of the patient and risk to the mode of transfer if the patient again becomes acutely disturbed. Full discussion between those who will provide the transport and those caring for the patient is essential.

When do you stop?

SEDATION ASSESSMENT TOOL (S.A.T.)

	RESPONSIVENESS	SPEECH	SCORE
+3	Combative, violent, out of control	Continual loud outbursts	+1 to +3 Agitation
+2	Very anxious and agitated	Loud outbursts	
+1	Anxious / restless	Normal / Talkative	
0	Awake / calm	Speaks Normally	ZERO
-1	Asleep but rouses if name is called	Slurring or slowing	-1 to -3 Sedation
-2	Responds to physical stimulation	Few recognisable words	
-3	No response to stimulation	Nil	

Figure 4: Sedation Assessment Tool

Bibliography

Bolton JM, Spiwak R and Jitender S. 2012. Predicting suicide attempts with the "SAD PERSONS Scale". *J Clin Psychiat* **73**: e735–e741. Available at doi:10.4088/JCP.11m07362. PMID 22795212.

National Institute for Health and Clinical Excellence. 2005. Violence: the short-term management of disturbed/violent behaviour in in-patient psychiatric settings and emergency departments. NICE clinical guideline 25.

National Institute for Health and Clinical Excellence. 2015. Violence and aggression: short term management in mental health, health and community settings. NICE clinical guideline 10.

Patterson WM, Dohn HH, Bird J and Patterson GA. 1983. Evaluation of suicidal patients: the SAD PERSONS scale. *Psychosomatics* **24**: 343–345, 348–349. Available at doi:10.1016/S0033-3182(83)73213-5. PMID 6867245.

Saunders K, Brand F, Lascelles K and Hawton K. 2013. The sad truth about the SAD PERSONS Scale: an evaluation of its clinical utility in self-harm patients. *Emerg Med J* **31**: 796–798. doi:10.1136/emermed-2013-202781. PMID 23896589.

Taylor D, Paton C and Kapur S. 2012. *The Maudsley Prescribing Guidelines in Psychiatry*, 11th Edn. ISBN: 978-0-470-97948-8. Hoboken, NJ: Wiley-Blackwell.

Wright NM, Dixon CA and Tompkins CN. 2003. Managing violence in primary care: an evidence-based approach. *Br J Gen Pract* **53**: 557–562.

Chapter

9

Remote General Medical Practice

Malcolm Valentine

Section 1 — The Approach to General Medical Practice

Introduction

General Medical Practice sits at the core of the provision of Primary Care to a typical population. This could be a general population as may typically be found in a certain geographical area, comprising a general spread of population, or it may be more atypically found within a remote environment, comprising a more diverse or non-standard population such as a remote work site or remote populated facility.

The issue that binds all these different potential care scenarios together is that General Medical Practice, in the context of Primary Care, is in effect the day-to-day healthcare provision that is being made available. This provider will typically act as the first point of contact for medical care and is likely to be the main coordinating influence in terms of any further care that a patient might need e.g. secondary or even tertiary care (WHO, 2018).

In fact, the WHO itself goes further in its definition of General Medical Practice, stating

> The specificity of the general practitioner is that he/she is: "the only clinician who operates at the nine levels of care: prevention, pre-symptomatic detection of disease, early diagnosis, diagnosis of established disease, management of disease, management of disease complications, rehabilitation, palliative care and counselling" (Atun, 2004).

However, General Medical Practice continues to evolve and is no longer the singular provision role of a medically qualified General Practitioner (GP). The front-end provision of General Practice is as likely now to be by a Nurse Practitioner, Physician Assistant, Pharmacist or Paramedic. A critical key to this diversification of workforce is adequate training and calibration.

Within WHO analysis of the merits of a Primary Care approach, the available evidence demonstrates some advantages for health systems that rely relatively more on primary healthcare and general practice, in comparison with systems more based on Specialist Care in terms of better population health outcomes, improved equity, access and continuity and lower cost. This argument can apply not just to established communities, but also to more atypical and remote communities. Specialist Care is by definition expensive, whilst Primary Care is immensely efficient for what it delivers.

Illness Behaviour and Influences to Consult

There are many influences on health behaviour and the seeking of healthcare and advice. These will inevitably be influenced environmentally by culture (both in terms of past culture and current cultural specifics), family expectations and ideas, resources, availability, etc. But it remains a complex issue. Gochman has written extensively on this singular issue and defines illness behaviour as

> those personal attributes such as beliefs, expectations, motives values, perceptions and other cognitive elements, personality characteristics including affective and emotional states and traits; and overt behaviour patterns, actions and habits that relate to health maintenance, to health restoration and to health improvement (Gochman, 1988).

This is a more complex way of stating that an individual's response to perceived illness will inevitably vary according to the individual and the situation that they find themselves in. At individual level, this will vary from more extensive use of scant resources for perceived, rather than real illness, through to limited use of a clinical resource when it would be more appropriate to have done so. Situationally, the response will depend on the scope of the provision of medical care in that a welcoming and well provisioned facility may well be more attractive for use than a poorly provisioned and unwelcoming or difficult to access facility.

This is illustrated well in many remote environments where naturally there are many influences on consultation behaviour beyond the statement above. There is great potential influence from colleagues and peers within the immediate environment. The 'culture' regarding health and accessing healthcare will always be influential. It is important, both for the provision of care for perceived illness or injury and for the promotion of health and well being, that any Primary Care medical facility is able to strike a balance between availability and the proper use of such a facility.

Additional issues arise. Many remote healthcare facilities will have been provided for a discreet work population where there are no alternative suitable medical facilities. This then raises the ethical and moral issues that arise when help is sought by those near the facility not necessarily covered by the remit of the facility. This issue has been debated before (Quinn and Jablonski, 2013), where the issue of either non-contracted workers or local populations accessing healthcare facilities is debated. It is not a clear-cut matter — the conclusion is that individual practitioners in any remote location must reflect on their ethical responsibilities when deciding whether to provide care or not. Liability issues also need to be considered.

Contrasting General Practice and Secondary Care

Many models have been explored over the years to define the differences between the approach to General Medical Practice and Secondary (Specialist) Care. Some aspects of the differing approaches to clinical diagnosis and management will be explored in the section dealing with the consultation itself. However, some of the differences can be summarised in Table 1 (Fraser, 1992).

Therefore, it is important to recognise the tasks that exist within a remote Primary Care/General Medical Practice environment and accept these responsibilities as the strengths of what is possible within the medical facility provided. It is equally important to realise the part that engagement with a Secondary Care facility can play in supplementing the care of the patient. Both systems complement each other. But understanding the structural, functional and attitudinal differences will maximise the best care of the patient. Referral to a Secondary Care facility

Table 1:   Differences between General Practice and Secondary Care

General Medical Practice	Secondary Care
Usually small, defined population	Large undefined population
Patients have direct access	Access by referral or transfer (prior triage)
Close to patient cohort	Potentially distant to patient cohort
Potential variability between Primary Care facilities	Defined environment
Holistic patient care	Specialty focussed care
Undifferentiated problems or disease	Organised or triaged referral
Common diseases, problems	Complicated disease entities
Selective and focussed use of technology	Extensive use of technology
Continuing responsibility for patient	Episodic responsibility
Anticipatory and preventative care	Disease or task focussed care
Ability to use time as a diagnostic tool	Time sparing — 'need to know'
Doctor–Patient relationship important	Outcome more important
Continuing care when no absolute 'cure'	If no 'cure' patient will be discharged
Patients perspective and autonomy incorporated	Patient autonomy less important

(particularly in an urgent referral scenario) should never be viewed as a patient 'dump' or a way of absolving responsibility. Referral in any circumstance should be with an explicit expectation and also with a view to then providing continuing care for the patient as a follow through once that episode of secondary intervention is completed. This applies in any circumstance or location — remote or otherwise.

The consultation

The consultation within the context of General Medical Practice whether in mainstream Primary Care settings or in remote care settings is really at the heart of clinical care. The patient's journey will be defined by the competency by which the consultation is carried out or otherwise. The consultation is there to define the primary reason for patient presentation and from that will spring everything that then follows in terms of patient care. That may well be the management of a perceived rather than a real problem, the management of a problem within the context of the immediate care facility — or engaging with external sources of advice — or onward referral.

A number of tasks have been described as challenges within a GP consultation and a systematic approach to these tasks will ensure that the practitioner is practising with an enhanced level of clinical competence. By adopting a systematic approach, it is also then possible to engage meaningfully with other sources of advice or to make onward referral with a coherent and well communicated rationale to do so.

Much has been written over the years about the nature of the GP consultation and surprisingly little has changed since the fundamental tasks were identified. Stott and Davis (1979) identified four basic tasks:

- Identification and management of presenting problems
- Management of continuing problems
- Opportunistic anticipatory care
- Modification of the patient's help-seeking behaviour

If we accept these as the basic tasks, not all of them will be essential in equal measures in all consultations. Further work was rapidly undertaken to establish the core content of these basic task headings (Pendleton et al., 1984) and much of this section is influenced by these authors and also by Neighbour's subsequent book 'The Inner Apprentice' (Neighbour,1999)

Neighbour takes the four basic tasks and not just expands these numerically to six tasks but also adds much more detail to what should be achieved. He lists six tasks that need to be achieved in the consultation:

- Discover why the patient is bringing an issue to your attention
- Define the clinical problem
- Address the patient's problems
- Explain the problem to the patient
- Make effective use of the consultation
- Achieve reasonable outcomes

Taking each of these tasks in turn:

1. Discover why the patient is bringing an issue to your attention

The key critical issue here is to listen to the patient describing the problem. This is not cursory — but requires a process of active listening such that you are concentrating on what is being said and how it is being said. This really is an important issue. It has been shown over and over again (particularly in video analysis of GP consultations) that if the patient is given time to explain their problem, in their own words and without the practitioner pushing them, then the patient will indeed paint a more holistic picture of the problem being presented — both the nature of the problem and the context for it. Thus it is vital to give time for this to occur and concentrate on being 'patient focussed' rather than 'practitioner focussed'

It has been previously mentioned that in the consultation it is important to look for 'cues' both verbal and non-verbal. This means that within the way that a patient explains a problem, there may well be parts of the presentation that are either mentioned repeatedly — or in fact parts of the conversation that are noticeable in their absence. Both can be important. There may be parts to the patient's story that seem irrelevant to the practitioner — but again they can be cues to issues that are of importance to the patient. In addition, there is a need to be sensitive to non-verbal cues. Embarrassment is one of the most obvious. This may be in relation to the patient's own perception of the problem being presented — or may be reflective of their societal or cultural values and beliefs. All these matters are important.

'Hearing' what is said infers a more active listening process. It infers not just that information is being picked up by the practitioner — but that the information is being absorbed, synthesized and sorted in an active way into what is important and what may be of lesser importance in interpreting the presenting problem. Add in the recognition of non-verbal cues and you can start to understand that this part of the consultation is perhaps more complex than at first might be assumed.

If there is an active process of hearing and recognition of visual cues going on, then it is equally important to reflect on these cues. In other words, it may be necessary to verbalise what is happening and gauge the response i.e. "You seem embarrassed when you said ….." or "You have now mentioned …… three times. What does it mean to you?" Visually, it could be along the lines of "When you mentioned …… you seemed to pause a bit and looked down. What were you thinking about?".

Thus this part of the consultation is vitally important and spending a little time here can in fact save much time later if it avoids practitioner-led assumptions and actions. Getting this bit 'right' will dovetail into later elements of the consultation.

Most consultations in General Medical Practice will result at some point within the consultation in formation of a 'hypothesis' about the issue being presented. This will be fully explored in the next section — but mentioning it here is important too. There is evidence over the years that in mainstream General Practice, an experienced GP may well have formed a working hypothesis around the presentation by about 30 seconds into the consultation. From what has been said here, there is clear merit in *delaying* the hypothesis in the interests of possibly gathering more relevant information.

Beyond the presentation of the patient's perception of the initial problem, it is vital to collect contextual information. Whilst this suggests a reversion to practitioner-led enquiry, questioning should be open and again, time and listening techniques should be applied. Contextual information includes:

- Relevant social and occupational information — it is important particularly in remote environments to understand what may be important collective and job pressures on the patient's presentation.
- Home life. Whilst in a remote environment this may not be perceived as important, in fact it is likely to be highly influential on the individual's intention to present and issue — or not. There may have already been family contact influencing illness behaviour — but there may also be significant concerns e.g. loss of income subsequent to any diagnosis or treatment. This information should be used to inform your management plan.
- Health understanding. Whilst the practitioner may have a working hypothesis developing, it is important that the level of understanding of basic health and human body issues is established. There is a great danger otherwise of over anticipating understanding when it comes to explanation. Also, there are significant cultural issues that will inevitably have influence here, with risk that the practitioner applies their own value set without understanding and taking into account the patient's.
- Ideas, fears, concerns and expectations. These are all wider contextual points but nevertheless are important in defining likely success from an intervention or plan. Simply asking the patient what they think may be the main issue will reveal much about their ideas, fears and concerns. Follow this up with some

exploration of what they are expecting from the consultation — it is essential that the patient is agreeable with whatever you might then propose.

- Enquire about other problems. This seems obvious, but it is essential that the main presenting problem is considered in the context of other ongoing health or other problems affecting well being. This may involve taking into account some more significant extant diagnoses (e.g. diabetes, blood pressure problems, etc.) but it may involve something more subtle that would still be influential on your treatment plan. It may also be that it is an opportunity to identify hitherto neglected health issues.
- Chronic issues. Extant medical conditions have been mentioned — but other information is important too e.g. allergies — drug or non-drug, medications already being taken for their risk of interactions or side effects and also the risks of poly-pharmacy interactions if your treatment plan is going to involve prescribing more medication.

2. Define the clinical problem

Having gained all the information you can regarding the patient's presentation, the next challenge is to define the clinical problem. Again, a number of tasks arise.

It is important to obtain any further information that may be necessary about critical symptoms or influential factors within the medical history of the patient. This is where the consultation acquires a more clinical focus where it is relevant to do so. If it has already been established *why* the patient is presenting their clinical problem, then this part of the consultation is more about the 'what'. Hence it may be necessary to be more clinically focussed with more 'closed' questioning (yes or no answers) specifically targeted at symptoms and signs that may be consistent with the working hypothesis.

Gathering this targeted information is essential for 'safety netting'. In other words, it may be that a reasonably accurate hypothesis has emerged, but it is important that in testing against it, other possibilities have been considered and discounted. This is called safety netting. As this focussed clinical questioning progresses, the emergent information should either be consistent with your hypothesis — or may be starting to raise doubt about the hypothesis. Both facets are important and need to be considered. However, if the flow of information is consistent with the emergent hypothesis, it may be that shortcuts can then present. It is not essential to go through the history and physical examination in its entirety if it is patently obvious what the emergent problem is. Also, this clinical enquiry is flexible and modifications can be made to your intended plan as information emerges if it is appropriate to do so.

Clinical examination is relevant at this point — but again this can be different in General Practice compared to more analytical environments e.g. Secondary Care.

In other words, clinical examination can be targeted and carried out in order to provide useful information. Elements of the clinical examination that are not likely to provide useful information can be discarded. But never forget the therapeutic nature of clinical examination. Patients will often have the expectation of examination and may well find this of reassurance even although you may by this stage feel that clinical examination may not reveal any new useful information. The main expectation in examination is that it will contribute towards supporting or refuting your emergent hypothesis and consequent to this, your working diagnosis.

In terms of the working diagnosis, this can either be a specific formulation, likely disease-based — or it may be just as important to maintain it as a more flexible concept. A classical example of this might be the feeling of a need to define a presentation as 'appendicitis' rather than leaving the concept as an acute abdominal presentation. There is a risk that if a closed diagnosis is achieved at too early a stage, then this becomes an over-riding belief among the healthcare practitioners involved rather than them maintaining independent objectivity. This can be a significant problem especially in remote locations — so adopting flexibility with the diagnosis of the patient may in fact be more relevant.

Approaches to defining the clinical problem can in fact be quite variable in their complexity. Examples include

- Hypothesis testing. This is essentially the approach that has been described in this section. It sits well with the psychometric approach to General Practice. Sometimes called 'hypothetic-deductive thinking', it is a highly efficient way of taking unrefined information and converting it into a working hypothesis. As discussed, a hypothesis is formed and then through a process of deduction, that hypothesis is tested until it becomes the most plausible explanation — or that the hypothesis needs changed. This is what GPs do — they take undifferentiated symptoms and signs and turn them into a plausible possibility that they then either seek to resolve or explore in more depth.
- Analytical approach. This is almost the opposite of hypothesis testing. It is often what happens in Secondary Care environments and emergency rooms. This approach requires the application of a rigorous and structured set of questions, a structured clinical examination and the applications of often a broad range of investigations. From this is then analysed any pattern of abnormality and from that a likely (or definite) diagnosis is made. It is time and resource intensive — but in fact likely retains high merit as the preferred approach in secondary or emergency situations. This approach seeks to address questions in full and to leave minimal uncertainty.
- Pattern recognition. This is relevant when applying standard or sometimes routinised care. For instance, in a fracture clinic or wound dressing clinic,

it will be clear what the issue is that needs addressed and departures from a standard pattern can easily be recognised. This will tend to be more reliant on the experience of a practitioner within a narrower field of clinical care and is less likely to be able to assess undifferentiated symptoms.

- Clinical algorithm. These have become more prevalent in recent years. Initially established to help support non-medical practitioners to deal with undifferentiated symptoms, they engaged a flow chart comprising mainly yes or no responses to specific questions. Initially, whilst helping to define clinically important versus less important clinical presentations, they were limited in their effectiveness. Generally, someone would need to go somewhere along the line to re-check or continue management of the patient. Many out-of-hours services in Primary Care around the world have successfully adopted clinical algorithms as a way of streaming patients towards appropriate assessment and management. More recently, with the use of ever more sophisticated IT, Bayesian Probability testing has been incorporated into the use of algorithms. So now, by feeding back outcomes into the clinical algorithm programme, the programme and the algorithm intelligently modify themselves to reflect changes in probability. Thus the algorithms become naturally more complicated, with the ability to absorb more variables and in theory, outcomes are more accurate.

Finally, as mentioned above, there is the need to accept whether it is possible to make a clinical diagnosis or not. It may be that by adopting a more open concept about the patient's status and any dynamic change, a better plan can be constructed than might have occurred with a closed diagnosis. There are merits in all these approaches. Fundamental to General Medical Practice however, is the ability to accept and cope with uncertainty. Not all patients will culminate in having a clear diagnosis and defined course of clinical management. Practitioners that can cope with high levels of uncertainty will tend to do well in General Medical Practice.

3. Address the patient's problems
This is perhaps the more straightforward task in a GP focussed consultation, reverting to clinical management of the hypothesised issue needing to be addressed. It may be that an obvious solution is apparent if there is a clearly defined clinical entity. There will generally be either a clear evidence base for the management of a specific problem that is presented, or if the problem is less well defined, reversion to basic medical principles of management will help guide the practitioner.

However, in order to move on with this stage, it is still essential to assess the severity of the presenting problem. There are two facets to this. Firstly, there is the objective assessment of that problem and its severity relative to the practitioner's knowledge and awareness. Secondly, there is the patient's perception of severity. That perception can be variable — the patient may well seek to minimise the severity of the problem, for various reasons, or may seek to exaggerate the severity of the problem for equally various reasons. It is important that the practitioner can bring some objectivity to this assessment and negotiate that through with the patient. This issue may also transcend the patient's illness behaviour, as has already been discussed.

In addition, the presenting problem may not be the one that is initially presented and considered. Considering the earlier discussion of verbal and non-verbal cues earlier, the true problem may be the issue that the patient raises when they state "While I am here, can I ask you about......". In other words, addressing the patient's problems may well require some sophistication in being able to sort and agree what problems are truly being presented and the order of importance with which they should be dealt with. This all requires a good level of clinical judgement with a flexible approach to synthesis and thinking.

Choosing an appropriate form of management will primarily depend on the practitioner's knowledge and skills, modified by experience. It is into this knowledge and skill base that evidence-based practice needs to be incorporated which is significantly improved now by many online resources. Examples of these resources are widespread (www.patient.info/patientplus) and there are now well researched guidelines for the management of various conditions (www.nice.org.uk). It is well established now that a balance has to be struck between such evidence *dictating* clinical practice or *informing* clinical practice. In many situations, in General Medical Practice, the clinical situation may well be less fully defined than in a Secondary Care situation and so the use of guidelines to inform, rather than dictate practice can be argued as more effective. Internal protocols for management of specific conditions may also exist within a remote healthcare site. Deferring and incorporating established protocols and evidence will always have the benefit of risk mitigation, which again needs to be balanced against an excessively cautious or defensive approach, which may not ultimately be in the patient's best interest.

Finally, it is always essential to engage the patient on the management plan — to an appropriate extent. This will mean openly exploring options and seeking feedback on them. It will mean explaining what is and what isn't feasible within the context of the available medical facility. It will mean ensuring that the patient understands what is being proposed is in their best interests. However, this is all worthwhile because in part, it shifts the balance of control a little and reduces practitioner centred behaviour and focus. It engages the patient in a partnership in seeking a treatment or solution — which will inevitably result in better compliance with the proposed care and hopefully a more successful outcome.

4. Explain the problem to the patient

Explanation of the nature of the defined diagnosis — or working hypothesis — is essential for the patient to then be meaningfully engaged into resolving the issue. This has been touched on before — but is addressed more fully here.

It is important to be able to share your findings meaningfully with the patient, in a way that they understand as much as possible, of the nature of the problem and your negotiated intervention. This will mean a carefully tailored explanation of the working diagnosis. It may be essential to be clear that the diagnosis can change, if it is not clear at this stage that it is definitive. A careful explanation of the management options is essential. The patient may have their own beliefs about what treatment would be better and this needs to be taken into account as well as your own thoughts and ideas. It is essential to explain the possible effects of treatment — beneficial effects and side effects — and the time frame that treatment might need to be effective. In a remote environment, this may well also involve at this stage an explanation of why and how you might seek another opinion on the problem and an explanation of the appropriateness of doing this.

Any explanation or negotiation at this stage must be tailored to the needs of the patient that are relevant at this point. There is a risk of causing alarm if an excess of information is given, as much as there is the fundamental need to ensure that adequate information is given. As ever, it is important to establish a good balance. Whatever information you decide to impart or negotiate, your manner and language should be appropriate. It is important to be professional — but approaching this communication with empathy and in a supportive manner, will go a long way to help reassure someone and give them confidence that they have someone acting in their best interest. Avoid jargon — many practitioners hide behind medical jargon — but this is more likely to convey doubt on your part than to convey reassurance. Use simple explanations where possible and always check with the patient their understanding of what you have said and seek to answer any questions arising. Link the explanation to the patient's beliefs whenever you can. In remote and distant workplaces, there are frequently different nationalities and otherwise diverse communities. The patient's own health beliefs will have been grounded in their own background and experiences (as has already been discussed) and any explanation or information that you are providing must be capable of fulfilling your own knowledge and skill base, modified by what is feasible in the context of the clinical environment in which you are practising, whilst also explaining why something the patient may desire may not be feasible. Thus your manner and language must be appropriate on a number of different levels if you are to ensure good communication.

Finally, it is important to ensure that the explanation provided is understood and accepted. This will mean deliberately taking serial opportunities to check that the patient has understood what you have said and understands what you interpret has been agreed. If not, then it may be necessary to ask again whether the patient has outstanding worries or concerns and seek again to address them. It is also important to keep in mind who the explanation is for. It can often be seen in consultations that the practitioner seeks to give a long and technical explanation more for self reassurance than to address the needs of the patient. It is important not to do this — the explanation is for the patients benefit. Check out serially what has been said, it is after all a two way process and patient compliance with management options will always be improved if the patient has been fully engaged into explaining the problem and agreeing the suggested treatment plan. If there is any residual doubt, or if you feel that the patient would benefit from understanding more regarding a possibly complex diagnosis, consider the use of online resources. The British website patient.info now has a translation tool that allows their many patient information leaflets to be instantly translated to a substantial number of different languages and this has revolutionised the way that information can be imparted and explained to patients virtually anywhere in the world (www.patient.info, accessed 2018).

5. Make effective use of the consultation

There are a number of different tasks to address if any consultation is to be used to its best effect. It goes without saying that the previous sections apply — accurately defining and addressing the perceived problem and explaining and negotiating with the patient. But within the consultation, there a number of 'resources' that can be brought into play that can enhance the effectiveness of what you are trying to achieve.

One of the most useful resources is of course time. It is vital that a balance be struck between efficiency and the proper use of time in any consultation to enhance possible outcomes. In the traditional clinical setting, the use of time is often spent 'doing' things. This can be anything from extensive examination to more active and direct patient intervention. Within general practice, there is a different use of time — more of it is spent on diagnosing and planning (including engaging with the patient) than mainly on direct patient interventions. It is from this proper use of time that a functional hypothesis will emerge around which a plan for intervention can be generated.

There is then the matter of utilising investigations in General Practice. These can be near patient tests — anything from urine screening through to D-Dimer, Troponin and other such analyses. Ultrasound is now commonly available — as will be x-ray and other facilities. But a fundamental rule applies in that all investigations should be done to help confirm or refute a working hypothesis. Investigations should not be done just for the sake of doing them. It is an emergent belief in General Practice that the person instructing an investigation is the person that then takes ownership of the result. Thus it would be wise to be certain that you would know how to interpret a result, or a set of results, in the context of the patient's presentation, before instructing investigations. Additionally, many investigations have cost implications and many can be uncomfortable for the patient. Whilst these matters should not prevent investigations being requested — they are another element that should be taken into account.

There is then the question of prescribing. Much will depend on what medication is available and what can be prescribed within the licensing restrictions that may apply in any particular environment. The decision to prescribe may well be necessary and protocol driven (e.g. management of acute coronary syndrome) but if it is a possibility that emerges from the consultation, then careful thought should be given to all aspects — potential benefit vs potential side effects, safety, efficacy, cost, etc. No prescribing decision should be made lightly. Once again, it is the prescriber that will have to take ownership of the decision to use a medication and should that subsequently cause any problems, then the individual needs to accept their fair liability for the decision in the first place. Practitioners should not prescribe or use medication outside of their knowledge and skill areas, although may have to accept a necessity to do so if advised in consultation with someone providing higher level advice or cover. The basic expectations of prescribing safely are well covered elsewhere and the British National Formulary remains a prime resource in this regard (www.bnf.org).

Making effective use of a consultation also requires consideration of what other health professionals can bring to agreed patient management. This is commonplace in mainstream general practice as it is often the case now that paramedical staff can take forward a number of interventions. Thus in establishing a hypothesis and agreed management plan, it may be that parts or all of this can be delegated to others to complete. This makes sense and represents best use of available resources. Even in a remote situation, there may well be other team members that can carry out agreed interventions or investigations.

But utilising other medical expertise will also apply to situations where interventions that are of a more expert nature are needed. This is obvious and can vary from engagement of a Physiotherapist where more expert assessment and physical therapy is needed, through requesting further advice from a peer (either directly or utilising media), through to requesting advice and guidance from someone who may be more senior or experienced but may well be more remote from the patient, to request an agreement for patient stabilisation and transfer urgently to a more specialised facility. A whole host of opportunities now exist to engage both direct advice and advice input in formulating and carrying through an agreed intervention. This is increasingly the norm, where advice need not necessarily be physically immediately at hand and providing good media links exist, then advice can be effectively sought from nearly anywhere in the world.

There are increasing examples of where traditional approaches to patient assessment are being 'turned on their heads'. By that, it might have been suggested that the traditional model of care — especially in remote areas would have been front end patient assessment and then hierarchical pursuit of further advice. Now, many models exist using media, where there is higher level initial assessment of the patient then supplemented by more targeted para-medical interventions. One such emergent system in the UK is the 'Telephone First' approach with GP-led triage which claims great success with access and workload (https://gpaccess.uk/) but at the time of writing, there is still debate as to the actual gains that can be achieved from using this system in mainstream populations (BMJ London, 2017). It remains in this author's opinion that there is as yet unexplored use of the approach in providing triage to remote communities — be they work site or otherwise — with ever improving media capability.

Finally, in making effective use of any consultation, the extended scope of the consultation should be explored. Always, where possible, utilise the opportunity to promote good health. Lifestyle challenges are rapidly threatening to overwhelm healthcare systems — mainstream or remote. Hence all opportunities must be taken to address weight, fitness, dietary, alcohol and smoking issues. This always needs to incorporate a realistic and balanced approach with realistic advice and objectives and always with positive reinforcement of even small efforts at improving personal health. Particularly in remote situations, the practitioner should recognise their inherent role in promoting good health and there may well be opportunities to engage patients in such efforts directly.

6. Achieve reasonable outcomes
In successfully achieving a consultation and subsequent intervention, the outcome should always be reasonable. It is not a matter of always achieving excellence — good or reasonable is all that anyone would normally expect.

It should be about achieving what is best for the patient — and this may mean standing up for this outcome in the face of commercial or other social pressures. Your responsibility is to the patient. You are the patient's advocate — particularly if they are unwell such that they require advocacy.

Your assessment and actions should be informed by safety matters and risk awareness. This particularly applies to any interventions or prescribing that you intend or authorise. You must avoid doing harm by your decisions.

As ever, a considered approach that engages with the patient as a partner in the management plan will avoid complaint and possibly worse.

Conclusion

The approach to General Medical Practice — or Primary Care Medicine has not changed significantly in terms of its focus on the consultation as being at the core of the clinical approach — but that consultation may now be delivered not just by a doctor but a diverse range of practitioners on a Primary Care platform. When taking into account remoteness, the use of novel online and communication technologies allows for far greater input into the consultation — so there is a necessity to continue to reflect on how all this fits together to maximise the outcome for the patient. It is obligatory that systems and technologies should progress and maximise what becomes available — whilst always questioning and ideally researching the gain from novel approaches.

Section 2 — A Clinical Approach

The Extended Scope of Primary Care

In terms of delivering a coherent Primary Care focussed medical service, how does this translate into service delivery to a remote community or workforce? For a remote workforce, the argument may be that the remote worker is in fact no different to anyone else in terms of their entitlement and expectation regarding their health needs and the necessity that this expectation is fulfilled by the companies responsible for the care of their employees when they cannot access what would be their normal Primary Care provision.

Whilst certain standards for fitness of remote workers currently exist (and the OGUK Medical Guidelines are as good an example as any), the fact is that they are designed for the assessment of workers to work mainly on installations on the UK continental shelf and its environs. However, this UK environment, especially for chronic condition management, is less 'remote' than many places in the world where workers may undertake much longer tours of duty and thus have less access to mainstream Primary Care.

The OGUK medical guidelines (OGUK London, 2009) have also become more 'enabling' i.e. less exclusive and more inclusive of workers with chronic medical conditions — potentially increasing the need for chronic disease management at the work site. This is not an unreasonable change. Why would you wish to exclude highly experienced, mature workers from complex workplace challenges when it should be possible to provide for their chronic health management? The result however, is that this fitness to work screening is revealing more chronic medical conditions that have to be considered in context and decisions made. This is also occurring in the context of more general health screening in the population anyway which is undoubtedly yielding increased prevalence of chronic health conditions — type 2 diabetes is a good case in point. There is also a maturing workforce. Life expectancy is increasing and whereas in the past, there may have been an expectation of tail off in the numbers of workers still active in remote work sites by their mid 50s, increasingly many workers are keen to continue to carry on their occupations well into their 60s. This increases the need for objective fitness assessment — but undoubtedly increases the need for a more Primary Care-led approach to the health management of these older cohorts.

Most of what has been written up until now regarding healthcare of remote work communities focuses on 'reactive' care. However, as mentioned above, more scope now exists for preventive activities. There is undoubtedly scope for a Primary Care philosophy at the remote work site to establish its own emphasis on the early identification of individuals at risk of future health problems (think obesity, exercise, diet, family history etc.) and then to actively develop good quality health screening. Consequently, there is scope also for active intervention on lifestyle issues, medication compliance, self-monitoring compliance, etc — and this is surely better use of the remote healthcare practitioner's capability than time-filling clerking duties etc.

How can this be delivered? Even now, the answer is probably still elusive. There have been many good examples of companies and their initiatives to promote monitoring and management of known chronic conditions (Mika *et al.*, 2014).

These initiatives are commendable and show just what can be done if there is a will to solve such challenges. The limitations of these interventions however are that they are very focussed on single entity monitoring and for a whole number of different reasons, are also unique to the employees of the company involved. Extension to a more 'blended' worker cohort with different nationalities, value sets and different employers would be a challenge.

It may be that there is yet much work to be done within the specialty of Remote Healthcare to define what is required in terms of Primary Care delivery. Only by agreeing what might constitute the core elements, would it then be possible to start building training around this. Numerous texts exist that define the core of Primary Care and indeed, in most General Practices in the UK it would be the norm to find a copy of the Oxford Textbook which defines this — at least in the context of UK General Practice (Simon *et al.*, 2014). This author would argue that whilst the Primary Care platform is a broader entity, the major part of the clinical delivery and indeed that which the RHCP would need also to deliver is defined within the recognised core content of General Practice.

Predictably, the core clinical elements might include appropriate levels of knowledge and skill within:

- Consulting
- Prescribing and poly-pharmacology
- Healthy living
- Chronic disease management

- Emergencies in general practice
- Dermatology
- Ear, nose, and throat
- Medical, including:
  - Cardiology and vascular disease
  - Respiratory medicine
  - Endocrinology including diabetes
  - Gastrointestinal medicine
  - Basic neurology
  - Infectious diseases
- Obstetrics and gynaecology, including:
  - Sexual health and contraception
- Ophthalmology
- Paediatrics and child health
- Mental health
- Musculoskeletal problems
- Urology

And as a skill set:
- Minor surgery

The depth to which knowledge and skill would need to be developed would also have to be defined. There are some clinical entities that would require more learning than others. But the point is to have a RHCP capable of providing safe clinical practice within the domain of General Medical Practice/Primary Care and especially to be able to provide this reasonably competently when required to very isolated work communities where tele-medical back up may be less consistently available.

There will still be many technical challenges to the incorporation of a greater Primary Care effort in remote work areas. For instance, there is a need to be able to record data achieved and then to be able to integrate that with other medical advisers — either those to whom the RHCP is responsible, or to the patient's own mainstream medical adviser. This is more problematical than it may at first seem. As soon as you get into personal data management, you have to then address the challenge of software and recording platforms, data transmission, data security, confidentiality etc.

Data also needs to be structured, searchable and retrievable. There are many existing tools — e.g. UK GP computing platforms — but unlikely to be much use internationally as they would not easily integrate — nor might the issue of different units of measure and different drug names be easily recordable. Thus there is another challenge for the international community — how do you select a clinical and recording standard from those that seem to apply in different countries?

There are further international inconsistencies in medication use e.g. from heavily evidence-based/heavily price conscious approaches to random choice (possibly still drug company influenced) with little or no attention to cost control. There are even basic challenges with consistency of lifestyle interventions — e.g. what dietary advice, what exercise advice and considerations of ethnicity-led influences on the advice that should be given.

Clinical Attributes Guide

Looking at the bulleted list in the first part of this section, the first four items have been referred to and explored in section 1 of this chapter. These can be referred to as 'Generic Attributes':

- Consulting
- Prescribing and poly-pharmacology
- Healthy living
- Chronic disease management

This then leaves the more focussed clinical attributes that would be needed to ensure competent delivery of a Primary Care-led remote healthcare service (Page and Valentine, 2008)

It was never the intention that this textbook, never mind this chapter, would provide an in-depth text on the entirety of the clinical approach to general practice — many textbooks of significant size and complexity have been written on this before. However, it is appropriate to consider the major knowledge and skill domains that would be essential to provide a reasonable clinical understanding at Primary Care level and if considered and targeted for learning and skill development, would ensure competency within the remote healthcare practitioner. These can be called 'Clinical Attributes':

- Emergencies in general medical practice
- Dermatology
- Ear, nose, and throat
- Medical, including:
  o Cardiology and vascular disease
  o Respiratory medicine

- o Endocrinology including diabetes
- o Gastrointestinal medicine
- o Basic neurology
- o Infectious diseases
- Obstetrics and gynaecology, including:
  - o Sexual health and contraception
- Ophthalmology
- Paediatrics and child health
- Mental health
- Musculoskeletal problems
- Urology

And as a skill set:
- Minor surgery

The following sections therefore comprise the recognised attribute guide that would be anticipated for someone practising in a remote environment. These attributes are not an exhaustive list. They will not be relevant to every situation. The level of knowledge and skill within each attribute will vary according to location and the complexion of the clinical care that is expected or feasible in that context.

Please note that the sections on Urology and Minor Surgical Skills have been absorbed into other knowledge and skill areas.

1. Generic attributes

History & examination

- Takes a proper clinical history
- Carries out a proper clinical examination incl. neurological, examination of the systems, rectal examination, vaginal examination, etc.
- Is proficient in the use of basic diagnostic tools, for example: stethoscopic examination of the heart, chest and abdomen, use of the sphygmomanometer, otoscope, ophthalmoscope, peak flow meter, pulse oximeter, etc.
- Proficient in the use of communication and tele-medicine utilities available
- Understands basic communication theory and consultation models
- Understands body language and cues
- Understands physical, social and psychological influences on illness behaviour
- Can assess accurately what the patient does and doesn't know
- Can communicate bad news sensitively and effectively
- Can communicate effectively with patients and relatives and work colleagues

Investigations

- Can initiate and arrange appropriate investigations
- Has a thorough understanding of the appropriate use of investigative techniques e.g.:
  — Indications for, carrying out and interpretation of ECGs
  — The use of chest and abdominal X-rays
  — The range and scope of laboratory investigations
  — The scope and use of ultrasound and various imaging techniques
  — The use of near patient testing facilities

Problem solving/making a diagnosis/management plan

- Has good problem-solving skills
- Has an understanding of how GPs think and work
- Can cope with uncertainty
- Reflects formatively on accuracy and inaccuracy in diagnosis
- Can assess the implications of the patient's ethnicity and social context

Prescribing

- Has a good understanding of the principles of prescribing and therapeutics including drug side effects, interactions and contra-indications
- Is aware of prescribing costs
- Understands the purpose and use of drug formularies

Record keeping

- Understands the structure of the clinical record
- Keeps regular, appropriately detailed, accurate records
- Understands medico-legal and risk management aspects of record keeping

Emergency care

- Understands how emergency medical care is organised
- Understands how unplanned care is organised and integrated including the role of the Remote Healthcare Practitioner, Clinical Cover, Evacuation and Support
- Can understand the presentation of, accurately assess and initiate a management plan for medical emergencies
- Can fully assess a patient in collapse/arrest, initiate and manage basic CPR, life support and use of the defibrillator

- Proficient in the assessment of the unconscious and/or very ill patient, stabilising them and initiating an action plan
- Proficient in establishing venous access and venous blood sampling

Works within limits of confidence

- Is aware of available and relevant guidelines, evidence and protocols
- Engages appropriately in critical self-appraisal
- Can engage team support appropriately
- Understands the nature of support staff and engages this appropriately

Maintains good medical practice

- Enthusiastically participates in and effectively contributes to learning opportunities
- Has a good ability to access and appraise medical literature
- Accepts and values constructive criticism
- Commits whenever possible to parallel training programmes
- Understands audit opportunities in remote healthcare
- Understands and is able to set quality standards
- Understands how audit feeds into quality assurance

Working relationship with colleagues

- Understands the roles of the wider healthcare team both locally and distant
- Respects and engages **all** team members' knowledge and skills
- Communicates accurately and effectively with team members
- Effectively engages with the whole medical team to ensure best outcomes for patient care
- Appropriately delegates and participates in care management
- Has competent telephone and tele-health capabilities
- Constructs good quality written communication
- Communicates accurately and effectively with wider healthcare involved individuals keeping them informed about their patients

Relationship with patients

- Has a good basic understanding of human rights
- Understands basic personal needs of patients, respects their dignity and minimises discomfort
- Can illustrate patience and tolerance

- Copes with and defuses confrontation
- Uses language appropriate to patient, relatives and work colleagues understanding
- Takes appropriate responsibility for initiating communication with patients and others involved
- Has an understanding of ethnic influences on patient care

Teaching and training

- Willing to participate in teaching and training responsibilities
- Willing to develop basic training skills and attributes
- Appropriately supervises/mentors more junior colleagues and can motivate others
- Provides honest feedback on colleagues when requested

Probity

- Understands what constitutes acceptable and unacceptable ethical practice
- Understands and maintains professionalism at all times
- Seeks help early if concerned about their own performance or that of others
- Understands how to handle complaints
- Understands the legal requirements and how to handle e.g. death certification, mental health certification, fitness to drive, notifiable conditions and other statutory requirements
- Understands and is committed to medical confidence
- Understands rights regarding access to information
- Ensures punctuality and availability when on duty
- Understands principles of time management
- Understands the need for high levels of honesty and trustworthiness in medicine including when financial transactions are involved
- Ensures that information relating to medical services is given clearly and objectively
- Never exploits patient vulnerability especially in terms of financial issues
- Always declares and withdraws from issues with conflict of interest

Health

- Is aware of health issues that may affect personal ability to work safely
- Is aware of work issues that might affect personal health
- Understands stress effects on doctors, patients and colleagues
- Manages personal causes and effects of stress

- Has an awareness of strategies for coping with stress
- Understands and tolerates other personality types
- Maintains as high a level of personal health and fitness as possible
- Has an awareness of the scope of Occupational Health services

2. Emergencies

Clinical acute presentation & management

Cardiac resuscitation	Adult major trauma	Acute general surgery
Acute medicine	Orthopaedic trauma	Gynaecology
Problems in the elderly	Soft tissue injury	ENT conditions
Paediatric medicine & surgery	Wound management	Eye conditions
Paediatric trauma	Maxillo-facial trauma	Psychiatry
Pain control	X-ray interpretation	Dealing with difficult patients
Legal/ethical issues	Dealing with distresses/bereaved relatives & colleagues	

Clinical skills — resuscitation

Basic life support	Needle cricothyroidotomy	Intraosseous access*
Oral airway	Heimlich manoeuvre	
Nasopharyngeal airway	Defibrillation	Chest drain*
Bag & mask ventilation	IV access in adults	Central venous line*
Intubation	IV access in children*	

Clinical skills — trauma

Fracture reduction	Spinal immobilisation	Log-rolling
Dislocated shoulder reduction	Limb splinting	Plaster backslab
Wound assessment, cleaning & debridement		Steristrips
Suturing	Wound glue	Dressings

Clinical skills — other skills

Digital nerve block*	Femoral nerve block*	Abscess I & D
Joint aspiration	Bladder catheterisation	Nasal packing

*These criteria are more specialised and may only be needed in more specific remote situations

3. Dermatology

Dermatological conditions

Eczema	Seborrhoeic dermatitis	Scabies and lice
Psoriasis	Hyperkeratosis & ichthyoses	Fungal infections
Acne vulgaris	Rosacea	Herpes simplex & zoster
Pigmented lesions &		Warts & molluscum contagiosum
malignant melanoma	Bullous conditions*	
Basal cell carcinoma	Alopecia*	Pityriasis versicolor*
Squamous cell carcinoma	Urticarias	Pityriasis rosea*
Solar keratosis	Pruritis	Lichen planus*

Dermatological skills

Dermatological examination	Skin scrapings etc	Use of topical preparations
Examination with UV light	Crytocautery	
Curettage and cautery*		

---

* These criteria are more specialised and may only be needed in more specific remote situations

4. Ear, nose, and throat

- Be able to use a light source, nasal and aural speculae, examination of the larynx and postnasal space, audiometer (if needed).
- Be competent to examine and recognise normal and abnormal ears, noses, throats and necks.

Be able to recognise and manage the following common conditions:

Otitis media	Vertigo	Tonsillitis
Otitis externa	Nasal polyposis	Epiglotitis & croup*
Discharging ears	Epitaxis	Hoarseness
Ear wax	Allergies of the nose & throat	Neck lumps
Glue ear	Sinusitis	
Deafness	Foreign bodies in noses & ears	

Be able to perform:

Nasal packing, anterior and posterior (including nasal tampons)

Nasal cautery
Ear toilet and dressing

---

*These criteria are more specialised and may only be needed in more specific remote situations

5. Medical issues

Be able to recognise and manage the following common conditions:

Acute Coronary Syndromes	Insulin & Non-Insulin Dependant Diabetes	Uncontrolled Diabetes & Ketoacidosis
Cardiac Arrest (CPR)	Asthma	COPD
Angina	Pneumonia	TB*
Heart Failure	Hypoglycaemia	Pneumothorax
Common Arrhythmias	Hypo/Hyperthyroidism*	
Hypertension	DVT & Pulmonary Embolism	
Dyspepsia	Headaches/Migraine	Osteoarthritis
Peptic Ulceration	CVA & TIA	Acutely Inflamed Joint
Acute GI bleeding	Meningitis & septicaemia	Gout
Diarrhoea	Epilepsy & Status Epilepticus	Jaundice
Inflammatory Bowel Diseases*	Acute Confusion	Coma
		Pain control
Renal Failure*	Overdoses	Parkinson's Disease*
Urinary obstruction	Anaphylaxis	Anaemia
Urinary Tract Infections	Alcohol & substance misuse	Multiple Sclerosis*
Urinary Incontinence*	Faecal Incontinence*	
Haematuria		
Testicular and scrotal abnormalities		
Bladder catheterisation		
Anticoagulation	Infectious diseases	Malaria
Hypothermia		

---

*These criteria are more specialised and may only be needed in more specific remote situations

6. Obstetrics and Gynaecology

Obstetrics

It would be rare for the Remote Healthcare Practitioner to have to deal with Obstetric problems — unless working in a planned and stable community. In which case, a much more substantive set of knowledge and skill attributes would apply, all RHCPs however should have basic, sound knowledge of:

- The routine procedures and screening used in modern antenatal care.
- The initial management of common obstetric conditions and emergencies.

Gynaecology

Gynaecological history, examination & investigations   Infections of the genital tract

External genital abnormality & infection   Female catheterisation

Issues relating to the menopause and HRT*

Contraception issues including complications (a working knowledge)

— Combined hormonal preparations	— Progesterone only	— Progesterone implants
— Intra uterine device/system	— Novel developments	— Injectables
— Barrier methods		

Miscarriage   Problems with menstruation*

Ethical & legal implications   Chaperoning   Age of consent

Sexual assault   Genital mutilation

Sexual health (including males)

— Chlamydia	— Gonorrhoea	— Syphilis
— HIV	— Hepatitis B and C	— Pubic lice
— Investigation of discharge or symptoms	— Urine sampling	— Swab sampling
	— Contact tracing	

---

*These criteria are more specialised and may only be needed in more specific remote situations

7. Ophthalmology

Be able to perform:

External examination of eye	Ophthalmoscopy	Visual field testing
Slit lamp examination (if available)	Visual acuity testing	Colour vision testing
Use of eye loupe	Fluorescein stain	Bengal red stain
Eye anaesthesia	Tonometry*	

Be able to recognise and manage the following common conditions:

Eye Injuries and Foreign Body	Vascular Haemorrhages and Occlusions	Chalazion incision and curettage*
Conjunctivitis	Amaurosis Fugax	Papilloedema and Optic Neuritis*
Blepharitis	Episceritis and Scleritis	
Styes and Meibomian Cysts	Iritis and Uveitis	Vitreous and Retinal
Corneal Ulcers and Keratitis	Hypertensive Retinopathy*	Detachment*
Glaucoma	Cataract*	Diabetic Retinopathies*

*These criteria are more specialised and may only be needed in more specific remote situations

8. Paediatrics and child health

This section is included as it will depend on whether a RHCP has direct responsibility for children — or as discussed earlier in the chapter, may find themselves having to manage children in the context of a local population seeking treatment.

- Ability to relate to children in illness and health, and to their parents, including parental anxiety and stress
- Prescribes safely and appropriately for children
- Basic awareness of developmental milestones, knowledge of normal growth and physical development and deviation from this. Awareness of the principals of nutrition and infant feeding*
- Recognise limitations of parents' ability to cope with illness and recognise deterioration
- Differentiate a well child, a well-ill child and an ill child and take appropriate action
- Knowledge of child vaccination schedules and ability to advise appropriately*
- Awareness of family interaction and dynamics*

- Ability to communicate with other doctors and other health professionals regarding the care of children
- These criteria are more specialised and may only be needed in more specific remote situations

Be able to recognise and manage the following common conditions:

Asthma	Recurrent abdominal pain	Possible child abuse
Eczema	Allergy	Diarrhoea & vomiting
Infections	Failure to thrive	
URTI (Croup, otitis media, tonsillitis)		Diabetes
Convulsions	Heart murmur	

Awareness of and ability to treat paediatric emergencies

Asthma	Removal of foreign bodies	Convulsion
Injuries & poisoning	Unconscious child	Epiglottitis/stridor
Meningitis	Dehydrated child	Acute abdomen
Diabetic coma & hypoglycaemia		Torsion of testis
Able to resuscitate children and neonates		

9. Mental health

- Understand the doctor-patient relationship & its therapeutic value
- Consultation skills — listening, recognising clues & providing explanation
- Factors leading to mental illness
- Recognise deviations from the expected norms of development — mental handicap, dyslexia, behavioural and personality disorders*
- Liaison with social services*
- Impact on family of mental illness*
- Formal procedures e.g. Mental Health Act*

---

*These criteria are more specialised and may only be needed in more specific remote situations

Clinical skills:

Taking a psychiatric history	Mental state examination	Safe stabilisation &
Prescribing drug treatment		transfer
Referral for specialist advice	Advising relatives	

Knowledge and understanding of mental and emotional disorders:

Acute life-threatening disorders & appropriate management

Schizophrenia*	Substance misuse	Bereavement/grief reactions
Early depression	Postnatal depression	Dementia*
Manic-depression illness	Phobias	

Treatment:

Basic pharmacology of drugs used in psychiatry

Non-pharmacological treatments available for psychiatric disorders

Sedation prior to transfer

Acute drug management

10. Musculoskeletal problems

Good working knowledge of the common and/or important complaints:

Osteoarthritis	Acute neck pain	Fibromyalgia*
Rheumatoid arthritis*	Chronic neck pain	Chronic fatigue syndrome*
Ankylosing spondylitis*	Acute low back pain	
Reactive arthritis	Chronic low back pain	Acute shoulder pain
Psoriatic arthritis*		Rotator cuff syndrome
Infectious arthritis	Gout	Adhesive capsulitis
Epicondylitis	Plantar fasciitis	Bursitis
Tendonitis	Vasculitis*	Carpal tunnel syndrome
Polymyalgia Rheumatica	Temporal (Giant Cell) Arteritis	

Awareness of less common conditions*

SLE*	Sjogrens syndrome*	Ankylosing spondylitis*
Poly- and dermato-myositis*	Scleroderma*	Systemic sclerosis*

Practical skills: Joint injections

1st CMC (base of thumb)	Shoulder	Medial epicondylitis
Knee (including joint aspiration)	Acromio-clavicular	Lateral epicondylitis
Plantar fasciitis*		

---

*These criteria are more specialised and may only be needed in more specific remote situations

Conclusion

It would be impossible within the scope of this book to provide a detailed textbook of all aspects of the attributes listed above. However, the attribute guide should act as a prompt for reflection on knowledge and skills already gained and a means of identifying those that may need further study. The continuing professional development of the Remote Healthcare Practitioner (RHCP) is an ongoing obligation and it is up to each individual to ensure that they have an adequate knowledge and skillset to address likely scenarios that they will be confronted with. The above Attribute Guide is very generic in its nature. It does not incorporate e.g. location-specific knowledge or skill areas that may be essential for the RHCP e.g. providing healthcare in either a very cold or very hot environment or providing healthcare in an area of tropical disease prevalence etc.

Fortunately, now, there are numerous online resources that can provide both diagnostic aid and management aid and the best of these sites are both evidence-based and regularly updated. Whilst this pre-supposes good online access, it is increasingly normal to expect this. Additionally, many resources can now be retained electronically if online access in any area may be known to be limited. The RHCP should ensure that they are properly equipped and supported for the tasks that they are likely to face.

References

Ask My GP. Available at https://gpaccess.uk/. Accessed March 2018.

Atun R. 2004. What are the advantages and disadvantages of restructuring a health care system to be more focussed on primary care services? Copenhagen: WHO.

BNF Publications. Available at https://www.bnf.org/. Accessed March 2018.

Fraser RC. 1992. *Clinical Method: A General Practice Approach.* Oxford: Butterworth Heinemann.

Gochman DS. 1988. *Health Behaviour.* New York: Springer Science & Business Media.

Information for medical professionals. Available at https://patient.info/patientplus. Accessed March 2018.

Mika F *et al.* 2014. Integration of tele-cardiology in Saipem's health management system. *J Inst Remote Health Care* 5: 11–17.

National Institute for Health and Care Excellence (NICE). Available at https://www.nice.org.uk. Accessed March 2018.

Neighbour R. 1999. *The Inner Apprentice: An Awareness-Centred Approach to Vocational Training for General Practice.* London: Routledge.

Oil and Gas UK (OGUK). 2009. Medical aspects of fitness for offshore work: Guidance for examining physicians — Issue 6.

Page J and Valentine M. 2008. *Attribute Guide for General Practice*. London: JCPTGP.

Patient. Available at http://patient.info. Accessed March 2018.

Pendleton D *et al*. 1984. *The Consultation: An Approach to Learning and Teaching*. Oxford: Oxford University Press.

Quinn J and Jablonski M. 2013. Duty of care in remote medicine: burden of care or opportunity for best practice. *J IRHC* **4**: 17–23.

Telephone first consultations in primary care (editorial) (2017). *BMJ* (*BMA London*) **358**: 4345.

Simon C *et al*. 2014. *Oxford Handbook of General Practice*, 4th Edn. Oxford: Oxford University Press.

Stott NCH and Davis RH. 1979. The exceptional potential in each primary care consultation. *J RCGP* **29**: 201.

World Health Organization (WHO). 2018. Main terminology. Available at http://www.euro.who.int/en/health-topics/Health-systems/primary-health-care/main-terminology.

10

Delivering Pharmaceutical Services in Remote Locations

Brian Wells

Introduction

The purpose of this chapter is to provide an insight into how to establish an efficient and defensible pharmaceutical service provided by healthcare professionals (HCPs) working in remote locations. These could include offshore installations, onshore oil sites, ships, or scientific expedition sites in remote areas. This is of importance as dealing with administration and supply of medicines is an integral part of daily duties of the remote HCP. The chapter examines the benefits of the traditional pharmaceutical service in developed countries, the legal framework for the provision and use of medications, management of medicines at remote locations, supplier selection, shipment issues, medical room facilities for storage of pharmaceuticals, the administration and supply of medicines to patients, how to deal with personnel who bring their own medicines on site, useful pharmaceutical information sources, as well as references to pharmaceutical records and training.

In summary how to transfer the benefits of the traditional pharmaceutical service to the remote environment in a legal and safe manner.

Traditional Pharmaceutical Service

In developed countries the normal model is that prescribers (usually physicians) diagnose and prescribe and pharmacists dispense to patients. The pharmaceutical service provides:

- A suitable range of licensed medicines
- Correct storage conditions
- Timely provision of medicines to patients
- Patient safety

- Efficiency
  - — Detailed assessment of the prescription regarding:
  - — Dosage
  - — Contra-indications
  - — Compatibility with existing medication
  - — Interactions
- Suitable counselling of patients relating to the medication

Legal Aspects

Introduction

Medicines are subject to strict regulation in most jurisdictions and it is important to be aware of this when planning a remote medical service. Rules vary from country to country, but basic principles exist. Put simply, some medicines are normally only available on prescription, whilst others are allowed to be purchased by the public.

For the purpose of illustration, the following sections provide a brief overview of the UK system, which is in compliance with EU legislation.

UK medicines regulatory system

In the UK, medicine production and distribution is controlled by the Medicines and Healthcare Products Regulatory Agency (MHRA).

Its objectives are:

- To safeguard public health by ensuring that all medicines on the UK market meet appropriate standards of safety, quality and efficacy.
- Safety aspects cover potential or actual harmful effects; quality relates to development and manufacture; and efficacy is a measure of the beneficial effect of the medicine on patients.

In the US these functions are undertaken by the Federal Drugs Administration (FDA).

UK medicines legislation

The main laws relevant to medicines in the UK are:

The Medicines Act 1968 and associated Human Medicines Regulations 2012 which are policed by MHRA and;

The Misuse of Drugs Act 1971 and associated Misuse of Drugs Regulations 2001, which are policed by the UK Home Office.

Medicines Act licensing system

The Licensing System protects the public by requiring that the manufacturing and distributive chain conform to defined standards and operating procedures.

Licences issued:

- Marketing Authorisation for individual medicinal products
- Manufacturer's Licence (required by all companies that produce medicines)
- Manufacturer's Assembly Only Licence (required by companies which package and label medicines)
- Wholesale Distribution Authorisation [WDA(H)].

Marketing authorisation (previously known as product licence)

In most jurisdictions, before a medicine can be placed on the market, it must be given a marketing authorisation by a medicine regulator (in the UK this is the MHRA). Before granting a licence, the regulator must be satisfied that the medicinal product works well and is acceptably safe.

Only when the regulator is satisfied that a medicine meets high standards of safety and quality, and that it works for the purpose intended, will the licence, a marketing authorisation (formerly known as a product licence), be granted. This is denoted by a marketing authorisation number shown on the label of the product prefixed with the letters "PL".

The marketing authorisation is specific to each individual product. Where a product is made by several different manufacturers (e.g. paracetamol tablets), each will have its own unique marketing authorisation. The marketing authorisation defines the product in its entirety including amongst other details:

- Composition (i.e. active and inactive ingredients)
- Method of manufacture
- Presentation (e.g. tablets, capsules, injection suppositories etc.)
- Licensed uses
- Licensed dosage
- Contra-indications, warnings, special precautions, interactions.
- Pharmaceutical precautions
- Legal category

- Packaging
- Storage conditions

UK licence holders are required to produce a "Summary of Product Characteristics" (SmPC) for each of their licensed medicines, which details important information about the licensed use of product.

In the UK most of these can be found in the Electronic Medicines Compendium [eMC] (Medicines.org.uk, 2019), others can be accessed via the MHRA "Medicines Information: SPC & PILs" search facility (MHRA, 2019). This topic is expanded on later in this chapter when the eMC is discussed as a reference source.

It is important to note that any use of a medicine outside the parameters stated in the marketing authorisation, as shown in the SmPC, is classified as being used "off-licence". This would be the case where a medicine was used for a medical condition, not included in the list of indications in the licence (and SmPC). Similarly, use at dosages differing from those defined by the manufacturer, diluting IV injections with diluents not approved by the manufacturer, storage outside the defined temperatures, use for those for whom it is contraindicated or, who are taking medicines with which it adversely interacts would also be classified as "off-licence". In such cases, and in the event of a problem occurring, the manufacturer is entitled to state that it is being used outside their recommendations. In the event of a predictable adverse event occurring following use outside the conditions defined in the licence, a failure to take due account of the licensed information included in the SmPC, could be used as evidence in a negligence case.

It is worth noting that in certain (exceptional) circumstances, medicines may be used "off-licence". However, such use is subject to strict conditions and includes a need for patient consent and would normally only be undertaken by specialised personnel when there is no licensed alternative. In the remote healthcare situation, the general rule should be that "off-licence" use of medicines should be avoided.

Wholesale Distribution Authorisation [WDA(H)]

Sale by wholesale, as far as a medicine is concerned, means supply to a person or company, who purchases it for use in his trade business or profession. This includes oil companies and others who provide remote medical facilities. Those who supply medicines to such customers, must hold WDA(H) and are subject to inspection by the MHRA for compliance with Good Distribution Practice (GDP).

Wholesalers may only source medicines from licensed sources (e.g. other licensed wholesalers or licensed manufacturers) and they may only supply persons who may legally purchase the medicines in question. Similar rules apply in other jurisdictions (e.g. USA).

Competence is required in the following areas:

- Validation of sources
- Validation of customers
- Procurement
- Storage and temperature control
- Stock rotation
- Dispatch and shipment
- Dealing with customers' returns
- Procedures to avoid falsified medicines (i.e. counterfeit and diverted medicines)
- Emergency product recall procedure

If falsified medicines — that is counterfeit or diverted (e.g. stolen or those from unlicensed sources) are stocked on any site, then patients are put at risk. New systems to prevent this are being introduced in many developed countries in 2019. Remote sites should always check that their supplier has measures in place to prevent this problem.

It is worth mentioning that with respect to product recall, WDA(H) holders are required to have a system of notifying their customers of the recall. Products are recalled when there is a safety concern caused by either a manufacturing problem or a pharmacological safety issue. A good remote pharmaceutical supplier, should target product recalls to those establishments, which have been supplied with the products in question. If a remote site receives such a recall notification, the supplier should advise the action to be taken.

It is important to note that in the UK and European Economic Area (EEA), businesses operating solely as retail pharmacies are not permitted to sell by wholesale.

Legal classification of medicines in UK

General sales list (GSL)

These are medicines which are considered safe for the public to purchase from a variety of retail outlets (e.g. antiseptic creams, simple antacids, small packs of analgesics, common cold remedies). GSL medicines are labelled with very specific instructions.

Paracetamol Tablets 500mg Pack of 16 — General Sales List Medicine

day lewis

500 mg

Paracetamol

500mg Tablets

Caplet-shaped tablet

16 tablets

Effective pain relief

Uses
For the relief of headache, migraine, neuralgia and rheumatic aches and pains. Also for the relief of symptoms of colds and influenza.
Tablets for oral use.
Swallow with a drink of water.
Dose
Adults, the elderly and children over 12 years:
Take one or two tablets up to 4 times a day, or as instructed by your doctor.
Children 6 to 12 years of age:
Take half to one tablet up to 4 times a day.
Not recommended for children under 6 years of age
The dose should not be repeated more frequently than every 4 hours and not more than 4 doses should be taken in any 24 hour period.
Do not take more medicine than the label tells you to. If you do not get better, talk to your doctor.
Each tablet contains paracetamol 500mg.
KEEP OUT OF THE SIGHT AND REACH OF CHILDREN.

Protect from heat, light and moisture.
Please read the leaflet enclosed before taking this medicine.

Do not take anything else containing paracetamol while taking this medicine.
Talk to a doctor at once if you take too much of this medicine, even if you feel well.

PL 20416/0186
PL Holder:
Crescent Pharma Ltd.,
Polhampton Lane, Overton,
Hants, RG25 3ED
Distributed by:
Day Lewis Medical Ltd.
Croydon, Surrey, CR0 4UQ

GSL

5 060376 360004

Note: The label includes specific dosage instructions and also cautionary labelling about maximum dosage of Paracetamol.

Pharmacy medicines (P)

Pharmacy medicines have a higher perceived risk than GSL and may not be sold to public without a pharmacist being able to intervene in the sale (e.g. larger packs of analgesics, sedating antihistamines, some antimalarials, more potent cough and cold remedies). These are also labelled with very specific instructions and relevant counselling and cautions.

Prescription only medicines (POM)

These are normally supplied on practitioner's prescription via a pharmacy. Parenteral administration is only allowed by a prescriber or under direct medical supervision. POMs have less specific labelling than P or GSL. They are not required to show cautionary labelling or specific dosage instructions. An acceptable dose instruction on a manufacturer's POM container is "to be taken as directed by the doctor" (or similar). This is unhelpful to the remote healthcare professional as reference works may need to be consulted to determine dosage information as well as important warnings and counselling information (e.g. take before food, may cause drowsiness etc.).

Paracetamol Tablets 500mg Pack of 100 — Prescription Only Medicine

Paracetamol 500mg Tablets

100 tablets

500 mg

Tablets for oral use.

To be taken as directed by the doctor.

Do not take more medicine than the label tells you to.

If you do not get better, talk to your doctor.

Each tablet contains paracetamol 500mg.

KEEP OUT OF THE SIGHT AND REACH OF CHILDREN.

Protect from heat, light and moisture.

Please read the leaflet enclosed before taking this medicine.

Do not take anything else containing paracetamol while taking this medicine.

Talk to a doctor at once if you take too much of this medicine, even if you feel well.

PL 20416/0123

PL Holder:
Crescent Pharma Ltd., Polhampton Lane, Overton, Hants, RG25 3ED

Distributed by:
Day Lewis Medical Ltd, Croydon, Surrey, CR0 4UQ

[POM]

Note: Dosage instructions are non-specific. Also there is no cautionary labelling about maximum dosage of Paracetamol. This is because a patient specific "dispensing" label will be affixed by the dispensing pharmacy.

From the examples shown above it can be seen that the legal classification of Paracetamol depends on the pack size in which it is supplied i.e. GSL for packs of 16, P for packs of 32 and POM for packs of 100. It is also the case with several other medications that legal category varies dependant on pack presentation (e.g. chloramphenicol eye drops, acyclovir cream).

Controlled drugs (CDs)

The rules relating to CDs in the UK are detailed in the 2001 Misuse of Drugs Regulations pursuant to the Misuse of Drugs Act 1971.

The Regulations control:

- Manufacture
- Import
- Export
- Possession
- Safe custody
- Sale or supply
- Administration
- Dealing with addicts
- Record keeping

CDs are also subject to the same licensing requirements as other medicinal products.

Controlled Drugs (CDs) are divided into five Schedules:

Schedule 1 — no medicinal use e.g. Cannabis plant, LSD
Schedule 2 — very addictive, but useful drugs e.g. Morphine, Diamorphine, Pethidine
Schedule 3 — Less addictive e.g. Buprenorphine, Barbiturates
Schedule 4 (Part 1) — Benzodiazepines (diazepam, lorazepam, zolpidem, etc.)
Schedule 4 (Part 2) — Anabolic steroids
Schedule 5 — Low risk — diluted preparations of certain Schedule 2 drugs, to such an extent that they pose a much-reduced risk of misuse.

In the US controlled drugs have similar categories to those in the UK.

All controlled drugs solely included in Schedules, 2, 3 and 4 are also POMs. The Schedule 2 CDs also included in Schedule 5 may either be POMs or Pharmacy Medicines dependent on amount in each dose unit. Examples of Schedule 5 CDs which are classified as POM include, Dihydrocodeine tablets 60mg and Codeine tablets 15mg, 30mg & 60mg. Examples of Schedule 5 CDs which are classified as pharmacy medicines (P), such that they may be sold in pharmacies, include combination analgesics containing lower doses of codeine phosphate (e.g. tablets containing Paracetamol 500mg with Codeine 8mg), also cough remedies (e.g. Pholcodine Linctus).

It is likely that remote sites will stock CDs in Schedules 2, 3, 4 (Part 1) and 5.

Storage

For UK organisations stocking CDs, it is required that Schedule 2 and most (but not all) Schedule 3 controlled drugs are kept securely in a controlled drugs cabinet. However, in a remote situation, the safe approach is to keep all controlled drugs (except Schedule 5) in a controlled drugs cabinet or safe.

Records

A controlled drugs register must be used to record details of any Schedule 2 controlled drugs received or supplied.

For CDs received, the following must be recorded:

- Name of the drug received including strength and dose form
- Date supply received
- Name and address from whom received
- Quantity received

For controlled drugs supplied, or administered, the following must be recorded:

- Name of controlled drug supplied (or administered) including strength and dose form
- Date supplied
- Name and address of recipient
- Details of authority to possess (e.g. prescriber's name)
- Quantity supplied or administered.

The register should also keep a running total of stock holding to facilitate audit.

Any unexplained discrepancy in stock level is a serious matter which must be reported to law enforcement authorities. In the UK this is the police and the Home Office Drugs and Firearms Licensing Unit.

Exempted persons

The previous sections show that the normal situation in the UK is that, GSL medicines for minor ailments may be purchased at any retail outlet, Pharmacy (P) medicines may only be purchased from pharmacies, with a pharmacist in a position to intervene in the sale and POMs and controlled drugs (Schedules 2 to 4) may only be obtained on the prescription of a suitable practitioner (usually a doctor). If this were always the case, then it would be impossible for ships, offshore installations remote sites and their healthcare professionals (HCPs) to obtain and use medicines to treat the personnel in their care.

Schedule 17 of the Human Medicines Regulations (UK Government, 2012), includes a number of exemptions from the restrictions on administration and supply of medicines of all legal categories. These exemptions enable, those to whom they apply ("exempted persons") to supply or administer medicines as part of their trade business or profession, subject to any conditions or restrictions listed in the exemption. Exempted persons may purchase the medicines they can legally use from a licensed wholesale dealer in medicines (WDA(H) Holder).

Those exemptions of relevance to remote healthcare provision are shown below:

a) Persons operating an occupational health scheme
An occupational health scheme is one which is set up by an employer to provide healthcare to his employees, who may be injured or become ill at work. Medicine stocks may only be used in the course of the occupational health scheme, such that treatment is not available to non-employees. In such a scheme, treatment must be provided by a doctor or registered nurse. The nurse may administer, or supply GSL and P medicines, but POMs may only be supplied or administered

(parenterally) in accordance with written instructions from a doctor "as to the circumstances in which POMs of the description in question are to be used in the course of the occupational health scheme". The registered nurse may order GSL, P and POM medicines from a WDA(H) holder. However, controlled drugs should be ordered by a doctor employed within the scheme. Requirements relating to licensing and safe custody requirements should be established with the appropriate regulatory authority (in the UK this is the Home Office Drugs Branch). This exemption for occupational health schemes applies to activities within the UK, but provides an example of best practice, which can be of use when setting up remote clinics.

b) The owner or master of a ship

These persons may order medicines of any legal category. The medicines may only be used to treat those on board the ship. In practice, ships are also required to adhere to standards imposed by Merchant Shipping Regulations and guidance.

The master of a ship may also order controlled drugs to be held on board. In the UK, for a foreign ship in a UK port, additional requirements apply.

c) Persons employed as qualified first-aid personnel on offshore installations

These persons may supply or administer (including parenterally) GSL, P and POMs. CDs required as sickbay stock must be ordered by the offshore installation manager (OIM).

Other statutory obligations or recommendations relevant to remote sites

Statutory requirements relating to the provision of healthcare exist for certain remote locations.

Offshore installations

In the case of UK offshore installations, companies are required to comply with The Offshore Installations and Pipeline Works (First-Aid) Regulations 1989. This requires companies to make appropriate arrangements in terms of sickbay facilities, medications, consumables, equipment, site healthcare professionals as well as medical supervision of offshore healthcare. Interpretation of the regulations is assisted by an "Approved Code of Practice and Guidance" (Health and Safety Executive, 1989) which sets out recommended standards. The Code of Practice itself is not part of the Regulations, such that a failure to follow it, is not, in itself, an offence. However, in the event of a prosecution for a breach of the Regulations, failure to comply with the Code of Practice may be used in evidence.

The Norwegian and Dutch governments have similar statutory obligations for installations operating in their sectors of the continental shelf.

Merchant ships

UK Merchant Shipping Regulations require provision to be made for the medical treatment of crew members. Guidance is produced in a Merchant Shipping Notice "MSN 1768" (UK Government, 1995).

Similar arrangements exist for most jurisdictions and it is important that those who operate vessels make sure that they are aware of the requirements. Several countries have their own recommended list of medical conditions which should be catered for and also the recommended medicines to be stocked. The World Health Organization also publishes a recommended list of ship medical stores in the *International Medical Guide for Ships*, 3rd Edition (World Health Organization, 2007).

Management of Medicines at Remote Locations

The purpose of a medicines management system is twofold:

- to ensure that an adequate range of medically approved, pharmacologically appropriate and pharmaceutically safe treatments is available in sufficient quantities to cater for the medical conditions which may be encountered on site; and
- to ensure that those treatments are used safely and defensibly in the correct circumstances in accordance with medical opinion.

The management tools required to fulfil these objectives are an inventory list to define the stocks of medicines and written instructions as to the circumstances in which those medicines may be supplied or administered to patients. Both the inventory list and written instructions will most likely be produced by the medical management team, but it is of value to remote site HCPs to be aware of the processes involved. Also, when reviews take place the views of onsite HCPs should be carefully considered.

Selection of medical conditions to be catered for

The first stage of establishing a medicines list should be to decide which medical conditions are to be treated on-site. Many factors should be evaluated in making this decision. Omitting treatments or classes of products from a list is as important a medical management decision as including them.

The following factors must be taken into account:

- Compliance with relevant statutory requirements (e.g. offshore healthcare regulations and merchant shipping regulations)

- Industry recommendations and informed guidance
- Local risks (e.g. endemic diseases)
- Population requiring care (workers only, families, local personnel)
- Local healthcare infra-structure (for in-country projects)
- Ease and transit time of evacuation — stocks of emergency medicines (e.g. oxygen and iv fluids) will need to be increased where delays in evacuation are likely.

Selecting inventory list medicines

Once it has been decided which medical conditions are to be catered for, the next stage is to select which individual medicines are to be included in the inventory. The factors that need to be considered are detailed in the following sections.

Pharmacological factors

Pharmacological "safety" is an important factor when selecting individual products. For instance, it is reasonable to exclude potentially soporific remedies for minor, self-limiting ailments from a list to be used on a hazardous site (e.g. offshore installation), where sedation may be (or could later be claimed to have been) a safety hazard. In some cases, products may be selected because their interaction profile is safer than that of an alternative. For instance, if a H2 receptor blocker is included, Ranitidine is preferable to Cimetidine because of the impairment of hepatic metabolism of other agents by the latter.

Environmental factors

In very hot climates medicines with anticholinergic properties may reduce sweating and present a risk of hyperthermia (e.g. Chlorpromazine).

Pharmaceutical factors

Pharmaceutical factors can be of importance in product selection e.g. shelf life — whilst this is a matter in the hands of manufacturers, in some cases a different brand of the same product may have a longer expiry (e.g. Adrenaline 1:10,000 injection). Remote site operators should ask suppliers to provide goods with the best shelf life possible. However, it should be recognised that manufacturers and pharmaceutical wholesalers are required as a condition of their licences to rotate stock in order.

Lists should always specify manufacturers' original packs for medicines (this is particularly important with "in-country" suppliers). The manufacturers of medicines which have been re-packed and labelled by pharmacists may not retain full product liability as their material is no longer in its licensed and tested packaging. In the United Kingdom re-packing and labelling of medications by pharmacists for supply to oil companies (and others) is not permitted in the terms of a Wholesale Dealing Authorisation.

Inventory lists should define pack size and presentation. It is preferable if "patient packs" (i.e. packs which contain a full course of a particular treatment for one person e.g. 21 × Amoxicillin Capsules) are used, as these facilitate supply by HCPs and provide patient information via pack labelling and leaflets. Single dose sachets are preferable in the case of antiseptics for reasons of hygiene. Similarly, single dose eye drops are preferable to multiple dose containers in those cases, where the products will be administered as just one or two single doses, rather than a course (e.g. local anaesthetic eye drops). Over the counter (otc) packs (although more expensive) may be more convenient for the HCP as they are ready-labelled for the recipient.

It is costly to ship products requiring special ("cold chain") storage conditions and in some cases, it is possible to use alternatives which avoid the problem. An example is Chloramphenicol eye drops which require storage and shipment between +2°C and +8°C. This can be replaced with other antibacterial eye preparations without cold chain requirements (e.g. Gentamycin 0.3% eye drops).

Similarly, in the case of flammable products hazard packing and paperwork required for freighting can be avoided by picking (chemically) safer alternatives (e.g. aqueous, rather than spirit-based antiseptics).

Restrictions on movement of particular medicines

Certain classes of medicine may be subject to special import restrictions, in some countries this applies to narcotics and psychotropic drugs. A good supplier will be able to advise remote healthcare providers on the procedures for these products.

It is important to be sure that medical lists do not include products which are prohibited in destination countries (e.g. codeine in Indonesia, tramadol in Egypt and pseudoephedrine in Japan). The presence of these in a shipment can prevent all of the consignment from reaching its destination.

Pharmaceutical input

Advice from suitably experienced pharmacists is of value, when producing inventory lists. Areas of expertise should include advice on medicines which have unfavourable side-effect profiles, alternative products where interactions may be an issue, advice on more cost-effective inclusions, most suitable pack presentations, products requiring cold storage and potentially (chemically) hazardous products.

Too often, lists are produced without pharmaceutical input and need to be corrected later (my personal experience).

The resultant list

The steps above should create an inventory list for the site in question. The range of stocks should be suitable for all anticipated eventualities and should meet the standards of statutory and informed official guidance. The site should stock only the medicines included on the list, except in exceptional circumstances (e.g. lack of availability of a particular product). Ideally, the list should be presented as a sortable document, such that products can be displayed in alphabetical order or under therapeutic headings. Also, it is good practice to also show the legal classification of the listed products. If UK designations are used, these will include POM, P. GSL, CD2, CD3, CD4-1. In oil industry lists, when the classification is based on US designations, these are often shown as over the counter (otc) medicines, prescription medicines (Rx), and for controlled drugs Rx, (schedule II. III or IV).

It is worth looking at an inventory list as a whole, products should complement each other, antidotes should be included where appropriate.

Stock audit and ordering schedules

Inventory lists should define stock holding requirements for individual medications, based on operational experience, lead times for re-supply etc. It is the responsibility of onsite medical staff to maintain stocks at these levels. This should involve a full audit of stocks at agreed intervals, including an examination of expiry dates, storage conditions and packaging. The lack of a medicine is at least an inconvenience and at worst a serious issue of relevance to patient care. Similarly, having only a date expired medicine available for use in an emergency places the HCP in an impossible position. It is worth mentioning that particular attention should be paid to checking the expiry dates of medicines included in emergency bags and kits. From personal experience, these can often be overlooked, such that single ampoules of emergency drugs may be well out of date when needed.

The medicines in Table 1 are taken from the 2013 IRHC "Remote Healthcare Guidance Document for Energy and Associated Maritime activities". In this example the legal class is based on the US system. The "Category" column refers to the circumstances in which individual medicines may be issued (e.g. whether medical advice is required — explained in Section 4.3 below). Many remote sites add additional columns to include expiry dates etc.

Table 1:   Potential Layout for Inventory List

Item	Description	Legal Class	Pack Size	No Packs Stocked	Category
	Analgesics				
1	Co-Codamol Tablets 8/500 Tablets (or Effervescent Tablets)	otc	32	6	A
2	Codeine phosphate 30 mg tablets	Rx	30	2	B
3	Diclofenac Emulgel (or similar)	otc	30g	6	A
4	Diclofenac Injection 75mg/3ml	Rx	10	1	C
5	Diclofenac Tablets 50mg	Rx	84	2	C
6	Entonox cylinder size D	Rx	Size D	4	B
7	Ibuprofen, 400 mg tablets	otc	48	5	A
8	Lemsip Sachets (or similar cold remedy)	otc	16	10	A
9	Migraveve Pink and Yellow Tablets (or similar otc migraine treatment)	otc	24	3	A
10	Paracetamol. 500 mg tablets	otc	16	30	A
11	Tramadol Inj. 100mg/2ml (alternative to Morphine)	Rx Schedule 3	10	1	B
12	Tramadol Tablets 50mg	Rx Schedule 3	60	1	B
13	Voltarol (Diclofenac Sodium) 50 mg suppositories	Rx	10	1	C
14	Morphine Sulfate Injection 10mg/1ml	Rx Schedule 2	10	3	B

Written Instructions

It has been observed that in the case of occupational health schemes in the UK, the issuing of POMs by a registered nurse should be in accordance with written instructions from a doctor "as to the circumstances in which prescription only medicines of the description in question are to be used in the course of the occupational health scheme". Also, the original UKOOA Guidance notes to the Offshore installations and Pipeline Works (First-Aid) Regulations 1989 recommended that medicines should be issued in accordance with "standing orders" or on the directions of a medical practitioner (who may be onshore).

The nature of the written instructions/standing orders varies considerably between organisations, with some providing detailed clinical guidelines and categorising medicines to identify which may be issued on the authority of the on-site HCP and those which require authorisation from a topside doctor. The system will vary depending on the location, the level of training of HCPs and communications.

A common system of categorisation of medicines is:

Category A
Can be prescribed by a healthcare professional on his own authority

Category B
Can be given, when indicated, in an emergency by a healthcare professional without contact with a supervising doctor. However, the use must be reported to the doctor as soon as possible.

Category C

Must not be supplied or administered without first contacting a supervising physician.

It is helpful to site medical staff for the inventory lists to be annotated to show the categories.

Medicines which may cause sedation or impair judgement

Wherever possible, products with sedative side effects should have been omitted from the inventory list, for safety reasons. However, in some cases no alternatives exist and so, it is a good idea to include in written instructions a cautionary statement of the type below:

> If it is necessary to use any sedative product, it is essential to have due care for the safety of the recipient and those around him or her. In particular, individuals must not be allowed to operate in hazardous areas or on tasks that may affect safety if they have received a potentially sedative product. Furthermore, in the event of an evacuation or safety drill, those who have received sedative products should be escorted if necessary.

> Arriving and departing personnel must be warned about the dangers of driving, operating machinery or engaging in any activity where sedation would (or could) prove hazardous. They must also be warned of the increased risk if alcohol or other sedatives are also consumed.

Good medical practice requires that the healthcare professional documents in the patient's medical file that the necessary warnings have been given.

What can go wrong with the system

Effective governance at a remote site relies on medicines being used in accordance with protocols determined by the supervising medical officers. This can only be properly achieved by the use of written instructions relating to a specific list of medications as described in this chapter. Where additional medications are stocked outside the agreed medicines list, without the knowledge of medical advisors, then no associated current written instructions would exist. Clearly, this can prove problematic in the case of POMs, but can also be an issue in the case of otc medicines (e.g. the introduction of potentially soporific cough and cold remedies).

There are a variety of ways in which additional medicines, not covered by currently valid written instructions can be part of sickbay stocks. These include:

- Orders being placed for non-inventory products, which are supplied without the supplier first checking with the responsible medical department or topside provider.

- Introduction of a new inventory list and written instructions without removing discontinued products, which may continue to be ordered and supplied. This can happen when a medical department or topside provider amends the existing inventory list, or when a new topside provider takes over.
- Supply of alternative products by a supplier. This may be due to stock availability issues or it could be that an overseas supplier is unable to obtain the precise products listed in the inventory.
- Compliance with a different country's regulatory requirements. This can apply in situations where a ship or mobile offshore installation changes the jurisdiction in which it is mainly operating.
- Imposition of particular extra requirements by a client. This can happen with ships or offshore installations, when a contractor company has its own inventory and written instructions, but is told that it must stock certain additional products for the client company. I have come across this situation more than once and it can lead to an unnecessary "widening" of the stock holding with "me too" products.

The situations above can be largely avoided if change is managed properly. Suppliers should be aware that non-inventory medications should not be supplied without first checking with, and receiving approval from, the appropriate medical advisors. This would also apply in cases where alternatives can be offered in place of unavailable inventory products. Also, when a list is changed, suppliers should be informed and be aware that orders for discontinued products must not be supplied.

In those cases where an "in-country" supplier is used, inventory lists should be rewritten specifying pharmaceutically approved equivalent medicines available in the jurisdiction in question. I have done this on a number of occasions in collaboration with medical departments.

When it is necessary to comply with a different set of regulatory requirements, it may also be necessary to amend the inventory list and written instructions to reflect this on a site-specific basis.

In those cases, where a client imposes a condition that certain particular medications be stocked, it may be necessary for these to be separated out for audit purposes, whilst the inventory approved by the contractor's own medical advisors is routinely used.

Procurement, Supply & Logistics

Efficient initial supply and re-supply is important for any remote site. Any failure of the supply chain may lead to individuals being placed at risk. For this reason, it is desirable (if not essential) for the operator, medical supplier and freighting agent to agree on a system of procurement and supply to remove avoidable delays. The supplier should also be aware of those items authorised for the location (i.e. those on the company inventory list), so that any additions may be queried with the medical department. This can be a valuable second check to avoid the accumulation of unauthorised products.

At the planning phase of any new project it is essential to establish precisely what is required to get initial and subsequent re-supply shipments to the work site with minimum hindrance. A schedule should be established detailing who is responsible for which aspects of the shipment. Depending on the location and the nature of the consignment, any of the following (and more) may be necessary:

- Import licences
- Export licences
- Certificates of origin
- Certificates of quality/conformance
- Hazard data sheets
- Special packaging
- Special invoicing requirements for destination country
- Special packing note formats
- Miscellaneous declarations

The supplier will also require documentation to confirm that the customer may lawfully be supplied with the medications requested.

Careful planning of paperwork can greatly assist transit times. In particular, where permission to import medications is required, the purchaser should ensure that the in-country authorities have full details of the items to be shipped well in advance so that goods do not wait in customs for a prolonged time whilst paperwork is completed.

Additionally, any "in-house" paperwork requirements should be shared with the supplier earlier rather than later. Similarly, arrangements for freighting any refrigerated goods and hazardous items should be established. A policy for dealing with unavoidable part shipments should also be agreed.

Working with a fixed inventory list can facilitate shipment time as documentation requirements should be on record, which may not be the case with a series of ad-hoc requests.

Assistance with paperwork requirements for particular destinations is available from reputable international freighting agents and suitably experienced pharmaceutical suppliers. Audit of the procurement process is of value and should be undertaken to identify and address any issues causing delays in the system.

Supplier selection

It is clear that a good supplier can be of great benefit to any project. Organisations should seek out suppliers with pharmaceutical expertise and a good track record of dealing with remote health facilities. Suppliers can bring a great deal to the table at the planning stage and those with experience of providing input to inventory list production can be of great use. Sourcing of suppliers can be undertaken using databases or by word of mouth from other organisations. UK and EU suppliers must be licensed wholesalers (WDA(H) holders) as observed in Section 3.6 (above) and remote site operators should require proof of this. Some UK and EU licence holders can liaise with "in-country" suppliers to assist overseas organisations with producing achievable lists of supplies in difficult areas.

A competent supplier can assist remote healthcare compliance by following policies with respect to adherence to inventory lists and in cooperation with organisation medical management.

The eventual supplier should be under contract and should be able to ship (or arrange shipment) of medicines in manufacturers' original packs, with a good shelf-life and in accordance with manufacturers' label storage conditions. This is particularly important in the case of "cold chain" medicines which require shipment and storage at temperatures between +2°C and +8°C.

A good supplier should be able to offer a point of contact for the provision of pharmaceutical information to those operating the remote site or to their medical advisors.

Shipment to site arranged by remote site company

Some remote site operators select their own preferred shipping agents as this enables consolidation of a wide range of products. If this is the case, it is important that they have a contract with the shipper to ensure that any medicines are shipped in accordance with the storage conditions shown on their labels. It is also important that medical supplies are not held in hub warehouses for prolonged periods during transit. In the UK this is defined as 36 hours or more.

Medicines arriving on site, which have been subjected to temperatures and/or storage conditions outside those defined on their labels are "off-licence" and can be classed as "damaged".

It is important that every effort is made to ensure the integrity of the product arriving on site.

Receipt of medicines on site

Medicines should be unpacked and checked immediately on arrival. Incoming shipments should never be exposed to external weather conditions. Stocks should be stored within the sickbay as soon as possible and any damaged goods or discrepancies reported to the supplier as soon as possible.

On-Site Storage of Medicines

Sickbay general arrangements

The sickbay or clinic should be a dedicated space under the control of a site HCP. It should be maintained in good order and should be clearly identifiable. It should be available at all times and should only be used for medical purposes and the duties of the HCP.

The sickbay should be lockable and should be kept locked at all times when not in use, with the keys preferably in the possession of the HCP in charge. There should be a system in place to obtain access in an emergency (possibly with additional keys held by the person in charge of the site, installation or vessel in question).

The sickbay or clinic, should be easily identifiable with a sign on the door. There should also be clear contact details for "out of hours" or emergency contact.

There should be suitable communication equipment in the sickbay (computer, telephone, radio) for the HCP to get contact to additional medical advice etc.

The facility should contain suitable furniture and storage provision for medical supplies. Medicines should be stored separately from consumables and equipment.

There should be some form of temperature control and air conditioning system to maintain temperature within suitable limits for storing medicines.

In terms of storage temperature, the medicines likely to be included on a site inventory list, fall into two main categories:

- Those requiring storage at ambient temperatures generally considered to be room temperature (in the US defined as being between +15°C and +25°C)
- Those requiring refrigerated storage (between +2°C and +8°C).

These are considered further in the following sections.

Ambient medicines

Ambient medicines should be stored in shelved cupboards or cabinets attached to the wall of the room. The sickbay should be locked and ideally, the cupboards should also be lockable see (Figure 1).

When a medicines storage area is being set up, it is important to ensure that the temperature is suitable. It is suggested that an initial "temperature mapping" exercise is undertaken to identify any hot or cold spots in the storage area (this procedure is mandatory for UK pharmaceutical wholesalers). This can be undertaken using data loggers which can be downloaded onto a PC. In general, it is to be expected that high shelves will be warmer than lower ones. This exercise should be undertaken when the temperature control system (air conditioning/ heating) is operational, so that settings can be adjusted accordingly.

Once set up, temperature of the storage area and cabinets should be continuously monitored and recorded to ensure that ambient products are stored between +15°C and +25°C. Again, the best method of doing this is to use calibrated data loggers. These can be set to show deviations from the acceptable range. It is best for a sickbay to define this as a lower temperature of 15.5 °C and a higher temperature of 24.5 °C, to allow for errors in the data logger. Temperatures should be ideally downloaded daily and saved on a PC. Figure 2 shows a sample temperature graph.

Within the cupboards or cabinets, there should be ample room to accommodate stocks of medicines. Ideally stocks should be laid out in the order in which they

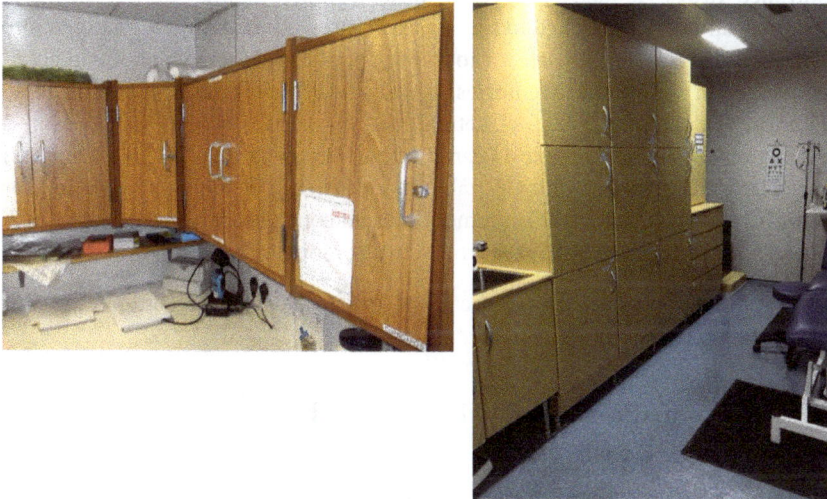

Figure 1:   Examples of Sickbay Storage Cupboards on two Offshore Installations

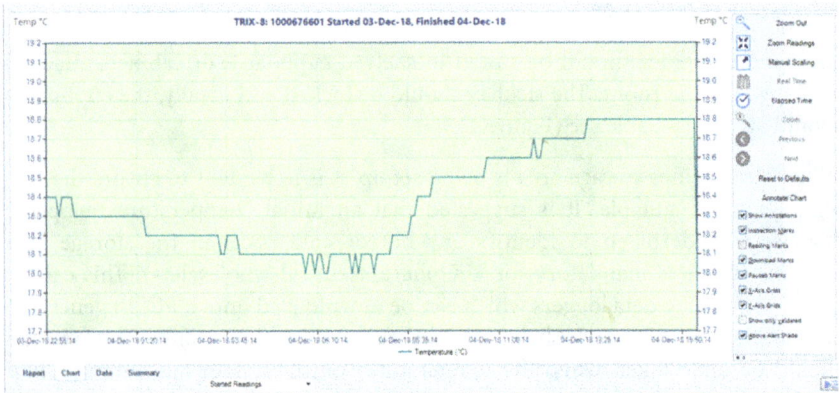

Figure 2:   Downloaded Temperature Graph From Data Logger in Storage Area for Medicines Requiring Ambient Storage Conditions +15°C and +25°C

Note: The data logger also produces a summary of maximum and minimum readings as well as a record of every temperature measurement. Data loggers also have an alarm function to show when a maximum or minimum (user defined) temperature is breached.

appear on the inventory list to assist with stock management. The addition of shelf edge labels showing the position of each product can also be helpful.

Controlled drugs on remote sites should be stored in a strong safe or dedicated controlled drugs cabinet, either as a lockable inner cabinet, or one which is separately and firmly attached to a wall (see Figure 3). Based on UK classification, controlled drugs requiring safe custody within a CD cabinet, which are likely to be included in remote site inventories, include those in Schedule 2 (e.g. morphine, diamorphine, pethidine, fentanyl, ketamine) and some (but not all) in Schedule 3 (e.g. buprenorphine). Schedule 4 (Part 1) controlled drugs (e.g. benzodiazepines) do not require storage in the CD cabinet. However, it is strongly suggested for administrative purposes, that on remote sites all controlled drugs in Schedules 2, 3 and 4 (part 1) are kept in the controlled drugs cabinet.

A good pharmaceutical supplier can be of assistance in recommending or providing suitable storage facilities.

Cold-chain medicines requiring storage between +2 °C and +8 °C (35°F to 46°F)

There should be a lockable refrigerator of sufficient capacity to house medicines requiring storage between +2°C and +8°C (35°F to 46°F).

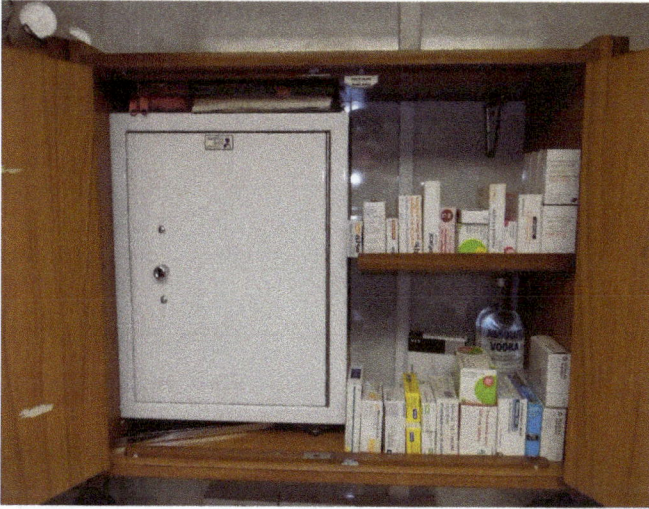

Figure 3:   Offshore Installation Controlled Drugs Cabinet within a Locked Outer Cupboard in Sickbay

The refrigerator should have an alarm set to alert staff to temperature excursions. There should be a method of recording maximum and minimum temperatures. The best way of doing this is to use a calibrated USB data logger, which will plug straight into a computer. Readings should be downloaded daily. Again, the loggers should have an alarm to show deviation from the acceptable range. For a refrigerator, this should be set a lower temperature of 2.5°C and a higher temperature of 7.5°C, to allow for errors in the data logger. Temperatures should be ideally downloaded daily and saved on a PC (see Figure 4).

The Department of Health "Green Book" Immunisation against Infectious Disease Chapter 3 "Storage, distribution and disposal of vaccines" (UK Government, 2019), advises that "Specialised refrigerators are available for the storage of pharmaceutical products, and must be used for vaccines and diluents. Ordinary domestic refrigerators must not be used". This is good advice, because the motor on a pharmacy refrigerator cuts in and out more frequently than that of a domestic refrigerator, maintaining a narrower temperature range.

The refrigerator should also have grille type shelving — to enable air movement, fan assisted cooling, automatic defrost and should either be directly wired to the mains or otherwise have a notice saying "Do Not Switch Off" attached to plug and fridge.

Refrigerators should not be overloaded with products and should not include non-medicinal items (e.g. food and drinks). Pharmaceuticals should be well spaced and

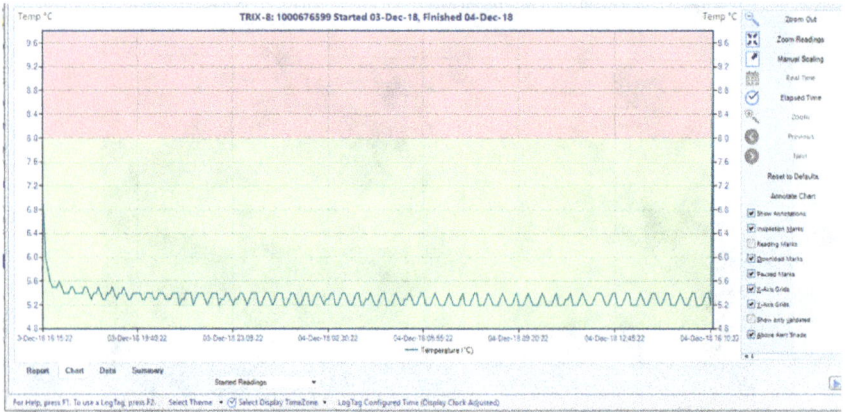

Figure 4:   Downloaded Temperature Graph From a Data Logger in Storage Area for Medicines Requiring Refrigerated Storage Conditions +2°C and +8°C

Note: The data logger also produces a summary of maximum and minimum readings as well as a record of every temperature measurement. Data loggers also have an alarm function to show when a maximum or minimum (user defined) temperature is breached.

not allowed to touch the walls as this may result in freezing. Figure 5 provides an example of a well-packed refrigerator.

Dealing with temperature excursions

Loss of temperature control is a problem that can occur in any location, but it is particularly challenging in a remote location, where re-supply is more difficult.

Loss of air conditioning in hot climates can lead to ambient medicines being exposed to temperatures well above those defined on the manufacturers' labels. In most cases, this will accelerate deterioration of the product, reducing shelf-life. It is not possible to give a generic solution to this problem, other than to say for prolonged exposure to excessive temperatures professional advice should be sought (e.g. from the supplier). Sending a data logger file showing the extent of the excursion is always of great value.

In cold climates, loss of heating can result in freezing of medicines. If that is the case all injections should be quarantined and regarded as unsafe for use. This is because micro-cracks can occur in ampoules and compromise sterility. Any medicine with "Do Not Freeze" on the label will also be unusable. These medicines should be quarantined for destruction and re-ordered.

In the case of cold-chain medicines, refrigerator failures are problematic and there should be an emergency plan. If a refrigerator temperature is set too low and freezing occurs, the product should not be used and must be discarded.

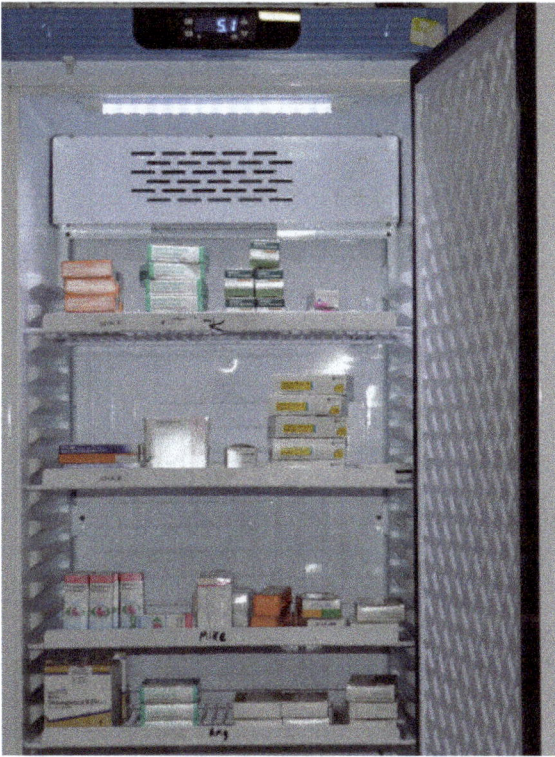

Figure 5:   Example of a Well Packed Refrigerator

Note: The refrigerator is not overloaded with stock, products are placed well apart and are not touching the walls. Also, there are no non-medicinal products present.

If the refrigerator ceases to function, such that the temperature will rise above +8°C. then the cold-chain medicines should be moved to another refrigerator and be kept separate from any other contents. A data logger should be placed with the medicines to monitor temperature conditions. Preparation for such an eventuality can be made by designating another (if necessary non-medical) refrigerator on the site for this purpose and checking that it maintains temperature between +2 °C and +8 °C.

If the problem is that all refrigerators are not working (e.g. power cut) then the cold-chain products should be left in the original refrigerator until it starts working again. The refrigerator and its contents should be quarantined at this time. Pharmaceutical advice should be obtained (usually from the supplier) and this will be assisted by emailing the information from the data logger during the excursion. The pharmaceutical advice will involve contact with manufacturers to establish the extent to which the excursion has compromised the products. It should be noted that if manufacturers advise that the excursion has not adversely affected the stability of the products, any subsequent administration will be "off-licence".

Pharmaceutical Waste

In UK pharmacies and pharmaceutical wholesale premises, date expired and damaged pharmaceutical products must be disposed of safely. This is done using dedicated pharmaceutical waste containers, which are sealed when full and collected by specialist waste contractors. It is important that any unusable medicine is removed from active stock, so that it cannot be accidently supplied or administered. In the case of offshore installations and ships, contracts with pharmaceutical waste contractors can be established and, in some cases, arrangements can be made for unwanted pharmaceuticals to be returned to the supplier who will arrange for safe disposal via a specialist waste contractor. Clearly, in some remote locations this will pose problems and local arrangements will need to be made. However, it is an important issue and if no local arrangement is feasible, the best course of action may be to store the waste medications until they can be returned to a supplier.

In the UK unwanted controlled drugs (e.g. date expired or surplus) in Schedules 2, 3 and 4 must be destroyed according to Home Office guidelines by denaturing in the presence of an authorised witness. For UK Offshore Installations and Ships, CDs for destruction should be returned to an authorised recipient (usually the supplier) for destruction. The removal of the stock must be recorded and witnessed in the CD register and inventory amounts adjusted accordingly.

CDs returned to a supplier for destruction, from a remote site must be sent by a secure courier. The method of return must be established between the remote healthcare provider and supplier. Where it is not possible to return controlled drugs for destruction (e.g. a very remote site overseas), then it may be acceptable for the destruction to be undertaken by the on-site healthcare professional in the presence of a suitable witness (e.g. senior site manager, installation manager or Captain). Both persons should sign the CD register to record that destruction has taken place.

Reference Sources

When choosing medicines from the site inventory list for patients, HCPs must be able to provide treatment as safely as possible.

Additionally, it is also important that any medication brought on site by personnel should be assessed (this is considered in more detail in Section 8). For these reasons, it is important that HCPs have access to suitable reference sources for pharmaceutical information. The following sections describe briefly suitable reference works and their uses.

British National Formulary (BNF)

The BNF (BNF London 2019), (published twice a year) is probably the foremost reference book used by UK healthcare professionals for information on the choice, uses and properties of medicines. There is information about common medical conditions, together with suitable medicines to treat them. The notes on medicines are divided into sixteen chapters, each of which is related to a particular system of the body (e.g. Chapter 2, Cardiovascular System) or to an aspect of medical care (e.g. Chapter 5, Infections).

Within the chapters are sections relating to particular classes of drugs, providing information on uses, dosage, contraindications, side-effects and references to relevant appendices. The beginning of sections relating to a class of drugs (e.g. Non-steroidal anti-inflammatory drugs or Beta-adrenergic receptor blockers (systemic)) includes information (including warnings etc.) which is common to all of the individual drugs in that class. For this reason, in addition to reading individual drug monographs, HCPs should also always read the information at the beginning of the section relating to that class of drugs.

In particular, due account must be taken of each of the following:

Indications

The general rule is that a medicine must only be used for medical conditions for which it is indicated in its BNF monograph.

The use of medications for unlicensed purposes may present legal problems in the event of a mishap.

Contra-indications

Medicines must never be used for patients in whom they are contra-indicated. For example, it is never safe to use diclofenac or ibuprofen in a patient who has shown previous hypersensitivity to aspirin or any other NSAID.

Cautions

In a remote location, the general rule should be not to use medicines in patients to whom cautions may apply. Where a HCP feels that, having taken due account of the BNF caution, use of a particular medicine may still be appropriate, he or she should seek authorisation from a topside doctor before use.

Side effects

Due account must be taken of side effects and information about them should be always included in the patient counselling which accompanies supply of medication. In remote and hazardous areas side effects can be of considerable importance. For instance, persons working in hazardous conditions can be put at considerable risk from medication with sedative side effect.

Often the condition with which a patient presents may be a side effect of medication, e.g. diarrhoea with antibiotics, nausea from NSAIDs etc, and it may be that withdrawal of the causative agent is preferable to treatment of the symptom.

Drug interactions

Any medication being considered by a healthcare professional must be checked for interactions with existing medication being taken by a patient. Appendix 1 in the BNF lists drug interactions, together with their significance. Some interactions are very minor and are more of academic interest. It is very useful, therefore, that the Appendix 1 annotates most interactions as follows:

[Severe] — the result may be life threatening or have a permanent detrimental effect.

[Moderate] — could cause considerable distress or potentially incapacitate a patient, but unlikely to be life-threatening or result in long-term effects.

[Mild] — unlikely to cause concern or incapacitate the majority of patients.

[Unknown] — predicted interactions where there is insufficient evidence to predict outcome.

The Appendix also advises the basis for the classifications as follows:

[Study] — based on a formal study, including other drugs with the same mechanism of action.

[Anecdotal] — based on a single or limited case reports.

[Theoretical] — predicted based on sound considerations.

Dose

Medications must only be employed within the dose range listed in the BNF for the indication in question.

Counselling

Recipients of medication should always be counselled about their treatment. Advice should ensure a clear understanding of the reason for use of the product, the dosage, and information about side effects.

Also, advice should be given about relevant cautions. This information can be found in Appendix 3: "Cautionary and advisory labels for dispensed medicines".

This is extremely useful information for remote site HCPs. It has been noted earlier in this chapter that in the case of prescription medicines sourced in the UK and EEA countries, there is no requirement for cautionary labelling to be included on manufacturers' labels. Appendix 3, includes a numbered list detailing the cautionary and advisory wording (together with explanation) to be included on the labels of dispensed medicines in the UK. This list is also reproduced on a page near to the back of the book.

Directions on which wording should be used for individual medicines is included in the relevant drug monograph, next to the dose form in question. For example, in the case of Ibuprofen, where the dose form "Tablet" appears in the monograph, it states "CAUTIONARY AND ADVISORY LABELS 21".

Consulting either Appendix 3 (or the list at the rear of the BNF) shows Label 21 to be "Take with or just after food".

In pharmacies, computerised systems automatically add these cautions to the dispensing label on an individual's medicine container. However, in the remote situation, it may not always be practical to include such wording on labels, but HCPs can still use the content to counsel the patient about how to most safely use their medication.

Once a person has found his or her way around the BNF, it proves to be a mine of truly valuable information.

Electronic Medicines Compendium (eMC)

The eMC (Medicines.org.uk, 2019) contains up to date, easily accessible information about medicines licensed for use in the UK. The eMC has more than 10,600 documents, all of which have been checked and approved by either the UK MHRA or European government agencies (European Medicines Agency — EMA) which licence medicines.

Detailed information is included for each product as a Summary of Product Characteristics (SmPC). There are also links to pdfs of manufacturer's Patient Information Leaflets (PIL), which can be printed off.

The product information in each SmPC is much more comprehensive than that in the BNF monographs, and fully reflects the licensing of each individual medicine. The interactions section may be less easy to follow for non-pharmaceutical personnel, but still includes all relevant information.

Whilst the SmPC does not provide cautionary and advisory labelling, it will include information about precautions relating to safe usage.

Notes on SmPC sections

Each SmPC is divided into the sections shown below, most are self-explanatory and the eMC gives an excellent description of the sections on its website (Medicines. org.uk, 2019).

1. Name of the medicinal product
2. Qualitative and quantitative composition
3. Pharmaceutical form
4. Clinical particulars
   4.1 Therapeutic indications
   4.2 Posology and method of administration
   4.3 Contraindications
   4.4 Special warnings and precautions for use
   4.5 Interactions with other medicinal products and other forms of interaction
   4.6 Pregnancy and lactation
   4.7 Effects on ability to drive and use machines
   4.8 Undesirable effects
   4.9 Overdose
5. Pharmacological properties
   5.1 Pharmacodynamic properties
   5.2 Pharmacokinetic properties
   5.3 Preclinical safety data
6. Pharmaceutical properties
   6.1 List of excipients (inactive ingredients)
   6.2 Incompatibilities
   6.3 Shelf life
   6.4 Special precautions for storage
   6.5 Nature and contents of container
   6.6 Special precautions for disposal and other handling
7. Marketing authorisation holder
8. Marketing authorisation number(s)
9. Date of first authorisation/renewal of the authorisation

10. Date of revision of the text
11. Dosimetry (applies to radiopharmaceuticals only)
12. Instructions for preparation of radiopharmaceuticals

The SmPC also states the legal category of the medicine and indicates if the information on the medicine has been updated.

Drugs.com

Drugs.com (Drugs.com, 2019) is a useful US database on medicines and includes references to non-US products also. It provides information for both health professionals and lay persons using similar headings to the eMC. It also provides information on illnesses and suitable treatments.

The interactions checker is useful and allows the user to enter the name of a drug and find the major, moderate and minor interactions associated with it. For example (at the time of writing) the database revealed that Colchicine has some 113 major, 117 moderate and 162 minor drug interactions.

MIMS online

This is a subscription product, which provides information about medications in a concise form (Mims.co.uk, 2019).

Other useful sources

NICE evidence search

This is a useful additional information source, which includes information on the UK National Institute for Health and Care Excellence (NICE) Pathways, Guidance and Evidence services relating to the treatment of medical conditions (evidence. nhs.uk, 2019).

Importance of Assessing Medicines Brought On-Site by Personnel Before Selecting a Medication

It has been observed earlier in this Chapter that the choice of medication for individuals may be made either by an on-site HCP or by a topside doctor. In either case, it is important that the choice is made carefully, taking into account the person's medical history, known medical conditions, allergies and any purchased or prescribed medication which they are taking.

Assessment of medication

Those arriving at any remote location, should be required to declare all medication in their possession. The method by which this is done will vary between organisations, what matters is that the issue is addressed and that the system works. It is always good practice for incoming personnel to be asked about medications and also to be strongly advised, during initial safety briefings, of the importance of declaring them to site medical staff.

The site HCP should record details of the medication and then check in the BNF (or other reference work) to establish what the medicines are and their indications.

It may be that the medication is fairly innocuous for example a preventative nasal spray for allergic rhinitis. However, it is important that the details are logged so that the HCP can take it into account when prescribing.

It is also possible that an individual's illness could be the result of adverse effects from medication he has brought with him, or it may be that the HCP may discover, based on the declared medication, that the employee is suffering from a condition which may render him unfit to be on a remote site, or that a side-effect of the medication may adversely affect his ability to operate safely in that environment. In such situations the HCP should discuss the situation with a topside Doctor.

The following examples demonstrate the importance of assessing individuals' own medications.

Case Study 1. "Feldene Capsules"

- An individual arrives at the sickbay complaining of recently feeling sick. He is normally well, has no known allergies, but has a painful knee.
- Before offering any treatment for his condition, it is essential to find out if he is taking any medication and at what dose.
- This patient has just started taking Feldene Capsules 20mg — one daily, prescribed by his own doctor.
- Checking the BNF reveals that "Feldene" is a branded version of Piroxicam, which is a non-steroidal anti-inflammatory drug (NSAID).
- The BNF monograph for Piroxicam [SIDE-EFFECTS, FURTHER INFORMATION: Serious side-effects], refers the reader to information about serious gastro-intestinal side-effects relating to all NSAIDs.

- This information can also be obtained by entering Feldene in the eMC and looking at the SmPC — section 4.8 "Undesirable effects" (Medicines.org.uk, 2019).
- or Drugs.com — Feldene: Professional: Warnings and Precautions: Gastrointestinal Bleeding, Ulceration, and Perforation (drugs.com, 2019).

Discussion:

This patient's nausea is very likely to be a side-effect of his recently instituted Piroxicam therapy. In conjunction with topside medical advice, discontinuing this should be considered as a first step, rather than just using medications to treat the condition.

Case Study 2. Ibuprofen

- A worker attends the sickbay with a headache.
- He is taking the following medication prescribed by his own doctor:
  - Bricanyl (Terbutaline) Turbohaler — 1 inhalation four times a day when required.
  - Pulmicort 200 Turbohaler — 2 inhalations inhaled twice daily.

Is it best to give him Ibuprofen or Paracetamol (Acetaminophen)?

He has not taken any non-steroidal anti-inflammatory drugs previously.
- Checking the BNF monographs for both Bricanyl and Pulmicort suggest that the patient is being treated for asthma, which is confirmed by discussion.
- The BNF monograph for Ibuprofen [SIDE-EFFECTS, FURTHER INFORMATION: Serious side-effects] refers the reader to information about possible exacerbation of symptoms in asthma, relating to all NSAIDs.
- Warnings relating to asthma also appear in the eMC in SmPCs for various makes of Ibuprofen tablets [Section 4.4 Special warnings and precautions for use] as well as in Drugs.com [Ibuprofen: Professional: Warnings].

Discussion: Although problems with asthma do not result in every case, on balance, Paracetamol (Acetaminophen) seems a safer option in a remote location.

Case Study 3. Mefenamic acid

- A female employee reports to the HPC with diarrhoea. She has recently started taking Mefenamic Acid Capsules 250mg (Two capsules three times a day) for period pains.
- Checking the BNF reveals that she is taking the correct dose. Also, diarrhoea can be a side-effect of mefenamic acid and that should it occur, treatment should be immediately withdrawn and not be reintroduced.
- This information can also be obtained from the eMC, product SmPC [Section 4.8 Undesirable effects].

Discussion: With the agreement of the topside Doctor, as a first step it would seem logical to withdraw the mefenamic acid and see if the condition resolves. If it appears that mefenamic acid is the cause of the problem, then the patient should not take it in future.

Case Study 4. Uniphyllin Continus 400mg

- An individual who is allergic to penicillin arrives on site. He takes "Uniphyllin Continus" Tablets 400mg (one twice daily) to control his asthma.
- Checking the BNF and eMC SmPC for "Uniphyllin" reveal that the ingredient is theophylline and that the therapeutic dose of theophylline is very close to the toxic dose, such that changes in plasma half-life can be critical. Furthermore, 400mg twice daily is the maximum dose.
- The site stocks the following oral antibacterial medications: -

Amoxycillin Capsules 500mg
Ciprofloxacin Tablets 500mg
Clarithromycin Tablets 500mg
Co-Amoxiclav Tablets 625mg
Cefixime Tablets 200mg
Flucloxacillin Capsules 500mg
Penicillin VK Tablets 250mg
Trimethoprim Tablets 200mg

Consulting reference sources, reveals that the only one which should not prove problematic for our patient is Trimethoprim for the following reasons:

Product	Reason unsuitable for a penicillin allergic patient taking theophylline	Information sources
Amoxycillin Capsules 500mg	Penicillin antibiotic	BNF, eMC, Drugs.com
Co-Amoxiclav Tablets 625mg	Penicillin antibiotic	BNF, eMC, Drugs.com
Flucloxacillin Capsules 500mg	Penicillin antibiotic	BNF, eMC, Drugs.com
Penicillin VK Tablets 250mg	Penicillin antibiotic	BNF, eMC, Drugs.com
Cefixime Tablets 200mg	Risk of cross-allergenicity in penicillin allergic patients	BNF, eMC, Drugs.com
Ciprofloxacin Tablets 500mg	Increases plasma concentration of theophylline — may result in toxicity	BNF drug interactions (Theophylline). eMC Uniphyllin SmPC section 4.5 Drugs.com interaction checker
Clarithromycin Tablets 500mg	Increases plasma concentration of theophylline — may result in toxicity	BNF drug interactions (Theophylline). eMC Uniphyllin SmPC section 4.5 Drugs.com interaction checker

Discussion: This example demonstrates the importance of pharmaceutical information sources, clearly some medicines were ruled out due to penicillin allergy, but interestingly Clarithromycin, an apparent choice for the penicillin sensitive individual was not suitable because of a potentially serious drug interaction, which was also the case for Ciprofloxacin.

Case Study 5. Propranolol

- A remote site sickbay stocks Propranolol tablets 40mg.
- An individual arrives who uses a Ventolin (Salbutamol) Evohaler (in US Salbutamol is called Albuterol). Would it be safe for him to take Propranolol?
- Checking the BNF reveals that Propranolol is one of the Beta-adrenergic blockers (systemic) class of drugs.
- The information at the beginning of the Beta-adrenergic blockers (systemic) section in the BNF warns that this class of medicines is contra-indicated in those with asthma. This is because beta blockade can induce bronchospasm.

- This information is also available in the eMC SmPC for Propranolol Tablets 40mg (section 4.3 Contraindications) and Drugs.com [Propranolol: Professional: Contraindications]
- Also, the SmPC for Ventolin Evohaler includes a warning [Section 4.5 Drug Interactions] that Salbutamol and non-selective β-blocking drugs such as propranolol, should not usually be prescribed together.

Discussion: It is unwise for an asthmatic to be started on propranolol or other non-selective systemic beta blocking drugs.

Prescribed or Purchased Medicines which Raise Concerns

Any medicine which may impact on the safety of the individual should be queried.

The main category is potentially sedative medicines which include:

— Some cough and cold remedies (potentially sedative)
— Sedating antihistamines
— Antidepressants
— Tranquillisers
— Hypnotics
— Strong opioid analgesics (e.g. dihydrocodeine)

Any medicine which may indicate to the HCP that the worker may be unfit for remote site work should be discussed with a company doctor. Obvious examples include cardiac drugs, anti-epileptics, treatments for severe respiratory conditions, medicines for psychiatric disorders, insulin, stimulant drugs and cytotoxics.

Supplying Medicines to Individuals on Remote Sites

On a remote site, individuals will often receive single doses of medication in the sickbay under the supervision of the HCP (e.g. analgesics for headache). Additionally, there will be cases where individuals are given a quantity of medicine to take away for self-administration. Such medicines should be labelled in such a way that the recipient is clear on how to use them and, where appropriate, HCPs should provide additional counselling in the same way as a pharmacist would. This section considers the best way to supply medicines on a remote site.

Supply of an over the counter medicine in a manufacturer's original pack

In this case, there is no need for additional labelling as the supply is similar to that made when a person purchases a medicine from a pharmacy. HCPs should make sure that the recipient is aware of the importance of reading the enclosed patient information leaflet.

Counselling should be given as appropriate (e.g. with a pack of 16 Paracetamol, attention should be drawn to the dose intervals and maximum daily dose).

Dispensing medicines

When a quantity of a prescription only medicine (POM) is supplied to a person to take away from the sickbay for self-administration, whether in its manufacturer's original pack, or a smaller quantity which has been re-packaged, this constitutes dispensing, Similarly, if a quantity of an over the counter medicine is removed from its manufacturer's original pack and repackaged for an individual to take away, then this is also dispensing. Such activities are regulated in the traditional health service and standards are required for packaging and labelling.

Labelling of dispensed medicines

The labels of dispensed medicines in the UK are required to include certain particulars. Pharmacy computer systems automatically produce labels based on these requirements and ideally, remote sites should label dispensed medicines in a similar manner. The generally used particulars are:

— Name of patient
— Name and address of supplier
— Date of dispensing
— Keep out of the reach of children (or similar)
— The name of the medicinal product (including dose form and strength)
— Quantity in the container
— Directions for use
— Precautions relating to the use of the product (e.g. cautionary labelling)
— Additional, recommended notes
— Use only on your skin (if applicable)

Where medicines are split down from bulk into smaller containers, the Batch Number and Expiry Date should also be added. Where medicines are supplied in blister packed strips, the expiry date and batch reference will usually be stamped on each strip.

Dispensing a POM in a manufacturer's original pack

In this case, a dispensing label should be affixed, including the particulars listed in the section above. This is important because, it has been noted (see previously) that POMs are not required to include specific dose instructions or cautionary labelling on original packs.

Example: A patient has been prescribed Doxcline capsules 100mg
The dose label on the pack states "to be used as directed by a practitioner".

The dose prescribed by the topside Doctor is 200mg on the first day then 100mg daily. Consulting the BNF, eMC or Drugs.com will confirm this is within the licensed dose range.

Consulting the BNF monograph for Doxycycline (Medicinal Forms — Capsule) shows that it recommends the following cautionary labels: 6, 9, 11, 27.

Label 6: Do not take indigestion remedies, or medicines containing iron or zinc, 2 hours before or after you take this medicine

Label 9: Space the doses evenly throughout the day. Keep taking this medicine until the course is finished, unless you are told to stop

Label 11: Protect your skin from sunlight — even on a bright but cloudy day. Do not use sunbeds

Label 27: Take with a full glass of water

Doxycycline Capsules 100mg: Pharmacy Label
DISP KEEP OUT OF SIGHT AND REACH OF CHILDREN CHKD   DISP KEEP OUT OF SIGHT AND REACH OF CHILDREN CHKD
8 Doxycycline 100mg caps   **8 Doxycycline 100mg caps**
Take TWO on the first day then Take ONE daily   REMEDIES, IRON OR ZINC PREPARATIONS 2 HOURS BEFORE OR AFTER YOU TAKE THIS MEDICINE. SPACE THE DOSES EVENLY. KEEP TAKING UNTIL THE COURSE IS FINISHED, UNLESS YOU ARE TOLD TO STOP. PROTECT YOUR SKIN FROM SUNLIGHT. DO NOT USE SUNBEDS. TAKE WITH A FULL GLASS OF WATER DO NOT TAKE INDIGESTION
Mr Joe Bloggs   20/12/2018   Mr Joe Bloggs   20/12/2018 DayLewis Pharmacy 85 Newbegin Hornsea, East Yorkshire. continues   DayLewis Pharmacy 85 Newbegin Hornsea, East Yorkshire. HU18 1PA01964 532066   HU18 1PA01964 532066
▮▮▮ Day Lewis Pharmacy   ▮▮▮ Day Lewis Pharmacy

The BNF also includes the advice (which may be given verbally) under the heading "Directions for administration" that "Capsules should be swallowed whole with plenty of fluid, while sitting or standing. Capsules should be taken during meals." This is to avoid oesophagitis, which may occur if the capsules disintegrate before reaching the stomach.

Dispensing a quantity of medicine from a manufacturer's original pack into another container for a patient to take away from the sickbay

In this case a dispensing label (as previously) should be affixed to the container. This applies to any medicine, irrespective of legal category, which is not supplied in its manufacturer's original pack. In addition to the label, the patient information leaflet should be supplied. This can either be photocopied from the one remaining in the manufacturer's original pack, or downloaded for products listed in the eMC.

Example: Dispensing 14 Naproxen 500mg tablets from a pack of 28

There are two possible presentations of Naproxen 500mg in oral dose form, the tablet and the gastro-resistant tablet.

In both cases, the dose label on the pack states "to be used as directed by a practitioner", or similar.

For the purpose of this example, we will assume the dose to be 500mg twice daily. Consulting the BNF, eMC or Drugs.com will confirm this is an acceptable dose.

The difference arises with respect to the cautionary labelling:

Naproxen tablets 500mg
Consulting the BNF monograph for Naproxen (Medicinal Forms — Tablet) shows that it requires the following cautionary label: 21

Label 21: Take with or just after food, or a meal

Naproxen Tablets 500mg **Pharmacy dispensing label**	DISP KEEP OUT OF SIGHT AND REACH OF CHILDREN CHKD **14 Naproxen 500mg tabs** Take ONE twice a day TAKE WITH OR JUST AFTER FOOD, OR A MEAL. Mr Joe Bloggs 20/12/2018 DayLewis Pharmacy 85 Newbegin Hornsea, East Yorkshire. HU18 1PA 01964 632066 ///Day Lewis Pharmacy

Reason: This label required because naproxen can cause gastric irritation and nausea, this is less likely if food is in the stomach first.

Naproxen Gastro-resistant tablets 500mg

In this case, the BNF monograph for Naproxen (Medicinal Forms – Gastro-resistant tablet) shows that it requires the following cautionary labels: Labels 5 and 25

Label 5: Do not take indigestion remedies 2 hours before or after you take this medicine

Label 25: Swallow this medicine whole. Do not chew or crush

Naproxen Gastro-resistant tablets 500mg Pharmacy dispensing label	DISP KEEP OUT OF SIGHT AND REACH OF CHILDREN CHKD **14 Naproxen 500mg gast-res tab** Take ONE twice a day SWALLOW WHOLE.DO NOT CHEW OR CRUSH. DO NOT TAKE INDIGESTION REMEDIES 2 HOURS BEFORE OR AFTER YOU TAKE THIS MEDICINE. Mr Joe Bloggs 20/12/2018 DayLewis Pharmacy86 Newbegin Hornsea, East Yorkshire, HU18 1PA01964 532066 **Day Lewis Pharmacy**

Reason: The gastro-resistant tablets have a coating, which will not dissolve in the acid environment of the stomach, such that nausea is not a problem and there is no need for the tablets to be taken after food. However, if antacids are taken, the pH of the stomach is increased, such that there is a possibility that the coating will dissolve, such that gastric irritation and nausea may occur. Chewing or crushing the tablets would destroy the gastro-resistant coating and would also increase the risk of nausea.

These examples demonstrate the importance of carefully checking which pharmaceutical presentation of a product is being supplied.

When issuing either presentation of naproxen, it is wise to also verbally counsel the recipient and give a printed copy of the patient information leaflet which can be downloaded from the eMC (Medicines.org.uk PIL 6023, 2019; Medicines.org.uk PIL5822, 2019).

Producing labels on a remote site

It is a good idea to have the capability of producing labels with the remote site name and address on. This is best practice if any medication is taken off site (e.g. to enable an individual to complete a course of antibiotics).

It is appreciated that in a remote setting, without a pharmacy labelling system, including all of the information required for a pharmacy label can prove challenging. However, the cautionary labelling and administration advice can be passed on verbally to the patient by the HCP and attention drawn to the Patient Information Leaflet.

Containers

Remote sites should carry stocks of suitable containers for dispensed medicines. These should ideally, include small tablet bottles, cartons for dispensing blister packed tablets or capsules and small medicine bottles for liquid medicines if necessary. Also, plastic dispensing envelopes can be used for small quantities of "loose" tablets. It is also desirable to keep a stock of disposable medicine measures and spoons.

Records

It is important that proper records are kept of medications supplied or administered. In addition to the clinical records which are required, the following pharmaceutical information should be recorded for each individual receiving medication.

- Known allergies
- List of any other medication being taken by patient
- Name of medication supplied
- Quantity supplied
- Batch number
- Expiry date
- Dosage
- Whether medical advice was sought

Training

For HCPs to be able to do their job safely and effectively and to have fully meaningful conversations with supervising medical practitioners and other health professionals, they require a basic knowledge of the pharmaceutical and pharmacological aspects of their role. The best way for this to be achieved is for it to be included in their training and it is suggested that an understanding of the topics discussed in this chapter could provide a useful basis.

Also, it should be said that pharmacy topics in training courses for remote HCPs are best provided by pharmacists, who have the breadth of knowledge on the full spectrum of pharmaceutical care, such that remote HCPs may deliver benefits of the traditional pharmaceutical service to the remote environment in a legal and safe manner.

Bibliography

Committee JF. 2019. *British National Formulary. 77*. London: BMJ Group and Pharmaceutical Press.

Drug Interactions Checker. Available at https://www.drugs.com/drug_interactions.html/. Accessed on January 2nd 2019.

Drugs.com. Available at https://www.drugs.com/. Accessed on January 2nd 2019.

Electronic Medicines Compendium. Available at https://www.medicines.org.uk/emc/. Accessed on January 2nd 2019.

Feldene, Warnings and Precautions. Available at https://www.drugs.com/pro/feldene. html#s-43685-7. Accessed on January 2nd 2019.

Government of the UK. 2013. Storage, distribution and disposal of vaccines. In: *The Green Book*, Chap. 3. Available at https://www.gov.uk/government/publications/storage-distribution-and-disposal-of-vaccines-the-green-book-chapter-3. Accessed on January 2nd 2019.

HSE. 2016. *Executive Health and Safety: Health Care and First Aid on Offshore Installations and Pipeline Works. Offshore Installations and Pipeline Works (First-Aid) Regulations 1989: Approved Code of Practice and Guidance*, 3rd Edn. London: HSE Books.

Medicines Act 1968, Chapter 67. Available at http://www.legislation.gov.uk/ukpga/1968/67. Accessed on September 4th 2019.

Medicines Information: SPC & PILs. Available at http://www.mhra.gov.uk/spc-pil/. Accessed on January 2nd 2019.

MIMS.com. Available at https://www.mims.co.uk/. Accessed on January 2nd 2019.

Misuse of Drugs Act 1971, Chapter 38. Available at http://www.legislation.gov.uk/ukpga/1971/38/contents. Accessed September 4th 2019.

Misuse of Drugs Regulations SI 2001/3998 2001. Available at http://www.legislation.gov.uk/uksi/2001/3998/contents/made. Accessed on January 2nd 2019.

MSN 1768 Applying the ships' medical stores regulations 1995–2003. Available at https://www.gov.uk/government/publications/msn-1768-applying-the-ships-medical-stores-regulations-1995. Accessed on January 2nd 2019.

NICE Evidence Search. Available at https://www.evidence.nhs.uk. Accessed on January 2nd 2019.

PIL Naproxen Gastro Resistant Tablets 500mg. Available at https://www.medicines.org.uk/emc/files/pil.5822.pdf. Accessed on August 29th 2019.

PIL Naproxen Tablets 500mg. Available at https://www.medicines.org.uk/emc/files/pil.6023.pdf. Accessed on August 29th 2019.

SmPC Feldene, Section 4.8 Undesirable Effects. Available at https://www.medicines.org.uk/emc/product/2901#UNDESIRABLE_EFFECTS. Accessed on January 2nd 2019.

Summary of Product Characteristics. Available at https://www.medicines.org.uk/emc/glossary/#SmPC. Accessed on January 2nd 2019.

The Human Medicines Regulations SI 2012/1916 2012. Available at http://www.legislation.gov.uk/uksi/2012/1916/contents/made. Accessed on January 2nd 2019.

The Human Medicines Regulations SI 2012/1916 Schedule 17 2012. Available from: http://www.legislation.gov.uk/uksi/2012/1916/schedule/17/made. Accessed on January 2nd 2019.

The Offshore Installations and Pipeline Works (First-Aid) Regulations SI 1989/1671 1989. Available from: https://www.legislation.gov.uk/uksi/1989/1671/contents/made. Accessed on January 2nd 2019.

World Health Organization. 2007. *International Medical Guide for Ships*, 3rd Edn. Geneva, Switzerland: WHO Press.

Chapter

11

Occupational Health in Remote Environments

Finlay Dick and Will Ponsonby

Introduction

Workers employed in geographically remote locations are generally some distance from established health services. In addition, organisations may have operations in austere environments where climate, transport or security issues make the provision of any health service challenging. This chapter considers the scoping and delivery of occupational health services in remote or challenging environments.

Occupational health is that medical specialty concerned with the interactions between health and work (i.e. how health conditions may impact on fitness for task) and work and health (i.e. how workplace exposures may cause occupational disease and work-related illness). The role of an occupational health service typically includes developing occupational health policies and procedures, assessing workers' fitness for task, undertaking health surveillance for work-related illness (HSE, 2018) and providing advice on sickness absence management and employees' eligibility for retirement on medical grounds. In some countries large employers are legally obliged to provide occupational health services whereas in other countries occupational health services are either non-existent or limited to high hazard jobs and industries. An understanding of local legislative requirements for occupational health, including worker fitness standards and legally mandated health surveillance, is essential. Increasingly wellness and wellbeing (PWC, 2008) are also an important part of occupational health practice. The underlying aim of company wellness programmes is to improve the health and wellbeing of staff: this goes beyond the traditional model of occupational health (targeted at the prevention and management of occupational disease and provision of rehabilitation for illness and injury) to encompass the prevention of non-occupational disease and the promotion of health. This can be particularly challenging to deliver on remote sites, and for worker populations who are not familiar with the philosophy and concepts of wellness.

Examples of industries which operate in remote and/or austere environments include the merchant navy, deep sea fishing, mining, logging, oil and gas industry, military, diplomatic missions, scientific research (e.g. polar research stations) and non-governmental organisations. While some sectors, such as the upstream oil and gas industry, have well-established occupational health services (Niven and Macleod, 2009) other industries such as agriculture, fishing and forestry may have limited access to occupational health support (Liebman *et al.*, 2013). Developing countries may pose additional challenges beyond those of geographical isolation (Jones, 2000) but recall that even in highly developed countries such as Canada, Australia and the United States of America, there are large areas which are sparsely populated with limited transport links. Indeed, even in Western Europe, providing occupational health services to offshore oil and gas installations, ships and fishing vessels can present significant challenges. Many remote regions are economically disadvantaged and some have an extreme climate. Low population density, economic deprivation, poor transport links and limited health infrastructure all pose challenges to the delivery of occupational health services.

Health Risk Assessment

When an organisation is planning to develop a remote site, the first step is to carry out a health risk assessment (HRA). Ideally, occupational health specialists, occupational hygienists and human factors specialists should be involved early on in the project scoping and design process. The output of the health risk assessment will define the required occupational health support for that facility or project, including the need for fitness for task assessments and health surveillance.

The purpose of a health risk assessment is to systematically identify health hazards, assess the risks posed by these hazards and then to determine appropriate control measures. Bodies such as the UK's Health and Safety Executive (HSE) and the European Agency for Safety and Health at Work (EU-OSHA) have produced guidance on how to undertake workplace risk assessments. (HSE, 2014; EU-OSHA, 2016) However, the challenges of work in remote areas are such that industry groups including the International Petroleum Industry Environmental Conservation Association (IPIECA) and the International Council on Mining and Metals (ICMM) have produced their own industry-specific guidance on health risk assessment. (IPIECA, 2008; ICMM, 2016).

The terminology used for health risk assessments may differ between organisations but the underlying principles applied in health risk assessment are:

i)   hazard identification — physical, chemical, biological, psychological, ergonomic
ii) risk assessment
iii) risk prioritisation (where organisational resource is focussed first on high probability, high severity events)

iv) application of the hierarchy of control measures — elimination, substitution, engineering controls, administrative controls, information, instruction and training and lastly, personal protective equipment.

v) identification of recovery measures (e.g. a medical emergency response plan) should existing controls fail to prevent an untoward event.

The output from a health risk assessment should inform the organisation's Health Plan, and the approach to exploration, facility design and construction, site operation (including process and plant modification), and ultimately, asset decommissioning and environmental remediation. Each of these steps will require either a de novo health risk assessment or the review and updating of an existing health risk assessment.

An initial health risk assessment is required during the exploration phase of a project for the extractive industries such as mining or oil and gas (IPIECA, 2008). Once it is established that the project is viable then the next phase is scoping the design of the facility and its subsequent construction. During the design phase there is an opportunity to apply the learning from other, similar, facilities to optimise workplace control measures through a health risk assessment. Equally, data from published occupational health research should be considered when designing new facilities. For example, a 2006 United Kingdom Health and Safety Executive analysis of manual handling incidents in the UK upstream oil and gas industry found that 13% of the 126 incidents identified were deemed to have their root cause in poor workplace design. The authors concluded that poor design was "*at the core of many manual handling incidents*" (HSE, 2006). The involvement of ergonomists, human factors specialists and industrial hygienists at the concept development and design stages should identify best practice and, through applying best practice, design out many occupational health risks.

Large infrastructure projects may have design offices, construction sites and project management offices in different locations around the world. While most of the work will be delivered by the principal contractor and their sub-contractors the client's representatives are likely to be deployed to the contractors' facilities for extended periods to supervise design and construction. This will require significant business travel; appropriate health insurance and repatriation arrangements should be in place, and communicated to all relevant personnel (deployed personnel, their line managers, Human Resources and HSE professionals) lest employees become ill or suffer injury when on deployment or travelling.

The construction phase of large industrial projects can involve thousands or even tens of thousands of workers. The number of workers required often greatly exceeds the capacity of the local labour market: workers then have to be brought into the area for site construction. These migrant workers need to be accommodated in construction camps, floating hotels ('flotels'), trailer parks, private rented accommodation or hotels. There may be significant impacts on the local community owing to such projects including; distortion of the local labour market; a marked gender imbalance with consequent societal impacts; an increase in sexually transmitted diseases; an increase in substance misuse (alcohol, illicit drugs); increased crime; heavy traffic; increased pressure on local facilities; housing shortages; and increased demands for healthcare. Not all of the impacts are negative; there may be new, well-paid employment opportunities for local workers, and these workers can be trained in new skills and acquire new trades. A health impact assessment (WHO, 2018) is usually undertaken in advance of major projects to identify and ameliorate these issues so far as is practicable.

It is also important to communicate with the community honestly about the project and its economic impact. Jobs during the construction phase of a project may be short lived and the number of workers required to operate a facility will usually be significantly less than that required during construction. Therefore, the community needs to be able to benefit from the activity during the construction phase, but also needs to plan for the long term. This long-term planning should also include the eventual decommissioning and closure of the facility. Inevitably communities and the local economy will adapt to, and may become dependent on, a large employer in that area. The eventual closure of such a facility can cause significant economic and social dislocation in that locale.

Measures to reduce the impact of large numbers of travelling workers on the local health services may include setting up a primary care facility on site. The site health centre provides both immediate trauma care and primary care for the large numbers of construction workers living away from home. During plant construction, some, but not all, projects will also undertake occupational health surveillance of the principal contractor's workers at the site health centre. The project needs to carefully consider what medical services it will offer to the local community. It is important to recognise that healthcare provision for the local population is the responsibility of government. The project should aim to support the national health service rather than attempt to replace it.

For accommodation camps and barges ('flotels'), rigorous attention to food and water safety (HSE, 2011) is necessary as food and water borne illness can spread rapidly in such semi-closed communities. One recurring problem during site construction is that day labourers will come to work when ill with gastroenteritis, and so bring illness on site: the driver for their actions being the fear that if they don't come to work, they may lose a day's pay or even their job. Besides food and water borne diseases, Norovirus outbreaks can result in high numbers of casualties (>50% of workforce) that can, in extreme cases, result in cessation of operations. All food handlers should be medically fit for food handling duties (FSA, 2009). It usually falls to the site medic or a member of the wider health team to monitor food hygiene and water management on site: a good knowledge of food hygiene is required. Larger organisations may employ or retain environmental health specialists to undertake this important work. It is prudent for the occupational health team to have a plan to quarantine or remove those who are sick from site to minimise the spread of any outbreak and its impact on operations. Organisations ignore the potential for major outbreaks of food or water borne illnesses at construction camps at their peril. In addition to the obvious risk of delays to the project, the potential media coverage of such outbreaks carries the risk of reputational harm for the organisation. For example, in Haiti, following a major earthquake, relief workers brought cholera into the country which caused a major cholera epidemic and led to the deaths of over 10,000 people (BBC, 2016).

A health risk assessment review should be undertaken once the site is operational to ensure that workplace control measures are functioning as intended and that predicted occupational exposures are satisfactorily controlled. Where workplace exposure monitoring, biological monitoring or biological effect monitoring indicates that control is inadequate then additional controls should be instituted. The identification of pre-clinical occupational disease or indeed overt occupational disease in workers (staff or contractors) demands a review of the existing workplace controls to establish why such preventable disease has occurred (ICMM, 2016). In addition, significant changes to plant or processes require that the health risk assessment be revisited. Finally, when the time comes for abandonment of a site then the health risk assessment should be reviewed and updated prior to final decommissioning and site rehabilitation. From this it can be seen that while a health risk assessment is a formal process it is an iterative one which is continually evolving.

The health risk assessment will need to address:

- site location
- distance and time to medical care
- nature of the operation
- specific occupational health risks e.g. dust, noise, carcinogens
- occupational exposure limits (OELS) — which exposure limits should apply?
- health surveillance relevant to identified risks
- environmental hazards
- climate
- infectious disease and vector-borne disease
- drugs and alcohol
- food and water safety
- community health and prevalent diseases — some workers may be drawn from the local community — how will that impact on the operation?

- wider community health as the surrounding population may look to the site for medical care
- legislation — HSE, employment and fitness for work requirements (which may not be risk-based)
- company and industry standards — use the hierarchy of controls to decide which standards apply
- medical emergency response requirements

Health Plan

Following the health risk assessment, the next step is to develop a health plan. The scope of the site health service needs to be defined: specifically, who is to be covered by that service, e.g. expatriate staff / nationals / contractors / dependents / local residents /other foreign nationals and, if so, on what basis. The provision of occupational health services is generally restricted to workers. The usual approach, in the absence of an agreement to the contrary, is that each employer is responsible for arranging the occupational health provision for their own staff. A related issue is who will deliver the occupational health service and where? The options are an in-house occupational health service managed and delivered by the business' own occupational health department or alternatively scoping and overseeing the provision of an outsourced occupational health service delivered by a contracted occupational health provider. Whichever model is selected, an additional consideration is whether the service will be staffed by expatriate health workers (be they on a long-term deployment in country or international rotators), national personnel or a mixture of both. Government policy, either at regional or national level may mandate the use of local health staff to maximise employment in-country and to build local healthcare capacity. Among the advantages of using local healthcare staff are; that they are likely to be familiar with existing health infrastructure, understand national laws as they apply to healthcare and have a shared language and culture with local workers.

Who is at Risk?

The inverse care law: *"that the availability of good medical care tends to vary inversely with the need of the population served"* (Hart, 1971) also holds true in occupational health (Steege *et al.*, 2014). Occupational health services are most accessible to well-educated, high status, managerial staff employed by major organisations but, as a group, they are the least likely to be exposed to significant workplace risks.

Both occupational injury and illness tend to be commonest among unskilled or semi-skilled workers. Disadvantaged groups that are especially vulnerable include migrant workers (Biering *et al.*, 2017; Moyce and Schenker, 2018; Reid *et al.*, 2018), ethnic minorities (Franklin *et al.*, 2016) and those with limited education. Workers employed in insecure work, including those paid as day labourers or agency workers are at increased risk of workplace accidents (Michaels, 2015; Giraudo *et al.*, 2016) and are those least able to speak up when workplaces have poor health and safety practices (Landsbergis *et al.*, 2014). To address this all contracts should include clauses to specify terms and conditions of employment for the contractor's workforce as well as defining health and safety performance criteria. This is important as a recent systematic review of precarious employment and occupational accidents concluded that the evidence tends to support an association between precarious employment (having multiple jobs or work as an agency worker) and workplace accidents and injuries (Koranyi *et al.*, 2018). Women, at least in Europe, are over-represented among those in insecure employment (Campos-Serna *et al.*, 2013). There are also the ethical issues thrown up by contractors who are employed as day labourers — where no work equals no pay. The ethical challenge may arise of whether it is better to allow workers to be exposed to work which (while not illegal in that jurisdiction) may adversely affect their health or, alternatively, to suspend work and so leave these labourers with no pay until the issue is resolved.

There is no universally accepted definition of an expatriate worker: Jones has suggested the working definition of someone deployed, for at least six months, into a host country (Jones, 2000). Expatriate workers may be in accompanied postings where their partner and immediate family relocate with them to the host country or in unaccompanied ('single status') postings. A significant number of expatriate postings, especially first expatriate postings, end in failure, usually for psychosocial reasons (Truman *et al.*, 2011), often owing to health problems affecting family members, rather than a lack of occupational competence in the employee (Jones, 2000). Research into expatriate workers' health has tended to focus on those undertaking extended foreign postings of several months' duration. However, there are two other groups of workers who share some of the risks of the traditional expatriate worker. These groups are: i) the frequent business traveller making multiple short duration visits to other countries and ii) the international rotator who travels on a recurring basis into a country for periods but who is domiciled either in their home country or a third country. Rotating staff are often found working on sites such as offshore oil rigs or geographically remote mines and may be engaged on a 'fly in/fly out' work schedule. Each of these groups throws up its own challenges for the provision and delivery of healthcare. Frequent business travellers tend to be in senior roles within organisations and as such travel health, work pressure and fatigue management (IPIECA, 2007a; IPIECA, 2013) are the main issues. International rotators share many of the workplace exposures experienced by expatriates but may have a significant travel commitment (and consequent fatigue burden) on a recurring basis (IPIECA,

2015). In general, however, both international rotators and expatriates are in supervisory or managerial roles; although exposed to the hazards of transport to, and work in, remote or austere locations, they do not have the same degree of workplace exposures experienced by local staff and contractors. That said, personnel working in developing countries may experience higher occupational exposures to hazardous substances (e.g. asbestos, benzene) than in developed countries where exposures to such agents may be better controlled.

Occupational Health Services

The organisation has to decide what, if any, specialist occupational health services are to be delivered on site, remotely by telemedicine or at bases in regional centres. One issue which must be considered is the logistics of setting up and supplying remote site health facilities if these are to include occupational health services. *These issues are considered further in the chapter:* "Medical Co-ordination and Management".

These services must comply with national legislation, company and industry standards — whichever is the most stringent. In terms of liability, where you have international workers on site they may be covered by the legislation in their country of origin.

The health risk assessment should have identified the key occupational risks (e.g. noise, hand arm vibration, dusts, carcinogens, skin irritants/sensitisers etc.) and the groups of workers (sometimes termed 'Similarly Exposed Groups' or SEGs) requiring health surveillance. Defining Similarly Exposed Groups can be challenging where workers move between roles with differing exposures and especially when determining at pre-placement assessments whether a worker should be subject to health surveillance for a particular agent. The advice of an industrial hygienist familiar with the work site and the varying exposures on site (similar jobs on the same site, e.g. face workers in deep coal mines, may have differing exposures dependent on their work location) is essential in achieving accurate and meaningful allocation to the most appropriate Similarly Exposed Group.

The decision as to what, if any occupational health service is delivered on site will depend on many factors including local health and safety laws, the nature of the workplace exposure, the skill set of the site health staff, and the costs associated with whichever option for health surveillance is selected. Depending on national regulations, some health surveillance may only be delivered by approved health professionals e.g. in the UK health surveillance is legally mandated for specific occupational exposures including lead (HSE, 2002), ionising radiation (HSE, 2017) and asbestos (HSE, 2013). In that situation it may be impossible to deliver the required health surveillance on a remote site and instead staff will have to travel to the nearest approved medical examiner to undergo the required health checks. However, for other workplace hazards such as noise, skin or respiratory sensitizers then health surveillance may be delivered by any suitably qualified health worker. For these exposures the initial occupational health surveillance may be administered on site and the results reviewed. Abnormal or technically unsatisfactory results can then be repeated and if necessary, the worker reviewed by an occupational health nurse/physician at a regional centre. There is some evidence (Petsonk et al., 2013) from developed countries that occupational diseases which have been under satisfactory control (e.g. coal workers pneumoconiosis) are increasing, implying poorer workplace exposure controls, perhaps due to increasing mechanisation (Blanc and Seaton, 2016). Recently in Queensland, Australia a failure in the State-run health surveillance scheme resulted in the re-emergence of coal workers' pneumoconiosis (CWP) in Queensland, with 8 cases of CWP being identified over several months (Monash University, 2016).

The benefit of undertaking on-site occupational health screening is that the role of the site nurse/medic is enhanced; the employer may reduce downtime associated with health surveillance; and the employee gains by not having to attend a medical review outside of their scheduled work pattern. The downsides include the cost of purchasing, maintaining and calibrating medical equipment which may be under-utilised and the associated challenges of quality assurance of any health surveillance done at multiple remote sites. Standard operating procedures for health surveillance, training of all staff undertaking surveillance, standardised screening equipment, and standardised calibration and maintenance of equipment reduces the risks associated with undertaking occupational health screening at remote sites. Arrangements for secure data transfer that comply with local data protection regulations are required if health surveillance data is to be transferred either physically or electronically and especially if it is to be transferred to a third country.

Staffing

The requirements of country or state health licensing may make it difficult or impossible for expatriate clinical staff to practise in that jurisdiction. However, in some countries occupational health services are not well developed and recruiting local health workers with the required skill set may not be possible. Nonetheless, the need for proficiency in the language(s) used by staff at site, awareness of national and state legislative requirements, knowledge of prevalent health problems, and targets for employment of local labour, may make it preferable to employ local health professionals. In that situation investment in the professional development of local health staff, including suitable training in occupational health is key.

Sometimes this can be achieved by deploying one, or more, expatriate occupational health specialists as advisors to the local health team. In addition, there are distance learning, and web-based training courses available in occupational medicine.

Telemedicine and distance training facilities can also support the training and development of staff in remote locations.

However, businesses in developing suitable site health facilities should not seek to usurp the role of government in the development and provision of wider health services such as public health, primary care, secondary care and communicable disease control. In general, it is to the benefit of all parties for multi-nationals to support national or state initiatives rather than set their own public health agenda which may, or may not, coincide with the health needs of the local populace.

Particular consideration is required where postings to remote areas involve deployment into a high threat area e.g. conflict zones or areas having a high risk of kidnapping or terrorism. It has been shown that increasing deployment length in conflict zones or high-threat postings is associated with poorer psychological wellbeing both in military personnel (Buckman et al., 2011) and in diplomats (Dunn et al., 2015a.). Recent qualitative research (Whittaker-Howe et al., 2017) has highlighted that remote-area medics, working in Iraq, experience psychological difficulties owing to their extended deployment, professional isolation, inter-cultural issues and clinical under-load with the attendant risk of 'skills-fade'. While the evidence base favouring shorter deployments in health workers is limited it seems likely that long deployments in high-threat postings should be avoided where possible. One survey (Dunn et al., 2015b.) found that current policies around deployment length for diplomatic personnel in high-threat postings are not evidence-based. Deployment policies within organisations posting personnel to high threat regions should limit lengthy deployments and avoid unpredictable extensions to deployments.

Occupational Health Benchmarks

A decision has to be made as to what occupational health benchmarks (IPIECA, 2007b; ICMM, 2014) are to be followed by an organisation (national regulations/ industry standards/ 'best practice') with regards to fitness for task/health surveillance/exposure standards/occupational disease recording. In addition, should the chosen standards apply only to operations in that country or across all the company's sites worldwide? The delivery of standardised, quality, occupational healthcare across a range of operating sites requires arrangements for equipment calibration, regular maintenance of equipment, staff training, good clinical governance and medical indemnity arrangements.

Where national or state laws stipulate a specific approach to occupational health issues then organisations have to demonstrate compliance with that law. However, in many cases there is no legally mandated approach. For example, for the majority of chemicals no occupational exposure limits (OELs) exist (Deveau *et al.*, 2015) whether as mandatory or recommended limits. In contrast, a small number of chemicals have multiple OELs published by different organisations which may have different risk tolerances and may interpret the same scientific data in differing ways. In such cases an organisation needs to decide what standards they are following and why (Deveau *et al.*, 2015). By standardising occupational health policies and procedures (while still meeting all local laws) an organisation can better understand where in the business occupational health problems lie. However, even in developed countries, achieving a harmonised approach across multiple sites in a single organisation can be difficult.

Fitness for Task

One of the main roles of any occupational health service is determining workers' fitness; both their fitness for task and, in the case of services supporting remote sites, employees' fitness for deployment to remote locations. A key element of assessing fitness for task is ensuring that the individual is fit to undertake their task without risk to their own, or others', health and safety (Serra *et al.*, 2007). To determine fitness for task it is important to establish the standard against which an employee's fitness will be judged. Occupational fitness standards may be determined by national or regional governments and may require an assessment by any registered medical practitioner or a limited number of approved medical examiners. In the United Kingdom an example of the former group of medicals is the assessment of fitness to drive whereas the latter group includes pilot medical fitness, seafarers' medicals and fitness to dive assessments. In the absence of legally mandated fitness for task regulations the occupational health physician must look to either industry guidance e.g. OGUK medical fitness standards for offshore oil workers (OGUK, 2018) or to company specific guidance on fitness for task standards e.g. refinery fire-fighter fitness standards.

Occupational fitness assessments may, or may not, be evidence-based (Serra *et al.*, 2007) but in general pre-placement health screening lacks a good evidence base (Pachman, 2009; Schaafsma, 2016). Pre-employment screening by health questionnaire alone is not effective and has a low predictive value in detecting future health problems (Madan and Williams, 2012). Pre-placement health assessments should focus on functional capacity for the role and consider what workplace adjustments might allow the worker with a pre-existing health problem to safely undertake that posting. Pre-placement assessments are not a good predictor of subsequent sickness absence and should not be used for that purpose.

One of the challenges of assessing fitness for task is that whatever fitness standards are applied they may be either out of date or may not be directly relevant to that specific work situation. For example, updating primary legislation can be time consuming and as a result legally mandated fitness standards may not have kept pace with evolving medical treatments. Sometimes there are no local medical fitness standards and a decision has to be made as to whether other industry fitness standards are applicable. The UK medical fitness guidelines for offshore oil workers (OGUK, 2018) were developed for use on the UK Continental Shelf. However, these medical standards are sometimes applied to operations elsewhere in the world where climate, healthcare and prevalent medical conditions all differ from those in the UK.

Some countries may set rigid health screening requirements, in particular for communicable diseases, for expatriate workers. However, prospective expatriates coming from a low endemicity area may be at much greater risk of acquiring communicable disease from the local populace than vice versa. Note that to protect employee confidentiality the health assessment should be carried out early in the expatriation process and any employee deemed medically unfit withdrawn from the selection process without detriment to their subsequent employment or career progression.

Transport is a major hazard in construction as well as in mining, onshore oil and gas and other extractive industries. Poor safety standards and inadequate driver training are particular issues in developing countries. The International Association of Oil and Gas Producers (IOGP) has produced extensive guidance on this issue including advice on assessing driver fitness (IOGP, 2006). National standards for medical fitness of occupational drivers exist in many countries (e.g. NZ Transport Agency, 2014; FMCSA, 2017; DVLA, 2018) but (subject to equality legislation) this does not preclude organisations applying their own, more demanding medical fitness standards on high hazard sites such as opencast mines or petroleum refineries.

In general, fitness for deployment assessments should be done well in advance of the planned mobilisation to a remote site. This should give sufficient time to seek medical reports from attending physicians where there are specific concerns regarding the impact of the underlying condition, its treatment or prognosis. Stable medical conditions which are unlikely to decompensate acutely are easier to accommodate in remote sites than those conditions which can deteriorate rapidly and potentially need hospitalisation. Possible outcomes of fitness for task assessments include fit; fit with restrictions (such restrictions may be permanent or temporary), temporarily unfit and permanently unfit (Schaafsmaz, 2016). Despite published guidance on criteria for fitness assessments there is likely to be significant differences between clinicians when assessing the same worker, reflecting their prior experience, training, knowledge of local conditions and their risk tolerance. Many bodies which publish occupational fitness standards (e.g. UK Maritime and Coastguard Agency) have in place an appeal system to reduce the possibility that an individual is unreasonably denied a role owing to a pre-existing medical condition.

Legislation has been introduced over the last four decades in many developed countries (e.g. the Americans with Disabilities Act (ADA, 1990) and the UK's Equality Act 2010 to reduce the gap in employment opportunities for those living with impairments. As a consequence, workers with medical conditions (fixed or evolving) are now more likely to be working in remote areas than would have once been the case. In general, fixed impairments are easier to assess than evolving conditions as, other than the effects of normal ageing (which can lead to gradual de-compensation over time), any deficits are likely to be stable.

Another important aspect of fitness for work are the more acute health conditions that will not be picked up on a periodic medical. Such issues include:

1. Use of alcohol and illegal drugs
2. Prescription medications which can impair mental acuity
3. Fatigue
4. Mental health
5. Acute illness

There should be policies to govern the above, with clear guidelines on what is allowed, and when and where a worker should report any concerns. The supervisor should check workers at the beginning of each shift for obvious signs of impairment. This may include requesting drug and alcohol testing 'with cause' where an individual appears impaired or is clearly under the influence of alcohol of drugs. Failure to comply with company substance misuse policies may result in disciplinary action up to and including dismissal.

The final decision as to who is deemed fit to mobilise to a remote site should be made by health workers familiar with the worksite, the local healthcare facilities and local environmental conditions. Difficulties can arise where an employee with a pre-existing medical condition is offered a (potentially lucrative) posting to a remote site only to be deemed medically unfit for posting. That medical support in remote areas may be very basic and is not always appreciated by those working in developed countries used to first world healthcare and transport links.

Health Surveillance

Health surveillance in occupational medicine (HSE, 2018) is the systematic monitoring of workers' health to identify early (ideally pre-clinical) signs and symptoms of adverse health effects of workplace exposures. Health surveillance is a legal requirement for specified occupational groups in some countries (HSE, 2002; HSE, 2013; HSE, 2017). Agents subject to mandatory health surveillance include carcinogens, skin and respiratory sensitizers and other agents that may cause irreversible health effects or even death e.g. ionising radiation, lead (Pb), asbestos. There are many factors to consider before introducing a workplace health surveillance programme. The health risk assessment should have highlighted where residual risks to health exist. The advice of an experienced industrial hygienist can be helpful in identifying all personnel exposed at levels where health effects may occur. For example, cleaners and maintenance staff are sometimes overlooked when considering 'who is at risk?' On the other hand, it is important not to include personnel who have zero, or limited exposure to that agent, as this adds costs. In addition, it makes it harder to identify early warning signs from surveillance data by diluting the results for those workers truly exposed with data from people who are not actually at risk. The recurring costs of health surveillance should not be underestimated. In general, it is preferable to design out risks and improve workplace control measures rather than rely on expensive ongoing health surveillance.

Health surveillance needs to be well-designed, targeted at those who are truly at risk, effectively communicated to all interested parties (management, workers, trades unions, worker councils), supported by a health surveillance policy, regularly monitored and subject to quality assurance. Grouped, anonymised, feedback of the results of health surveillance should be given to site management, safety committees and exposed personnel (HSE, 2018). When done properly, workplace health surveillance, by detecting pre-clinical health effects of workplace exposures, can act as an early warning that existing controls are either inadequate or not functioning as designed.

Problems can arise where health surveillance is done badly (Monash University, 2016). For example, surveillance may be conducted without the support of an agreed health surveillance policy, workers with minimal exposure to the agent of concern may be inappropriately entered into the health surveillance programme 'just in case', inadequately trained health staff may undertake surveillance, measurements may be gathered using uncalibrated equipment or samples may sent to a laboratory without adequate quality assurance in place. In remote areas there can be difficulties in recruiting and retaining appropriately skilled staff, getting competent technicians to service equipment may be problematic (one option is to backload equipment for calibration to a regional centre but then either replacement equipment is needed or health surveillance must be suspended until the calibrated instrument is returned), and finally, a suitable laboratory with experience of occupational health bio-monitoring may be hard to identify. Resolving these issues can be both costly and time consuming.

Absence Management

Sickness absence can be defined as any absence, attributed to illness or injury by the employee, and accepted as such by the employer. Sickness absence can be sub-divided into short-term absence and long-term absence (NICE, 2009). Definitions vary but most organisations would deem any absence of greater than 28 days as being long term. Short term absence may occur either as an isolated episode or as part of a recurrent pattern of absences. Site health services will be involved in the immediate management of any illness or injury occurring on site and determining fitness to return to duty. However, where the worker is unfit for work for an extended period or requires hospital treatment, the subsequent review of fitness for work will more often be the responsibility of occupational health services off site. For example, Oil & Gas UK medical guidance (OGUK, 2018) advises that where a worker requires medical evacuation from an offshore oil platform they will typically (but not inevitably) need review by an Oil & Gas UK registered doctor before they can return to work offshore.

Site health professionals should monitor the attendance of workers at health facilities to identify patterns of illness in individual workers or work groups. For the individual worker, recurring presentations to the medical centre with similar symptoms may indicate a poorly controlled chronic medical condition such as migraine or asthma. In that situation the worker should be advised to seek review by their usual medical practitioner on their return home. The site clinician and their remote medical support should, however, first consider the possibility of an occupational aetiology for the worker's recurrent health problem before advising referral back to the employee's usual medical practitioner. Where a group of workers presents to the medical centre with similar symptoms either at the same time or within a few hours of each other then the possibility of a shared aetiology should be considered. Such a presentation, dependent on symptoms, might indicate communicable disease or the (real or perceived) effects of a shared workplace or environmental exposure.

Case Study 1

A medic on an offshore oil platform contacted their shore-based medical advisor: several of the drill crew had presented over a 48-hour period with hand dermatitis. The drill crew were using oil-based drilling mud but owing to poor personal protective equipment (PPE) they were inadequately protected from exposure. In addition, limited cleaning facilities meant that their exposed skin was not being adequately decontaminated. Improvements to work practices and personal protective equipment to reduce exposure together with better cleaning facilities were required.

Non-Occupational Hazards

In addition to occupational hazards there are a number of environmental, transport and psychological factors which, while not directly linked to work, can impact on the remote site and its operation. Work locations where environmental extremes such as excessive heat, severe cold or low atmospheric pressure (due to high altitude) can adversely affect worker safety and may influence workers' ability or willingness to use required personal protective equipment such as chemical resistant suits or self-contained breathing apparatus.

Transport safety is a major issue for any business but especially those working in the developing world where inadequate regulation, poor infrastructure, limited vehicle maintenance and poor safety culture increase the risks of transport accidents. Linked to transport safety is the issue of employee fatigue although this is one example of a hazard which in part arises out with the operational perimeter (owing to family commitments, lifestyle, young children, second jobs, inconsiderate neighbours etc.) and partly within the site's boundary (owing to inadequate sleeping accommodation on sites, poorly designed shift patterns, long hours of duty, insufficient staffing levels, frequent call-outs for workers on-call, an organisational culture which implicitly, or sometimes explicitly, demands long hours of managers and supervisors etc.). The oil industry has produced guidance on managing fatigue in fly in/fly out operations (IPIECA, 2015) which includes considerations of the timing of travel and rest breaks to ensure that personnel arrive at their destinations safe and well rested. Many mining companies have also developed fatigue management programmes as the costs of fatigue related transport accidents in large mines can be significant.

Culture shock can be defined as the anxiety and stress which may be caused by moving to a new and unfamiliar culture where communication and behavioural norms differ from the individual's home culture (Muecke et al., 2011). The greater the cultural 'distance' from the person's home culture the greater the challenges they face. On return to their home country the traveller then goes through a period of readjustment to their home culture which has been termed reverse culture shock (Stewart and Leggat, 1998).

Cultural norms shape everyone's expectations both of illness and of medical treatment. Poor cultural competence can adversely affect workers' health and effectiveness. A recent systematic review set in Saudi Arabia found evidence of poor cultural competence together with limited language abilities among expatriate health workers despite ongoing government orientation programmes for expatriate health workers (Almutairi, 2015).

Health Interfaces

There is an overlap between primary healthcare, public health and occupational health. The quality of, and access to, existing primary health services and public health issues can interact with, and impact on, occupational health practice. This issue relates both to fitness for posting decisions and the approach to the management of suspected occupational health illness. For example, a prospective expatriate (or their spouse/partner/dependant) may present at a pre-posting assessment with a health condition which the host country's health services cannot adequately support. In that situation the proposed deployment may not go ahead even though the individual is fit for task. Similarly, a worker with a communicable disease e.g. HIV infection may be fit for work but sovereign government public health requirements may bar them from even entering the country. In such cases it may be necessary to carry out pre-deployment testing. Such pre-deployment testing can identify those who might otherwise fail a government mandated test in-country, resulting in the trauma of arrest and deportation for the worker and significant costs for the company. It is important for all prospective travellers to be aware of what medicines are legally permissible in all countries in their travel itinerary including both their final destination country and all the countries they may transit through. In some countries illicit drug or alcohol use can be heavily punished: as a result, companies may decide not to undertake drug or alcohol screening in that country.

Summary

The delivery of occupational health services to remote sites poses many challenges. The occupational health support required by a remote site should be guided by the site's health risk assessment and implemented through a health plan. Any health risk assessment for a remote site needs to identify the health hazards (workplace, environmental, and non-occupational hazards), assess the risks, identify who is at risk and how, review the adequacy of existing workplace controls and determine what else needs to be done if these controls are inadequate to protect health, record the risk assessment and keep it under review so that it remains up to date. That health risk assessment will then inform the health plan which should define what the requirements are for occupational health support including, defining benchmarks e.g. for occupational chemical exposure standards, fitness for task assessments, health surveillance and the occupational health aspects of absence management. The provision of occupational health services may be delivered at site, partly at site and partly at regional centres or wholly at regional centres. This is dependent on many factors including the available health professionals' skills, the size of the remote site and the nature of the occupational hazards. Monitoring of occupational health performance against other company sites, the wider industry and national occupational health benchmarks will assist in determining what continuous improvement is required for that site.

References

Almutairi, Khalid M. (2015). Culture and language differences as a barrier to provision of quality care by the health workforce in Saudi Arabia. *Saudi Med J* **36(4)**: 425–431.

Americans with Disabilities Act (ADA). 1990, as amended. Available at https://www.ada.gov/pubs/adastatute08.htm. Accessed on March 6th 2018.

BBC. 2016. UN admits role in Haiti's deadly cholera outbreak, 19th August. Available at http://www.bbc.co.uk/news/world-latin-america-37126747. Accessed on April 30th 2018.

Biering K, Lander F and Rasmussen K. 2017. Work injuries among migrant workers in Denmark. *Occup Environ Med* **74**: 235–242.

Blanc PD and Seaton A. 2016. Pneumoconiosis redux — coal workers pneumoconiosis and silicosis are still a problem. *Am J Respir Crit Care Med* **193**: 603–605.

Buckman JE, Sundin J, Greene T, Fear NT, Dandeker C, Greenberg N and Wessely S. 2011. The impact of deployment length on the health and well-being of military personnel: a systematic review of the literature. *Occup Environ Med* **68**: 69–76.

Campos-Serna J, Ronda-Pérez E, Artazcoz L, Moen BE and Benavides FG. 2013. Gender inequalities in occupational health related to the unequal distribution of working and employment conditions: a systematic review. *Int J Equity Health* **12**: 57.

Deveau M, Chen CP, Johanson G, Krewski D, Maier A, Niven KJ, Ripple S, Schulte PA, Silk J, Urbanus JH, Zalk DM and Niemeier RW. 2015. The global landscape of occupational exposure limits — implementation of harmonization principles to guide limit selection. *J Occup Environ Hyg* **12**: S127–144.

Driver Vehicle Licensing Agency (DVLA). 2018. Assessing fitness to drive — a guide for medical professionals. https://www.gov.uk/government/uploads/system/uploads/attachment_data/file/670819/assessing-fitness-to-drive-a-guide-for-medical-professionals.pdf. Accessed on March 5th 2018

Dunn R, Kemp V, Patel D, Williams R and Greenberg N. 2015a. Deployment guidelines for diplomats: current policy and practice. *Occup Med (Lond)* **65**: 535–541.

Dunn R, Williams R, Kemp V, Patel D and Greenberg N. 2015b. Systematic review: deployment length and the mental health of diplomats. *Occup Med (Lond)* **65**: 32–38.

European Agency for Safety and Health at Work (EU-OSHA). 2016. Risk assessment tool: OiRA — Online interactive Risk Assessment. Available at https://osha.europa.eu/en/tools-and-publications/oira. Accessed on March 6th 2018.

Federal Motor Carrier Safety Administration (FMCSA). 2017. Driver medical fitness for duty. Available at https://www.fmcsa.dot.gov/medical/driver-medical-requirements/driver-medical-fitness-duty. Accessed on March 6th 2018.

Food Standards Agency (FSA). 2009. Food handlers: fitness to work regulatory guidance and best practice advice for food business operators. Available at https://www.food.gov.uk/sites/default/files/multimedia/pdfs/publication/fitnesstoworkguide09v3.pdf. Accessed on March 6th 2018.

Franklin P, Reid A, Olsen N, Peters S, de Klerk N, Brims F, Threlfall T, Murray R and Musk AB. 2016. Incidence of malignant mesothelioma in Aboriginal people in Western Australia. *Aust N Z J Public Health* **40**: 383–387.

Giraudo M, Bena A, Leombruni R and Costa G. 2016. Occupational injuries in times of labour market flexibility: the different stories of employment-secure and precarious workers. *BMC Public Health* **16**: 150.

Hart JT. The inverse care law. *The Lancet* 1971 **1**: 405–412.

Health and Safety Executive (HSE). 2002. *Control of Lead at Work Regulations 2002*, 3rd Edn. Approved Code of Practice and Guidance, L132, 3rd Edn. Sudbury: HSE Books.

HSE. 2006. Manual Handling Incidents Database: A Compilation and Analysis of Offshore Industry Reports. Research Report 500.

HSE. 2011. Offshore food essentials OFE 1: food safety and hygiene. Available at http://www.hse.gov.uk/pubns/guidance/ofe1.pdf. Accessed on March 6th 2018.

HSE. 2013. *Control of Asbestos Regulations 2012*. Approved Code of Practice and Guidance, L143, 2nd Edn. Sudbury: HSE Books.

HSE. 2014. *Risk Assessment: A Brief Guide to Controlling Risks in the Workplace*. INDG163, ISBN: 9780717664634.

HSE. 2017. *Ionising Radiation Regulations 2017*. Approved Code of Practice and Guidance. L121, 2nd Edn. Sudbury: HSE books.

HSE. 2018. Health surveillance. http://www.hse.gov.uk/health-surveillance/. Accessed on March 2nd 2018.

International Association of Oil and Gas Producers (IOGP). 2006. Land transport safety. Available at http://www.iogp.org/oil-and-gas-safety/land-transport-safety/. Accessed on March 5th 2018.

International Council on Mining & Metals (ICMM). 2014. Health and safety performance indicators. Available at https://www.icmm.com/website/publications/pdfs/health-and-safety/6613.pdf. Accessed on March 21st 2018.

ICMM. 2016. *Good Practice Guidance on Occupational Health Risk Assessment*, 2nd Edn. Available at https://www.icmm.com/website/publications/pdfs/health-and-safety/161212_health-and-safety_health-risk-assessment_2nd-edition.pdf. Accessed on February 5th 2018.

International Petroleum Industry Environmental Conservation Association (IPIECA). 2007a. Managing fatigue in the workplace. Available at http://www.ipieca.org/resources/good-practice/managing-fatigue-in-the-workplace/ Accessed on March 5th 2018.

IPIECA. 2007b. Health performance indicators: a guide for the oil and gas industry OCP Report number 393. Available at http://www.ipieca.org/resources/good-practice/health-performance-indicators/ Accessed on March 21st 2018.

IPIECA. 2008. Roadmap to health risk assessment. Available at http://www.ipieca.org/resources/good-practice/health-risk-assessment/. Accessed on February 5th 2018.

IPIECA. 2013. Performance indicators for fatigue risk management systems. Available at http://www.ipieca.org/resources/good-practice/performance-indicators-for-fatigue-risk-management-systems/. Accessed on March 5th 2018.

IPIECA. 2015. Fatigue in fly-in, fly-out operations. Guidance document for the oil and gas industry. Available at http://www.ipieca.org/resources/good-practice/fatigue-in-fly-in-fly-out-operations-guidance-document-for-the-oil-and-gas-industry/. Accessed on March 5th 2018.

Jones S. 2000. Medical aspects of expatriate health: health threats. *Occup Med (Lond)* **50**: 572–578.

Koranyi I, Jonsson J, Rönnblad T, Stockfelt L and Bodin T. 2018. Precarious employment and occupational accidents and injuries — a systematic review. *Scand J Work Environ Health* **44**: 341–335.

Landsbergis PA, Grzywacz JG and LaMontagne AD. 2014. Work organization, job insecurity, and occupational health disparities. *Am J Ind Med* **57**: 495–515.

Liebman AK, Wiggins MF, Fraser C, Levin J, Sidebottom J and Arcury TA. 2013. Occupational health policy and immigrant workers in the agriculture, forestry, and fishing sector. *Am J Ind Med* **56**: 975–984.

Madan I and Williams S. 2012. Is pre-employment health screening by questionnaire effective? *Occup Med (Lond)* **62**: 112–116.

Michaels D. 2015. Adding inequality to injury: the costs of failing to protect workers on the job. Washington, DC: US Department of Labor, Occupational Safety and Health Administration. Available at https://www.dol.gov/osha/report/20150304⊠inequality.pdf. Accessed on March 5th 2018.

Monash Centre for Occupational and Environmental Health and University of Illinois at Chicago School of Public Health. 2016. Review of respiratory component of the Coal Mine Workers' Health Scheme for the Queensland Department of Natural Resources and Mines: Final Report 2016. Available at https://www.dnrm.qld.gov.au/__data/assets/pdf_file/0009/383940/monash-qcwp-final-report-2016.pdf. Accessed on May 11th 2018.

Moyce SC and Schenker M. 2018. Migrant workers and their occupational health and safety. *Annu Rev Public Health* **39**: 351–365.

Muecke A, Lenthall S and Lindeman M. 2011. Culture shock and healthcare workers in remote indigenous communities of Australia: what do we know and how can we measure it? *Rural Remote Health* **11**: 1607.

National Institute for Health and Care Excellence (NICE). 2009. Workplace health: long-term sickness absence and incapacity to work. Public health guideline [PH19]. Available at https://www.nice.org.uk/guidance/ph19. Accessed on March 22nd 2018.

New Zealand Transport Agency. 2014. Medical aspects of fitness to drive. A guide for health practitioners. Available at https://www.nzta.govt.nz/assets/resources/medical-aspects/Medical-aspects-2014.pdf. Accessed on March 5th 2018.

Niven K and McLeod R. 2009. Offshore industry: management of health hazards in the upstream petroleum industry. *Occup Med (Lond)* **59**: 304–309.

Oil & Gas UK (OGUK). 2018. *Medical Aspects of Fitness for Offshore Work: Guidance for Examining Physicians* — Issue 6 including supplement A.

Pachman J. 2009. Evidence base for pre-employment medical screening. *Bull World Health Organ* **87**: 529–534.

Petsonk EL, Rose C and Cohen R. 2013. Coal mine dust lung disease — new lessons from an old exposure. *Am J Respir Crit Care Med* **187**: 1178–1185.

Price Waterhouse Coopers (PWC). 2008. Building the case for wellness. Available at https://assets.publishing.service.gov.uk/government/uploads/system/uploads/attachment_data/file/209547/hwwb-dwp-wellness-report-public.pdf. Accessed on April 30th 2018.

Reid A, Merler E, Peters S, Jayasinghe N, Bressan V, Franklin P, Brims F, de Klerk NH and Musk AW. 2018. Migration and work in postwar Australia: mortality profile comparisons between Australian and Italian workers exposed to blue asbestos at Wittenoom. *Occup Environ Med* **75**: 29–36.

Schaafsma FG, Mahmud N, Reneman MF, Fassier J-B and Jungbauer FHW. 2016. Pre-employment examinations for preventing injury, disease and sick leave in workers. *Cochrane Database Syst Rev*. Available at http://onlinelibrary.wiley.com/doi/10.1002/14651858.CD008881.pub2/full. Accessed on March 6th 2018.

Serra C, Rodriguez MC, Delclos GL, Plana M, Lopez LIG and Benavides FG. 2007. Criteria and methods used for the assessment of fitness for work: a systematic review. *Occup Environ Med* **64**: 304–312.

Steege AL, Baron SL, Marsh SM, Menéndez CC and Myers JR. 2014. Examining occupational health and safety disparities using national data: a cause for continuing concern. *Am J Ind Med* **57**: 527–538.

Stewart L and Leggat PA. 1998. Culture shock and travellers. *J Travel Med* **5**: 84–88.

Truman SD, Sharar DA and Pompe JC. 2011. The mental health status of expatriate versus U.S. domestic workers: a comparative study. *Int J Ment Health* **40**: 3–18.

Whittaker-Howe S, Brown G, Williamson V and Greenberg N. 2017. The psychological health of remote area medics in Iraq. *Occup Med (Lond)* **67**: 666–671.

World Health Organization (WHO). 2018. Health Impact Assessment (HIA). Available at http://www.who.int/hia/en/. Accessed on March 6th 2018.

Chapter

12

Industrial Medicine
and Remote Healthcare
in Russia

Sergey A Antipov, Andrey B Karpov
and Ergena R Badmaeva

Introduction

The problem of improving the public health protection system remains one of the main (if not the main) for the modern world. Scientific and technical progress, the development of industrial production, the emergence of new technologies and materials served as the starting point for the emergence of a huge number of factors of anthropogenic origin, which have a negative impact on human health and the state of the environment. The extreme degree of such influence is the development of occupational diseases that entail disability and reduced life expectancy. At the same time, it should be noted that production factors act together with environmental factors and lifestyle factors, causing more pronounced negative effects.

In this regard, special attention is being paid to protecting the health of the working age population, which is the most economically and socially active group of the population and is experiencing the main pressure of man-made factors. Among this group, workers at industrial remote sites should be singled out as a special group. Such sites are usually located in remote places with extreme climatic conditions (arctic shelf, mountain areas, deserts, etc.). In most cases, the energy and water supply at such facilities is autonomous. There is no social structure. Medical facilities have limited staff and a minimum list of equipment for diagnostics and emergency care.

Remote industrial facilities may be places where the staff works in shifts from several weeks to several months, or are oil refineries or mining facilities with permanent personnel. Despite the fact that work at remote industrial sites has been actively carried out for 40–50 years, there are very few publications on the results of scientific research devoted to assessing the effects of industrial and external environmental factors on the health workers of enterprise in Russia (and in the world). As a result, there are no standards for organizing medical care at remote sites and educational programs for training medical specialists.

In this section, we tried to summarize all the available Russian publications relating to industrial medicine and remote healthcare, as well as to present approaches to solving the main problems in this area, proposed by the Russian Institute of Remote Healthcare.

At the same time, it should be emphasized that for Russia the problem of remote healthcare is extremely relevant but not only in relation to the personnel of remote industrial facilities. The historical feature of the country's population distribution is its concentration in the western regions, namely in the European part. The border of Europe and Asia, passing through the Urals, divides the territory of the country into two huge zones, fundamentally different in terms of population density. In the European Union, the population density is 119 people per square kilometer. At the same time, in the Russian Federation, the average population density is 8.4 people per square kilometer. But if the population of the European part of Russia is on average 27 per square kilometer, then the value of the same indicator in the Asian part of Russia — 1.9 people per square kilometer, that is almost 14 times lower than in the European part and one of the lowest in the world.

Thus, the provision of timely and qualified medical assistance to the population of the eastern regions of Russia living in small towns at a considerable distance from cities and even more from large cities is a strategic problem with a pronounced socio-economic and humanitarian focus.

The History of Industrial Medicine in Russia

The organization of medical care for working people is one of the most important principles of health protection because the health status of workers determines the quality of labor force, labor productivity, the size of the gross domestic product (GDP) and the overall economic development of any state.

The historical development of medical care in industrial enterprises dates back to factory medicine, which originated in the second half of the 19th century and served the mine and factory workers. In June 1912, the Russian Empire passed the Law "On the Provision of Workers in Case of Sickness", where for the first time, compulsory insurance of workers in connection with illness was provided for. In 1918, the state healthcare system was created in the country, in which workers in industrial enterprises received the right to medical care. Accordingly, medical and paramedic health posts began to be developed. Industrial medicine worked in close alliance with the management of enterprises, the sanitary epidemiological service and other organizations interested in preserving and strengthening the worker's health, prevention of occupational diseases and injuries. During the first five years, a resolution of the Central Committee of the All-Union Communist Party of the Bolsheviks (b) "On Medical Care of Workers and Peasants" (1929) was adopted. Measures were taken to develop and staff the medical institutions in the main industrial centers of the USSR.

The first Medical Sanitary Units (MSU) at industrial enterprises were created in 1939, which were complexes of prevention and treatment facilities and included a clinic or ambulance station, in-patient department and health posts.

The Soviet system of worker's health protection was aimed at preventing epidemic outbreaks and preserving the level of worker's health during the Great Patriotic War. In the post-war years, the priority tasks were to provide industrial centers with a bed capacity, medical staff and consolidation of Medical Sanitary Units, health posts and shop floors (Zakharov, 1965).

In the period from 1950 to 1977, the number of MSUs increased two-fold. More than 1,000 MSUs of various departmental identity, over 1,500 Medical and 20,000 paramedic health posts operated by the beginning of the 1980's in the country. At this time, about 80,000 doctors worked in industrial healthcare, including more than 10,000 general physicians of the shop floors. The MSUs took measures to improve the working and living conditions of workers, prevent and reduce general and occupational morbidity and injuries, provide specialized medical assistance and dispensary observation. The organization of medical care in the Medical Sanitary Units was carried out on the shop floors, which were organized for every 2,000 workers, and in the chemical, coal, mining and petrochemical industries — for every 1,000 workers. Where there was no medical sanitary unit, a doctor of the shop floor was prescribed by the attached territorial hospital or polyclinic. During this period, it is necessary to note the active participation of industrial enterprises, especially town-forming enterprises, in the construction and repair of medical institutions, in equipping them with diagnostic equipment, in introducing new medical technologies. Thus, until the 1990s, industrial workers were serviced according to the production principle.

By the beginning of the 1990s, when introducing a system of compulsory medical insurance, the principle of universality and accessibility of medical care for the population was declared, regardless of social status, professional affiliation and residency. For several years, the process of transferring departmental medical institutions to municipal ownership took place, and only a small part of departmental MSUs managed to retain their independence and connections with industrial enterprises. It should be noted that the transformation of departmental MSUs into municipal healthcare facilities led to a reduction in the functions of protecting the health of workers. As a consequence, reduced quality of care occured with a sharp decrease in the preventive and rehabilitation components of medical care, since the budget-insurance model in healthcare was not directed or interested in financing the preventive component of medical care.

As a result of the transformation, enterprises of various forms of ownership appeared, many enterprises closed and medical care for workers was provided simultaneously by primary care physicians and shop floor doctors, which did not allow concentrating the entire medical as well as professional history of the patient in the hands of one attending physician.

As such, in 1994, the order of the Ministry of Healthcare of Russia No. 130 "On the organization of medical care for workers operating in industry, transport, and communications in conditions of compulsory health insurance" was approved. The order reflected the principles of the work of the treatment and preventive care establishments, the main directions of reforming the shop floor service and Medical Sanitary Units, and their integration into the municipal healthcare system.

The existing duplication of medical care for working enterprises shifted to the system of a single attending physician and medical institution. Order No. 130 introduced into the nomenclature the specialty and the position of the occupational physician, it established a regulatory framework that allowed the development of a network of Occupational Therapy Clinics in each of the Russian Federation regions. Since the release of the order in the country, about 80 clinics of occupational physicians in the regions have been created, and the training of specialists of "Occupational pathology" has been introduced.

From 1995–1996, the Ministry of Health of the Russian Federation approved new medical regulations for admission to the profession. This was due to the development of new production technologies and the implementation of preventive medical check-ups of workers who have contact with production factors (orders No. 280/88 dated October 5th 1995; No. 90 dated March 14th 1996; and No. 405 dated December 10th 1996). These documents updated the regulations for admission to the profession in connection with the development of new production technologies and the associated emergence of new damaging influences. A new procedure for conducting preliminary and periodic medical check-ups was introduced. Check-ups could be conducted only with the participation of the attending physician, performing the entirety of examinations and reviewing, if necessary, the outcomes with the clinical expert commission. The possibility of sending persons who had long worked with certain production factors to an in-depth medical examination at the Occupational Therapy Clinic was established.

In 1997, the Government of the Russian Federation approved the concept of the development of medical science and healthcare, based on a gradual transition to a single attending physician system. This is a general practitioner (family doctor), or a primary care physician of a medical institution, who is responsible for all medical aspects of prevention, diagnosis, treatment and rehabilitation of the patient, as well as for the examination of his professional suitability and admission to occupational activities related to exposure adverse factors or of increased danger to the worker or others.

In May 2007 at the 60th World Health Assembly, the necessity for a Global Plan of Action on workers' health and the creation of appropriate mechanisms and legal frameworks for their implementation, monitoring and evaluation were proclaimed.

An "Action plan for the improvement of conditions and occupational safety" was developed as part of the Presidential Decree No.1351 dated October 9th 2007 *"On Approving the Concept of the Demographic Policy of the Russian Federation for the Period until 2025"*. The main objectives of the program were reducing mortality and injuries from accidents at work and occupational diseases due to transition in the field of occupational safety to a system for managing occupational risks from the previous system for responding to insurance claims after a health incident.

Within the framework of the concept of long-term socio-economic development of the Russian Federation for the period up to 2020, (order of the Government of the Russian Federation No. 1662-p of December 17th 2008,) the government noted the need to improve the system of public health protection. This system included: promotion and formation of a healthy lifestyle and increase in the responsibility of the employer for the health of their employees and in the population for their own health.

In the "National Security Strategy of the Russian Federation until 2020" (Presidential Decree No. 537 dated May 12th 2009) a progressive labor force shortage was identified as one of the main strategic risks and threats to national security in the field of economic growth in the long term. In recent years, important steps have been taken to enhance the regulatory framework in the field of employee health, thanks to the efforts of the Ministry of Health of Russia, the Ministry of Labor of Russia and the Russian Federal Service for Surveillance on Consumer Rights Protection and Human Wellbeing (Rospotrebnadzor). Other orders also were introduced, e.g.:

- Order No. 302n of the Ministry of Health of Russia dated April 12th, 2011 "On approval of lists of harmful and (or) hazardous production factors and works, during which mandatory preliminary and periodic medical check-ups (examinations) are carried out, and the procedure for conducting compulsory preliminary and periodic medical check-ups (examinations) of workers engaged in heavy work and work in harmful and (or) dangerous working conditions"
- Order No. 417n of the Ministry of Healthcare and Social Development of Russia dated April 27th, 2012 "On approval of the list of occupational diseases"
- Order No. 543n of the Ministry of Healthcare and Social Development of Russia dated May 15th, 2012 "On approval of the Regulation on the Organization of Primary Healthcare Assistance to the Adult Population"

- Order No. 911n of the Ministry of Health of Russia dated November 13th, 2012 "On approval of the procedure for providing medical care for acute and chronic occupational diseases"
- Federal Law No. 426-FZ dated December 28th, 2013 "On special assessment of working conditions"
- Order No. 869n of the Ministry of Health of the Russian Federation dated October 26th, 2017 "On approval of the procedure for conducting dispensary observation of certain groups of the adult population"
- Order No. 494 of the Federal Service for Labor and Employment dated December 5th, 2016 "On approval of the procedure for analyzing the status and causes of industrial injuries and proposals for its prevention in the Russian Federation"

However, despite all the measures taken, the legal framework in the field of the worker's health protection still requires improvement.

Problems of Industrial Medicine

The country's medical and demographic indicators show a progressive decrease in labor potential — high mortality rates, general and occupational morbidity, a high level of disability, as well as industrial injuries.

Today, over 30% of Russians who die every year are citizens of working age. The mortality of the working age population exceeds the same indicator for the European Union by 4.5 times and is 2.5 times the average mortality rate in Russia. About 180,000 people die in the Russian Federation every year for reasons related to exposure to harmful and dangerous production factors. Adverse working conditions cause a high level of occupational injuries and diseases. About 200,000 people are injured at work every year, more than 10,000 cases of occupational diseases are registered, over 14,000 people became disabled as a result of industrial injury. At the same time, the official statistical observation covers less than 45% of workers. Annual economic losses are estimated at 500 billion rubles (1.9% of GDP) due to adverse working conditions. According to expert estimates, on average, up to 10 working days per worker are lost due to illness (in EU countries — 7.9 days). The number of workers, who work in conditions which does not meet appropriate sanitary and hygienic standards, increased from 17.1% in 1997 to 26.2% in 2008 (Order 586 Ministry of Health and Social Development, 2008).

According to OKVED (All-Russian Classifier of Economic Activities) oil producing industries are included in the section "Crude oil and natural gas production; the provision of services in these areas". According to the Federal State Statistics

Service the share of workers in the crude oil and natural gas production industry engaged in harmful and/ or hazardous working conditions is growing from year to year (Bakirov and Gimranova, 2016).

The reasons for this are technological deterioration of equipment at enterprises, reduction of capital and preventive maintenance of industrial buildings, reduction of labor protection services at enterprises, low level of professional training in labor protection, the lack of technical re-equipping of production, modern safe production technologies, a high level of many harmful factors of production, violations of sanitary legislation, the absence and non-use of individual and collective protection means, the lack of timely, full and high-quality medical care for workers, etc.

At the same time, it should be noted that the financial costs (expenses for insurance payments, early pensions and compensation) of the country are not aimed at preventive measures to reduce industrial injuries, occupational morbidity, but to eliminate their consequences. In this regard, it is necessary to move from the insurance case response system to a modern professional risk management system.

Occupational risk management is the process of identifying, evaluating, and selecting methods and tools to minimize risk. The role and importance of risk management systems in managing the country's economy is growing and becoming a global issue. This tool works well abroad and shows good results in the form of jobs without injuries and occupational diseases. However, in our country there are difficulties in solving problems of occupational risk assessment, which is caused by the dominance of the "zero risk" doctrine for workers over the past 80 years, or the "absolute safety" of work, provided that the regulatory factors of the working environment are achieved (Roik V, 2003).

However, since ratification (Federal Law No. 265-FZ of the Russian Federation of October 4th 2010) of the International Labor Organization Convention No. 187 "On the Basics of Promoting Occupational Safety and Health", Russia is obliged to comply with the principles for assessing occupational risks or hazards and for combating professional risks or hazards at their place of origin.

If we turn to the definition of occupational risk, it is the probability of causing harm to health as a result of exposure to harmful and / or hazardous production factors when an employee performs his duties under an employment contract (Trikman et al., 2016).

Risk identification is carried out according to the results of two main measures — a special assessment of the working conditions of workplaces, and an assessment of the state of workers' health based on the results of periodic medical check-ups. There are manifested and hidden risks. The manifested risk consists of industrial injuries, which may result in death, temporary or complete disability and occupational diseases that may result in complete or partial disability. The hidden risk causes a generally unhealthy employee and consists of occupational diseases associated with one or more factors of work activity, occupational diseases caused by several factors (both working environment and external) and common diseases that are not related to work, but are complicated by professional factors (Glushkov *et al.*, 2015).

> The individual professional risk of workers is determined on the basis of an integrated assessment of working conditions, indicators of the workers' health status, the age and length of service of an employee in harmful and (or) hazardous working conditions, as well as taking into account data on occupational injuries and occupational diseases in this workplace.

It is possible to further evaluate the professional risk of the organization as a whole based on the integral assessment of the professional risk of individual employees. At the same time, the assessment should be based on the results of calculating the levels of professional risk of at least 95% of the enterprise's employees" (Bashurin *et al.*, 2014). Currently, in our country, unfortunately, there is no generally accepted and approved methodology for assessing occupational risks. However, some approaches have been developed and proposed (Levashov, 2012).

Assignment of the type of economic activity to the class of professional risk (Government Decree No. 713 of December 1st, 2005). Occupational risk is calculated for each type of economic activity. It is defined as an integral indicator of the total amount of insurance costs and the size of the wage fund, on which insurance premiums for industrial accidents and occupational diseases are assessed. This assessment methodology was developed by the Social Insurance Fund of the Russian Federation.

Prior to replacement by a special assessment of working conditions, certification of workplaces revealed the presence of a health hazard, both from unfavorable working conditions and an increased level of injury. It also determined the localization of the increased risk; engaged in the development of specific actions aimed at reducing the risk, taking into account the reduction and multiplying factors. The certification of workplaces was a "screening" and "managerial" model for assessing occupational risk.

The methodology of the Scientific and Research Institute of Occupational Medicine set out in Guideline R 2.2.1766–03 (Chief Sanitary Doctor, Russian Federation, 2003) is based on a quantitative health risk assessment of the employee from the action of harmful and dangerous factors of the working environment and workload, taking into account the likelihood of health problems and their severity. On the basis of such a methodology, mathematical models are built for the calculation of occupational risk, taking into account the level of the factor, the duration of its impact, as well as indicators of the employee's health.

"Methods of an integrated assessment of working conditions in the workplace, taking into account the complex impact of production factors with different classes of hazard, safety assessment, and the provision of personal protective equipment" developed by the Klin Institute for Labor Protection. This technique is determined on the basis of an integrated working conditions assessment, health indicators of workers, age and length of service in harmful and (or) hazardous conditions, as well as taking into account data on occupational injuries and occupational diseases in the workplace. Injury rates are determined by coefficients that take into account the number of injuries in the workplace during the past year and the severity of the consequences of injury.

The existing variety of assessment methods of occupational risks indicates the different views of scientific communities and federal agencies on this issue. In this regard, it is necessary to improve the regulatory framework with creation of an integrated professional risk management model including a special assessment of working conditions and an assessment of hazards associated with the performance of job duties (Kursov, 2016).

Another problem in the implementation of the occupational risk management system is the lack of reliable statistical information on the state of working conditions, industrial injuries and occupational diseases at state level. Available data on the state of working conditions, occupational injuries and occupational morbidity, on the number of deaths in production, given by the Federal State Statistics, the Social Insurance Fund and the Federal Labor for Employment Service differ (Timoshkina, 2012). The output of the Federal State Statistics on the state and conditions of work are considered on the basis of the types of enterprises economic activity, rather than professions or professional groups of workers. This fact characterizes the general situation in this area, but does not allow analyzing of the causal relationships in the system of "professional activity — professional risk" (Glushkov et al., 2015).

There is no unified information database in the country (equipment failures, accidents, etc.) as to the incidents occurring in cases of violations of labor protection requirements, but which did not lead to accidents. In European Union countries there are statistics of injuries and occupational diseases with the issuance of sick leave, micro injuries — without clearance of sick leave (absence in the workplace for a short time) and various production events that did not lead to injuries of workers, but only affected production, comprised certain conditions and causes of injury (Trushkova and Kantsigov, 2015).

As the most effective mechanism of professional risk management, compulsory social insurance of workers against industrial accidents and occupational diseases and introduction of additional contributions by enterprises to the Pension Fund of the Russian Federation for work in harmful conditions can be considered in economic terms. These measures will play a stimulating role for employers to take measures to improve safety and working conditions. There are other professional risk management mechanisms. These comprise of funding preventive measures and the imposition of administrative fines for violations of regulatory requirements of labor protection (Mikhina, 2016).

In Russia, the identification of hazardous and harmful production factors is performed at workplaces by conducting a special assessment of working conditions, in accordance with Federal Law No. 426-FZ dated December 28th 2013 "On Special Assessment of Working Conditions" and the Federal Law No. 421-FZ dated December 28th 2013 "On Amendments to Certain Legislative Acts of the Russian Federation in connection with the adoption of the Federal Law "On Special Assessment of Working Conditions".

A special assessment of working conditions was carried out at 10,945,000 workplaces during a period from April 2014 to December 2016. By December 31st 2018, complete assessment of the working conditions of all 48 000 000 workplaces in the economy was plannned (Samara, 2017).

Unfortunately, workplace assessment is not performed at all enterprises, and it is not always carried out to the same high level of quality due to the lack of qualified personnel and the necessary laboratory facilities. It does not allow determination of the contribution of working conditions in the development of occupational pathology and establish the relationship of the disease with the occupation. Previously conducted certification of workplaces for working conditions was replaced by a special assessment of working conditions, as a result of which the assessment of injury risk was excluded from the assessment of working conditions. Such harmful production factors as physical, chemical, biological, etc. assessed in a special assessment of working conditions are not incorporated as sources of injury at work.

With the entry into force of the order No. 33n of the Ministry of Labor of Russia, January 24th 2014 "On the Special Assessment of Working Conditions" there was expectation of a worsening of the situation (Gurvich *et al.*, 2015). This will affect the adequate assessment and management of occupational hazards, the disconnection between the methods of identifying harmful and hazardous production factors and the assessment of working conditions used for the special assessment of working conditions and industrial laboratory control (R 2.2.2006-05). Due to the lack of a unified methodology, the same workplace in the same classification system can be evaluated with different results.

At the same time, the introduction of this law allowed use of a differentiated insurance premium rate paid by the employer to the pension fund of the Russian Federation (the more dangerous the working conditions, the higher the rate and vice versa). In addition, it made it possible to objectively identify violations at specific workplaces, establish classes (and subclasses) of working conditions, determine guarantees and compensations for workers who work in harmful or dangerous conditions.

The leading role in the prevention of occupational morbidity is carried out by conducting preliminary and periodic medical examinations of workers employed in work in contact with harmful and dangerous production factors. The current deficiencies in conducting a standard medical examination in accordance with the order No. 302n of the Ministry of Health of Russia dated April 12th 2011 "On approval of the lists of harmful and (or) hazardous production factors and work, in the performance of which mandatory preliminary and periodic medical check-ups (examinations) are carried out, and the Procedure for conducting mandatory preliminary and periodic medical check-ups (examinations) of workers engaged in heavy work and work with harmful and (or) dangerous working conditions" are:

— lack of training in occupational health and occupational pathology of specialist doctors,
— lack of consideration of factors affecting workers,
— lack of necessary equipment of medical organizations for diagnostic research,
— the lack of data transmission identified during the standard medical examination to the clinic at the place of residence,
— the absence of a medical card that allows you to track the dynamics of previously established diseases,
— lack of electronic medical cards to exclude duplication of medical care,
— insufficient patient coverage,
— the large composition of the commission, leading to a sharp rise in the cost of medical check-ups, that does not allow identification of professional and general morbidity in the early stages.

The registered level of occupational morbidity in our country does not reflect the true situation and the main part of occupational diseases is masked in the structure of general morbidity. Ermakova and Salnikov (2016) present the data of the international medical statistics analysis concerning the diagnosis of occupational morbidity among the working population in 2014. The proportion of occupational diseases per 10,000 people of the economically active population is: Belgium-164.2, Finland-52.2, USA-23.2, Germany-18.2, Great Britain-6.7, China-8.4, Russia-1.7. Some authors associate the high detectability of occupational diseases in a number of developed countries with the existing system of penalties for concealing occupational diseases, as well as the level of medical diagnostics of occupational pathology and the quality of standard medical examination. The trend of recent years in our country shows that workers with newly diagnosed occupational diseases have more pronounced clinical forms corresponding to a higher degree of disability. This is due to the reluctance of the company's administration to include their employees of harmful occupations into the survey at an earlier date, since this threatens to increase their insurance contributions to the Social Insurance Fund.

There is no interest among specialists of the medical organization conducting the medical check-ups. This is because if a large number of suspicions of occupational pathology are identified, the employer may not conclude an agreement to conduct periodic medical check-ups in subsequent years with this healthcare facility. It makes the administration and doctors economically co-dependent. In addition, some employees also try to hide the early signs of occupational diseases until the formation of permanent disability. Employees are afraid of dismissal and loss of material compensation in the event of illness.

The special assessment of working conditions and medical check-ups had their development in different state agencies, therefore they are carried out independently of each other. But they have a number of systemic deficiencies, since the results of occupational risk assessment at workplaces and the results of damage to workers' health and working ability are not combined into a single system, which reduces the efficiency in the use of their findings (Denisov *et al.*, 2011).

Early detection of occupational diseases is very important to prevent the development and possible onset of disability. The criteria for identifying disability should be based on early biochemical, morphological and functional shifts, when they are still reversible. In the future, identified diseases require systematic work to improve worker health, conduct rehabilitation activities, and provide high-tech medical care. However, paradoxically, sanatoriums, sports complexes, and health centers were eliminated in large enterprises in the emergent market economy.

It should be noted that the shortcomings of this law were discussed at the federal level and displayed in the conclusion N 13875-OF / D26i of the Ministry of Economic Development of Russia dated May 28th 2015 "On the examination of the order No. 302n of the Russian Ministry of Health dated April 12th 2011 On the approval of the lists of harmful and (or) hazardous production factors and work, during which mandatory preliminary and periodic medical check-ups (examinations) are carried out, and the Procedure for conducting mandatory preliminary and periodic medical check-ups (examinations) of workers engaged in heavy work and work with harmful and (or) hazardous working conditions".

It is noteworthy that the reason for the examination of this order was the written enquiries of OJSC "Surgutneftegaz", where reported difficulties in conducting medical check-ups due to the lack of definition of the terms "medical care facilities" and "significant disposal" in both order No. 302n and in the legislation of the Russian Federation.

As of 2019, reorganized MSUs in territorial medical care facilities have lost contact with enterprises, and are not able to carry out prevention of occupational diseases and dispensary observation of patients. Health posts in enterprises, that were previously part of the MSUs, are now owned by the employer, and they have also lost contact with medical care facilities. Health posts are practically the only structural element in the provision of medical care to workers at many industrial enterprises. They are not engaged in preventive work. Their tasks are reduced to the provision of first medical (prehospital) care. In addition, since most of the activities in terms of healthcare (a special assessment of working conditions, periodic medical check-ups) are now carried out by outside organizations, the employer does not have a holistic system of health protection.

Thus, today the system of an integrated approach to protecting the health of workers, which existed in the Soviet era, has been destroyed. Lack of funds and economic interest from employers do not ensure the preservation and improvement of the workers' health. Antipov, Sokolovich and Lugachev rightly observe that "the current responsibility of the employer in organizing medical care at the legislative level is limited to the list of required funded activities (medical check-ups and in some cases — providing emergency care)" (Antipov *et al.*, 2009).

Organization of the Healthcare System at Remote Sites

The health problems of workers in enterprises have been looked at in a number of studies (Gurinovich, 2009; Furman, 2009; Aliyeva, 2011; Averyanova *et al.*, 2012; Valeeva, 2013; Petrova *et al.*, 2014; Trikman *et al.*, 2016). However, analysis of the literature data showed that there are no studies reflecting the holistic system of organizing medical care for workers at remote industrial sites. Meanwhile the organization of medical care for workers in remote and underpopulated areas is a complex task. It should be noted that a number of factors complicate the provision of medical care in these places:

- extreme climatic conditions
- low transport provision
- shortage of medical staff and lack of qualifications
- poor medical equipment
- remote location of any accident from medical institutions
- poor communication support due to low commercial benefits of communication companies
- lack of a developed social infrastructure for living and working

Due to the above reasons, these territories are in an autonomous or semi-autonomous mode of existence most of the year.

Meanwhile, the oil industry enterprises, being a basic sector of the Russian economy, are mainly concentrated in the Northern regions. In the north of the Russian Federation more than 20% of GDP and 18% of electricity, 93% of natural gas, 75% of oil, 63% of gold, 83% of silver, 90% of nickel and copper, 100% of diamonds and platinum group elements, 43% of coal, 45% of export wood and 61% of fish are produced (Dudareva and Talykova, 2012).

Issues of workers' health are relevant in the Northern regions based on the significant contribution of workers in these regions to the country's economy. It is also worth considering a variety of factors affecting employees when organizing medical care. The "polar tension syndrome" was described and studied in detail by Kaznacheev V.P. and is known in the scientific literature. This is a condition of the body, characterized by deep disruption of processes at the cellular level. Changes are caused by a complex effect of the human environmental factors of high latitudes in the north area. This manifests in the form of a number of general pathological syndromes, which are characterized by early onset, non-specific symptoms and a greater prevalence of impaired functional state of the body. There is an early chronicity of inflammatory diseases of infectious etiology and rather rapid development of their complications compared with other climatic zones. Another author (Petrenko, 2014) noted that regular changes of rotational shift work and rest are also accompanied by chronic tension of the regulatory and adaptation systems of the body. Burnout and job stress cause negative somatic and mental states of workers and reduce their productivity in remote conditions due to monotony and long-term isolation from the usual socio-cultural conditions (Poletaeva, 2017).

In Russia 28,000 settlements do not have year-round access to transport and communications. All in all, 12 million people remain cut off from the transport infrastructure — mainly in the far North and similar areas. This is the entire territory of 13 and part of the territories of 10 subjects of the Russian Federation, which occupy 11 million km², or almost two-thirds of the territory of Russia. At least 20 million people live in these areas (Okulova, 2013).

In this regard, the use of air ambulance is the only way out when providing emergency medical care to an employee in remote areas with an undeveloped road network. It has been established that the result of many diseases directly depends on the time (the golden hour) during which key medical manipulations must be carried out.

Today, the air ambulance service in our country is underdeveloped due to the high cost of air transport, its operation and maintenance, the need for highly qualified staff for work and their training, the need to build appropriate infrastructure, and the organization of air traffic control (Lobzhanidze *et al.*, 2016). At the same time, in other industrialized countries (Canada, Australia, USA, Germany, Great Britain, Switzerland, Norway) medical helicopters play a significant role in providing pre-hospital care, for example, to trauma patients.

There are few publications on this topic in the Russian literature. Most of the studies support the use of helicopters in the provision of emergency community care to victims of severe mechanical injury in remote locations from a specialized trauma center at 75–100 km and more. Publications by a number of authors (e.g. Orlov *et al.*, 2016) indicate the important role of medical personnel in solving problems, including emergencies, at health posts at production facilities, remote from the transport and medical infrastructure. Telemedicine training was conducted for medical personnel at remote health centers on modern methods of emergency medical care, in which 300 medical workers who provide medical assistance to personnel of 48 enterprises were trained. The use of distance training allowed training of medical personnel at remote health posts without interrupting work, also to attract highly qualified teaching staff and to reduce the costs associated with travel expenses.

At the same time, a number of researchers (Radushkevich and Bartashevich, 2011) noted that medical personnel providing emergency assistance at remote sites should have special training and experience. Medical staff in conditions of limited diagnostic and therapeutic opportunities, have the necessity in a short time to determine the disease, the nature of the injury, to identify violations of vital systems, to organize the necessary medical care, including the evacuation of the patient to a hospital. It has been established that injuries and acutely developed cardiovascular diseases are often found in emergency situations. In this connection the doctors need training on Advanced Trauma Life Support (ATLS) and Advanced Cardiac Life Support programs (ACLS).

The skills that doctors should have in health posts serving the Continental Shelf, known as "remote doctors", were written in 1988 (Norman *et al.*, 1988). At first there were just first-aid training courses but then the requirements for "remote doctors" changed due to changes in the British law ("On the provision of medical care at facilities", adopted in 1980 and exchanged in 1993, 1995, 1999, 2015 with the abbreviation "OFAR 1989").

The legislatively approved "Code of Practitioners" contains recommendations and discussion of various issues, roles, responsibilities and qualifications of physicians at remote sites. Nurses and former military medical equipment engineers were recruited as first workers in this field. OFAR 1989 set the duration, the training program, the duration of practice for doctors at sea, as well as periodic retraining.

The high cost of medical evacuation can be reduced by introducing telemedicine technologies. Telemedicine plays an important role in providing medical assistance to oil rig workers. Remote doctor consultation using video conferencing improves the quality of offshore medical care and reduces the number of medical evacuations that can be avoided. Evacuation from remote sites located at a distance of several hundreds of kilometers by helicopter can cost 200–400,000 rubles per hour.

Therefore, telemedicine with equipment for remote monitoring and diagnostics becomes the preferred option if remote sites are equipped with internet or satellite communications. Medical specialists can conduct remote video consultations with diagnostic medical equipment integration. This allows them to make an accurate diagnosis with the help of a nurse or emergency doctor located at the remote site.

Telemedicine: History of Development and Current State

Telemedicine is widely used in countries such as Canada, Norway and Denmark with characteristic areas of low population density. The use of telemedicine for the Russian Federation is of particular importance due to the large number of territories with low population density, and differences in terms of providing medical personnel and equipment in central and peripheral areas. Telemedicine in Russia is at the stage of rapid growth, supported by the corresponding development of information technologies.

For Russia, 2017 was the decisive year in the development of the regulatory framework for health informatics and telemedicine. This is due to the adoption of the Federal Law No. 242-FZ "On Amendments to Certain Legislative Acts of the Russian Federation on the Use of Information Technologies in the Field of Health Protection" and also the draft Order of the Ministry of Health of the Russian Federation "On approval of the procedure for organizing and providing medical care using telemedicine technologies". There are also a number of State standards governing the requirements for telemedicine systems. However, there are problems: a lack of a comprehensive regulatory framework, financing mechanisms, staff training, standards, technical incompatibility of individual systems and a lack of infrastructure that does not allow the medical community to work in a single coherent environment.

The experience of using telemedicine is diverse and reflected in the following studies:

1. Teleradiology. Some authors (Smal *et al.*, 2017) showed not only the relevance of teleradiology in terms of personnel shortages in areas with low population density, but also revealed inaccuracies in the radiograph description by a remote expert and the doctor of the district hospital.
2. Distance learning of personnel. The experience of telemedicine technologies used in the form of video training, is presented as an optimal tool for training medical personnel in the remote sites of industrial companies (Levanov *et al.*, 2016).
3. Remote monitoring of chronic patients. The staff of the Slovene Gradec General Hospital monitored 280 patients with type 2 diabetes and 120 with

heart failure (measuring glucose, body weight, blood pressure, heart rate and oxygen saturation). Based on the obtained data, correction of therapy was carried out (Rudel *et al.*, 2015).

4. Teleconsultations. In 2014, 899 teleconsultations held at the "RB2-CEMP" 24-hour telemedicine center of the Republic of Sakha (Yakutia) were studied. A special need for teleconsultation was observed in the diagnosis and treatment of injuries and cardiovascular diseases (Begiev *et al.*, 2015).

5. Telesonography was used in emergency medicine in remote hospitals and in places with limited resources (Marsh-Feiley *et al.*, 2018).

6. Emergency telemedicine. The experience of using telemedicine technology in ambulance cars was reviewed (Rogers *et al.*, 2016).

The literature provides data on research of the cost-effectiveness of the introduction of telemedicine. In 2003, an economic analysis of the effectiveness of telemedicine consultations in the provision of surgical care to patients with bone and joint tuberculosis in the city of Irkutsk was conducted. According to the results it was established that the use of telemedicine has significantly increased the number of surgical interventions performed in this pathology compared with other methods without the use of telemedicine (Piven *et al.*, 2003). This article compares three treatment options for patients with bone and joint tuberculosis (providing surgical care to patients using telemedicine, without using telemedicine technologies and with the participation of invited specialists from other regions) in the city of Irkutsk, along with a cost-effectiveness analysis. According to the study, the greatest effect on the growth of surgical interventions by 27-fold, was achieved when using telemedicine. Fedyaev *et al.* (2014) in their work showed the economic feasibility of the possibility of using telemedicine as part of the clinical examination of people in difficult to access places (Fedyaev *et al.*, 2014).

There are additional studies on the relevance of the use of telemedicine in the enterprises of oil companies in the regions of the Far North of Russia (Teslya and Kryukov, 2018).

Conclusion

Thus, the analysis of the scientific literature showed that extensive research on these issues and generalization of existing practical experience in medical support performed at remote sites to date has not yet been properly conducted. This is despite the apparent urgency of the remote healthcare problem, including assistance standards, training programs, regulatory frameworks, etc.

We can once again formulate our main problems in the field of remote healthcare:

- lack of a clear regulatory and legal framework of medical activities at remote sites;
- lack of a system for training qualified personnel to work at remote sites.

This applies not only to the system of training medical personnel. It applies also to the lack of a holistic view of how a life support system should be built for people working at remote sites. It is necessary to prevent the development of not only professional but also the most significant diseases, reduce premature mortality and increase professional longevity;

The absence of permanent control of occupational safety and use of protective equipment means that it is expensive to maintain an industrial hygienist at the facility and so it is necessary to look for other approaches to ensure safe working conditions and reduce occupational hazards.

Currently as stated in Part 1, Russia has the following organization of medical care for personnel at remote industrial facilities:

- industrial companies form their own medical services, which assess and carry out health monitoring of workers;
- companies involve other medical organizations for medical monitoring of personnel.

When forming its own medical service, the company's management acts on the basis of its perceptions about the priority of certain activities, the education level and competence of medical service staff and the amount of material investment required in equipping medical departments, etc. This happens in many cases arbitrarily, without a clear understanding of the specifics of the activities and ways to achieve the main goals.

For example, the company's main requirement for the medical service is to reduce to a minimum (and ideally completely eliminate) the death of workers at a remote facility from acute diseases. Companies expand the ad hoc availability of medical facilities (for example, on offshore platforms) by various qualified specialists. However, they ignore: investment in research of morbidity and establishing rates of prevalence of the main risk factors, an adequate assessment of the initial health state and reserve capacity of the organization, as well as the development of targeted prevention programs for various categories of workers. This does not solve the true problem at all and moreover it is economically challenging.

Delegating to other medical organizations by outsourcing medical care also does not solve major medical problems. It does not reduce the number of complications from major non-communicable diseases, the number of medical evacuations, economic losses associated with morbidity, disability and premature mortality. This is connected with the desire of the company to minimize its costs associated with assessment of the health of workers. For example, many companies do not conduct a medical check-up before workers leave for a job, but they are satisfied with health certificates that workers receive at their own place of residence. But the analysis of the situation shows, such references can often be false or the state of health assessed according to non-relevant criteria.

However, given the lack of special training programs for specialists in remote healthcare and standards for assistance at remote sites, the initial state of health is frequently not assessed sufficiently. Doctors do not have enough special knowledge of the existing production risk factors and their effects on health, they cannot assess the level of psycho-emotional stress of workers, they are not competent in interpreting clinical data and data of instrumental and laboratory examination.

An important aspect of the remote healthcare system is conducting medical evacuations. It should be emphasized that there is no single medical evacuation system, nor any single fleet of medical transportation vehicles (airplanes, helicopters, ships) equipped with special medical modules in Russia. The Ministry of Defence has its own facilities and units to evacuate wounded and injured servicemen.

The All-Russian Disaster Medicine Service is a structure of a unified state system for the prevention and elimination of emergency situations. This system combines the Disaster Medicine Service of the Ministry of Health of Russian Federation, the Ministry of Defense of the Russian Federation, as well as resources of the Ministry of Transport of the Russian Federation and other federal executive authorities involved in emergency responses.

When evacuating from remote industrial or civilian facilities, air ambulance facilities with medical staff on board are used, but not necessarily equipped with specialized medical modules, which increases various medical risks for the sick and injured during transfer.

We analyzed the dynamics and structure of evacuations causes conducted by a company (Centre of Corporate Medicine, CCM) in the period from January [1st] 2017 to July 1st 2019. It should be emphasized that until 2017 there was no full auditing of the number or complexity of evacuations in the company. But since the organization of the Institute of Remote Healthcare (IRHC), this work has been systematized and a single database is being formed. This database is the basis for a serious analysis and conclusions that will determine the strategy for remote healthcare in Russia. It should be clarified that the increase in the number of evacuations indicates the expansion of the scope of our activity rather than an increase in critical situations at remote facilities under our supervision.

In 2016, the CCM company was a medical provider at about 60 facilities. In 2019, this number increased 1.5-fold. The results of the cause analysis of medical evacuations in the indicated period are of great interest. The bulk of workers in need of evacuation were over 30 years old. The lowest share was in the group of 60–69 years, which is natural, given that the main group of workers is in the age group of 20–49 years.

If we estimate the dynamics of the evacuations, with an increase in the volume of the analyzed data, it can be noted that the number of evacuations for medical reasons in the group of workers aged 20–29 years (persons without somatic symptoms) is one seventh of all evacuations. This number is increasing significantly (however, at the time of writing, the results of only the first 6 months of 2019 are available).

The main causes of evacuation of workers in remote industrial facilities are diseases of the cardiovascular system and injuries. In total, these reasons in the three consecutive years 2017–2019 were respectively 45.9%, 44.3% and 55.8%.

Table 1 and Figure 1 show data on the reasons for the evacuation of personnel at remote industrial sites in the study period. Taking into account the fact that the majority of workers are men, evacuation cases of predominantly males were analyzed.

It is logical that the frequency of evacuations grows with age, but the main thing is that in the group of 20–29 years old (as well as for injuries) the frequency of evacuations for cardiovascular issues was 18% in 2018 and 23% in 2019.

These statistics may indicate that the existing system of workers' health assessment at remote industrial sites requires significant modification and the introduction of diagnostic methods that allow evaluation of the reserve capacity of the body in non-standard conditions, such as psychological testing methods, etc. This will eventually make it possible to anticipate higher risk groups with possibilities for correction of detected health problems and subsequent monitoring.

There is no doubt that measures to reduce the number of evacuations for medical reasons should include:

- complete assessment of any existing employee diseases (medical history),
- full vaccination against infectious diseases,
- high-quality laboratory testing directly at an industrial site using modern laboratory technologies,
- carrying out measures to assess the health risks of working according to international standards (assessment of production factors, the biomarker levels of harmful chemicals, the quality of the used personal protective equipment, etc.).

It is obvious that without properly utilizing all the accumulated experience, conducting scientific research in a wide range of areas, and developing training programs for specialists in remote healthcare, we will continue to suffer high social and economic losses.

Table 1:   Causes of Medical Evacuation of Personnel at Remote Industrial Sites (from 01.01.2017 to 01.07.2019)

Age	Number of evacuations	Causes of medical evacuation		
		Cardiovascular diseases	Injuries	Others
2017				
20–29	5 (5.7%)*	—	1 (20.0%)	—
30–39	24 (27.6%)	3 (12.5%)**	4 (16.7%)	17
40–49	28 (32.2%)	11 (39.3%).	2 (7.1%)	8
50–59	31 (35.6%)	14 (452%)	3 (9.7%)	11
60–69	4 (4.6%)	1 (25%)	1 (25.0%)	1
Total	**87 (100%)**	**29 (33.3%)***	**11 (12.6%)***	**28**
2018				
20–29	63 (14.2%)	15 (23.8%)	13 (20.6%)	35
30–39	148 (33.3%)	24 (16.2%)	32 (21.6%)	92
40–49	119 (26.7%)	35 (29.4%)	16 (13.4%)	68
50–59	93 (20.9%)	35 (37.6%)	14 (15.0%)	44
60–69	22 (4.9%)	8 (36.4%)	5 (22.7%)	9
Total	**445 (100%)**	**117 (26.3%)***	**80 (18.0%)***	**248**
2019				
20–29	86 (13.6%)	16 (18.6%)	15 (17.4%)	55
30–39	186 (29.4%)	48 (25.8%)	33 (17.7%)	105
40–49	182 (28.8%)	102 (56.0%)	11 (6.0%)	69
50–59	155 (24.5%)	102 (65.8%)	10 (6.4%)	43
60–69	23 (3.6%)	14 (60.9%)	2 (8.7%)	7
Total	**632 (100%)**	**282 (44,6%)**	**71 (11,2%)**	**279**

Note: * — % of the total number of evacuations; ** — % of the number of evacuations in this age group.

An Illustration of New Ways of Working in Remote Healthcare

This section presents the experience of the Centre of Corporate Medicine (CCM) company in the field of remote healthcare and approaches which are now being used to solve emerging problems.

(person)   2018

(person)   2019

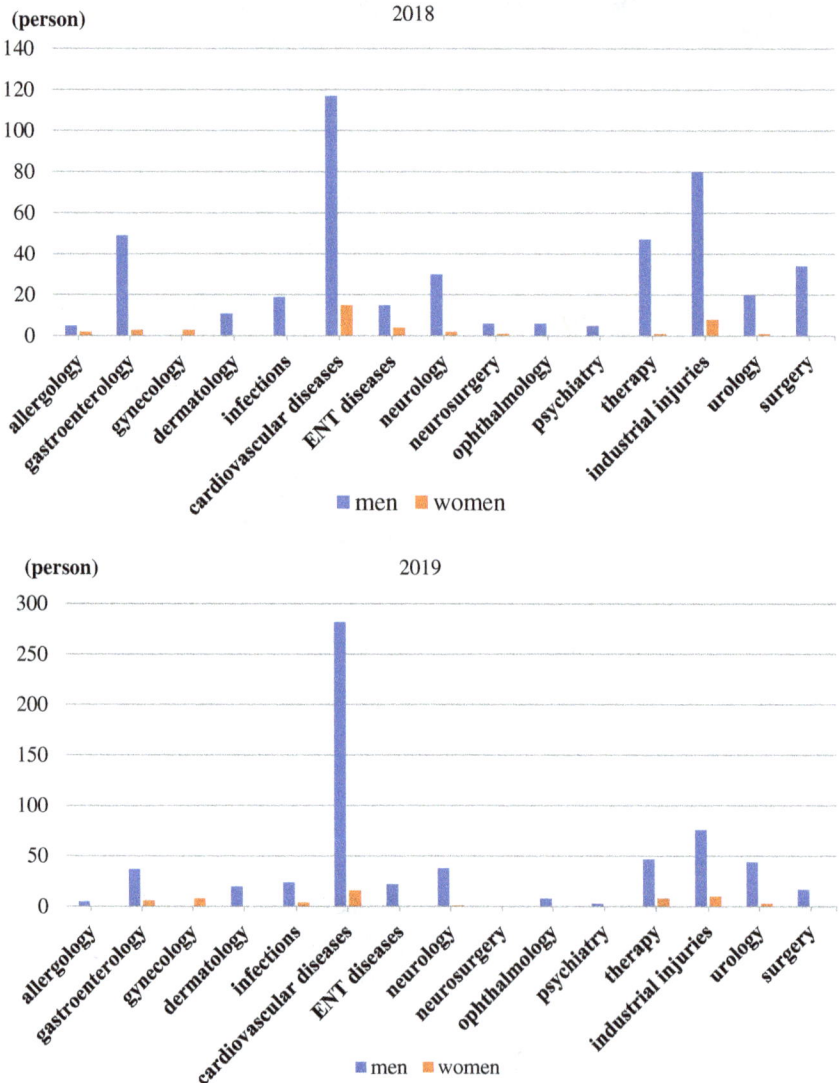

Figure 1:   Breakdown of the Causes of Evacuation

The company was established in September 2006. At the beginning, clinics in Strezhevoy and Tomsk were established to conduct preventive medical check-ups and assess the workers' health in oil and gas enterprises.

Between 2010–2011, the company began working at the Vankor Field in the Krasnoyarsk Territory. This was the company's first experience in remote sites.

From the end of 2011 to the present, the company expanded operations to the Yamalo-Nenets Autonomous District.

Since 2013, the company has expanded the area of medical services in the Krasnoyarsk Territory and since 2014, the company has been working on offshore projects.

From the beginning of 2015, the company began to work in the Nenets Autonomous District. From the same period, the company significantly expanded its presence in the Irkutsk region, and from the end of 2016, the company began working on Sakhalin Island and in the fields of the Khanty-Mansi Autonomous District, in Yakutia and on the Arctic shelf.

In 2017, the company's activities went beyond the borders of Russia when a representative office was opened in Vietnam.

Today the company employs over 600 people and operates at more than 90 remote health posts. The number of personnel serviced by remote industrial sites is about 300,000 people.

During the first 7–8 years of the company's activity, the range of medical services was limited to standard options:

- organization of medical centers and health posts,
- provision of emergency assistance at remote sites,
- conducting periodic medical check-ups,
- carrying out medical check-ups before shifts,
- prevention of occupational diseases,
- prevention of seasonal diseases,
- medical evacuation.

Today, remote healthcare has received new opportunities due to the rapid development of information technologies and in particular telemedicine. CCM now uses a telemedicine system, including the transmission of medical data (ECG, ultrasonography, etc.) in real time via secure communication channels even in the absence of the Internet. The system allows simultaneous connection of up to 250 users (participants) from anywhere in the world, any user to hold an emergency or scheduled consultation with a general practitioner or a medical specialist (cardiologist, neurologist, etc.) and organize a medical consultation. Consultations are more demanding in terms of technical equipment — broadband communication channels and specialized video equipment are used.

The coordinator of telemedicine activity is the 24/7 call center of the company, which unites health centers of industrial companies, medical consultants, emergency response services and other participants in the process of medical care.

At the present time there are about 50 highly qualified doctors in the main clinical specialties (cardiology, neurology and resuscitation). Neurology, psychiatry and some other specialisations have highly qualified specialists e.g. 3 specialist doctors, 12 candidates of sciences and 2 professors.

Along with medical consultations, the telemedicine system of the CCM company allows the following functions:

- Organization of distance learning for employees of industrial companies and conducting of sanitary and educational seminars and conferences.
- Regular professional development of the company's own medical personnel working at remote sites.
- Modernization and creation of mobile telemedicine complexes for emergency work at emergency sites and non-standard situations, land, air, sea transport.

Looking at the first and second bullet points, today we have a real resource for holding mass lectures, video seminars and conferences using telecommunication equipment. During classes, the teacher may have real time interaction with the audience. As a result of the use of such technologies, any specialist has the opportunity of continuing professional education without separation from the place of work.

Today, mobile telemedicine solutions and equipment are being further developed for work at accident sites. Small-sized mobile diagnostic systems can be used in the absence of telemedicine offices and centers, where the need arises, such as ambulance cars, remote hospitals, the brigade of disaster medicine and air ambulance.

The system was tested with a large partner of the CCM company at a remote site, where there is no Internet. Employees utilized satellite communications and achieved a speed of 4 megabits per second. The IT department of CCM is already working on the development of software and plans to develop a large-scale medical information system.

There follows a real case scenario that occurred on February 8th 2018 at one of the remote industrial facilities of the North, the medical provider of which is the company CCM. This case demonstrates the result of successful implementation of telemedicine technologies in the practice of remote industrial healthcare.

It should be emphasized that the scope of remote healthcare is not limited to issues of medical care. An important role in maintaining the workers' health at remote industrial facilities is played by a system for assessing working conditions, occupational factors, and risks of occupational and major non-communicable diseases. However, the constant presence of an industrial hygienist at the facility

Case Study 1

A 58-year-old employee of the enterprise (working as a machinist) appeared at 8 am in the medical center directly on the industrial site with complaints of pain in the upper abdomen and vomiting. The medical assistant of the medical center contacted the medical specialists of the CCM company and sent the patient to the medical center by car.

Upon arrival, the patient in the car had suffered cardio-respiratory arrest. Synchronous resuscitation, with indirect heart massage and artificial ventilation of the lungs were immediately started. Occurrence of ventricular fibrillation was recorded and defibrillation was performed. There was no effect.

Indirect cardiac massage and artificial ventilation of the lungs were continued for a further 2 minutes, after which the appearance of ventricular fibrillation was again registered. Defibrillation was made and adrenaline solution introduced into a peripheral vein. The supraventricular rhythm was restored, with the appearance of a pulse in the carotid artery, peripheral arteries and the appearance of spontaneous breathing. The patient opened his eyes, slurred speech appeared.

After consulting with a cardiologist provided by the call center and discussing the clinical situation, a collective decision was made to give intravenous Amiodarone hydrochloride injection. Tracheal intubation and mechanical ventilation were conducted. Thrombolytic therapy was started. 15 minutes after thrombolysis, ventricular fibrillation recurred and a third defibrillation was performed. After 1.5 hours from the moment of thrombolysis, ECG changes were recorded, indicating recanalization of the right coronary artery. The patient was taken to a helicopter by the resuscitation assistance car and then to the resuscitation department of the Salekhard clinical hospital, located 300 km from the location of the medical center.

The treatment tactics and medical evacuation were carried out with the support of a cardiologist provided by the call center of the CCM company.

The patient survived and continues to work after treatment and rehabilitation.

remains impractical, primarily from an economic point of view. In this regard, the CCM company developed its own program for training medical specialists in the basic rules for measuring the exposure of production factors and sampling, as well as informing about the main production factors specific to a particular industrial facility.

Measurement data online can be transmitted to the central office of CCM via the call center for risk assessment and monitoring of the production environment. Thus, we came to understand the need to create an integrated 'life support system' at remote sites, which includes the following basic components:

- risk assessment of the most significant diseases, taking into account the specifics of working conditions, climate and geographical, occupational and conventional risk factors,
- training of medical and non-medical specialists for the organization of an optimal life support system for personnel at remote sites,
- development and implementation of targeted programs for the prevention of the most significant diseases, taking into account the specific working conditions and the specifics of production activities.

An Association of Independent Experts — the "Institute of Remote Healthcare" was organized in September 2016 in Tomsk in order to fully implement identified tasks. The main activity is carried out in the following areas:

- educational activities,
- scientific research,
- consultancy.

Currently, an educational course "Occupational Hygiene and Occupational Risk Assessment" has been developed for postgraduate education in these topic areas, together with the Siberian State Medical University.

Along with this, experts of the Institute of Remote Health are developing programs for detailed workers' health assessment at remote industrial facilities with an increased risk of occupational and most significant non-communicable diseases (primarily oncological and cardiovascular). The results of periodic medical check-ups and the implementation of detailed health assessment programs are the basis for the formation of a personnel database of remote industrial facilities. This allows ongoing monitoring of the state health of personnel and improving large-scale epidemiological studies to assess the inter-dependence of morbidity and mortality from environmental conditions, industrial and endogenous factors.

References

Aliyeva LA. 2011. Study of lifestyle and health of workers of industrial enterprises. Moscow University: MedSc thesis abstract.

Antipov SA, Sokolovich EG and Lugachev VA. 2009. New model of the organization of medical care in enterprises in modern economic conditions. VIII All-Russian Congress "Occupation and Health". Moscow, November 25–27. Moscow: Delta Publishing House, pp. 17–18.

Averyanova TA, Poteryaeva EL, Trufanova NL and Chebykin DV. 2012. Medical staff health protection in the terms of healthcare modernization. XI All-Russian Congress "Occupation and Health". Moscow, November 27–29. Moscow: FSBI NII MT RAMS, pp. 473–475.

Bakirov AB and Gimranova GG. 2016. Priority areas of science in the extraction of oil, petroleum refining, petrochemical industries. *Occupational Medicine and Human Ecology* **3**: 5–10.

Bashurin AD, Kachalov IA and Salnikov AS. 2014. Methods of risk management. Science and education in the XXI century: a collection of scientific papers based on the materials of the International Scientific and Practical Conference, December 30, Part Y. Moscow: AR-Consult.

Begiev VG, Andreev VB, Potapova KN and Moskvina AN. 2015. Telemedicine to improve the advisory and diagnostic assistance of highly specialized centers in the conditions of the Far North. Proceedings of the I International Scientific and Practical Conference Belgorod, April 30, Part III. Belgorod: IE Tkacheva E.P., pp. 6–8.

Denisov EI, Prokopenko LV, Stepanyan IV and Chesalin PV. 2011. Occupational risk management: prognosis, causation and bioinformational technologies. Legal and methodological foundations of occupational risk management. *Occupational Medicine and Industrial Ecology* **12**: 6–11.

Dudareva AA and Talykova LV. 2012. Occupational morbidity and occupational accidents in Russia with emphasis on arctic regions, 1980–2010. *Biosphere* **4**: 343–363.

Ermakova SE and Salnikov AA. 2016. Opportunities to use international experience in managing the healthcare system, including public-private partnerships and outsourcing. *Russian Entrepreneurship* **17**: 811–822.

Fedyaev DV, Fedyaeva VK and Omelyanovsky VV. 2014. Economic justification for telehealth technology use for preventive medical examination of the population in remote regions. Farmakoekonomika. *Modern Pharmacoeconomics and Pharmacoepidemiology* **3**: 30–35.

Furman VY. 2009. Justification of the directions of improving the organization of medical care of workers of large industrial enterprises. Ekaterinburg University: MedSc thesis abstract.

Glushkov VA, Sayfutdinov RA, Nosova EV and Rodionova KA. 2015. System of social protection of the population in the field of social insurance. *Actual Issues of Modern Science* **40**: 56–65.

Gurinovich EG. 2009. Improving the organization of medical care for industrial workers. Kemerovo University: MedSc thesis abstract.

Gurvich VB, Kuzmin SV, Plotko EG, Roslyi OF, Fedoruk AA and Ruzakov VO. 2015. Analysis of the methodic approaches to the occupational risk assessment in the enterprises of the Sverdlovsk region. *Hygiene and Sanitation* **94**: 119–123.

Kursov OA. 2016. System of evaluation and management of professional risks: problems of legal regulation. J Lex Russica **10**: 182–188.

Levanov VM, Mamonova EY, Orlov OI and Kamaev IA. 2016. The use of telemedicine technologies for the purpose of remote training of medical personnel at health centers of a large oil and gas producing company. *Medical Almanac* **1**: 18–21.

Levashov SP. 2012. Occupational risks assessment in the Russian Federation and abroad. *Problems of Risk Analysis* **9**: 54–65.

Lobzhanidze AA, Yatsenko IB, Tkachenko OE and Barygin ME. 2016. Organization and evaluation of the functioning of the regional air ambulance service. *Scientific Notes St. Petersburg State Medical University* **23**: 21–25.

Mikhina TV. 2016. Economic mechanisms of professional risk management. *Mining Information and Analytical Bulletin* **6**: 222–230.

Marsh-Feiley G, Eadie L and Wilson P. 2018. Telesonography in emergency medicine: a systematic review. *PLoS One* **13**: e0194840, doi: 10.1371/journal.pone.0194840.

Norman JN, Ballantine BN, Brebner JA, Brown B, Gauld SJ, Mawdsley J, Roythorne C, Valentine MJ and Wilcock SE. 1988. Medical evacuations from offshore structures. *Br J Ind Med* **45**: 619–623.

Okulova VM. 2013. Problems in the development of regional air transport in the regions of Siberia and the Far East. Available at http://federalbook.ru/files 4.

Order No. 586 of the Ministry of Healthcare and Social Development of Russia of October 23, 2008. "Concept of the Federal Action Program for the Improvement of Labor Conditions and Safety for 2008–2010".

Orlov OI, Mamonova EY and Levanov VM. 2016. Organizational issues of distant trainings of medical personnel of remote health centers for emergency medical care. *Saratov Journal of Medical Scientific Research* **12**: 617–619.

Petrenko KV. 2014. The level of human resource health in the oil and gas producing regions of the North of Russia. *Omsk University Bulletin. Economy Series* **2**: 137–141.

Petrova NG, Teptin SE and Pogosyan SG. 2014. Health of the working population of a large agroindustrial oblast (according results of additional dispensarization). Problems of *Social Hygiene, Healthcare and Medical History* **3**: 15–19.

Piven DV, Koziakova ES and Tsoktoev DB. 2003. Evaluation of the economic efficiency of telemedicine in the provision of surgical care to patients with bones and joints tuberculosis. *Siberian Medical Journal (Irkutsk)* **40**: 79–82.

Poletaeva OV. 2017. Professional longevity and psychological health in the Arctic. *Bulletin of Kurgan State University* **1**: 118–122.

Radushkevich VL and Bartashevich BI. 2011. Emergency care in remote and difficult to access areas. *Ambulance* **4**: 41–48.

Rogers H, Madathil KC, Agnisarman S, Narasimha S, Ashok A, Nair A, Welch BM and McElligott JT. 2017. A systematic review of the implementation challenges of telemedicine systems in ambulances. *Telemed J E Health* **23**: 707–71, doi: 10.1089/tmj.2016.0248.

Roik V. 2003. Zero risk — chimera. Human resources — Professional risk: problems of analysis and management. Available at URL:http://www.rhr.ru/index.php/rule/social_work_and_PR.

Rudel D, Slemenik-Pušnik C, Epšek-Lenart M, Pušnik S and Lavre J. 2015. From a green field to a telemedicine service supporting 400 patients in one year: the Slovenian experience. *Journal of Telemedicine and e-Health*: 46–49.

Samara NA. 2017. The state of labor conditions and labor protection in modern Russia. *Labor Economics* **3**.

Smal TS, Zavadovskaya VD and Deev IA. 2017. Using telemedicine technology in radiology for low-density area. Journal of Social aspects of population health **53**: 1–9.

Teslya AB and Kryukov VK. 2018. Justification of the need for application of telemedicine technologies for workers of enterprises located in hard-accessed regions of the Russian Federation // *Scientific bulletin of the Southern Institute of Management* **4**: 100–106.

Timoshkina EV. 2012. Ways to improve the management of professional risks. *Occupational Safety and Safety in Industrial Enterprises* **1**: 21–25.

Trikman OP, Yushkova NG, Biryukova OA, Trikman EY, Karimova MV and Shikhta NA. 2016. Organization of medical care for industrial workers of Cate Zheleznogorsk. *Bulletin of the Clinical Hospital* **51**: 18–21.

Trushkova EA and Kantsigov BR. 2015. On the issue of the problems of transition to professional risk management. Proceedings of the International Scientific-Practical Conference. FGBOU VPO "Rostov State University of Civil Engineering", Union of Builders of the Southern Federal District, Don Association of Builders, pp. 87–88.

Valeeva ET. 2013. Scientific substantiation of the healthcare system for workers in the chemical industry based on an occupational risk assessment // thesis abstract for the DMedSc, Moscow, 2013.

Zakharov FG. 1965. Essay on the organization history of medical care of industrial workers in Russia and the USSR // thesis abstract for the degree of the DMedSc, Kharkov, 1965.

Chapter

13

Work and Experience of an Oil Industry Remote Medical Practitioner

Harry Horsley

Introduction

Remote healthcare is the means of delivering healthcare to remote communities, often in isolated and hostile environments. The name was probably first used by Memorial University, Newfoundland, where such a system of health was developed to serve the needs of the scattered population in that area (Norman and Brebner, 1988). The main limitations of providing health systems to such isolated populations are the need to rely on non-medically qualified personnel, so-called remote health practitioners, for the actual delivery of the care.

The following will describe some aspects of working as a remote health practitioner, and the associated issues of training, supervision, relationships and conflicts of interest, with special emphasis on providing healthcare to workforces serving the oil and gas industries.

The need to deliver healthcare in remote areas is not a new phenomenon, and regions such as Russia, Canada, Africa and Scandinavia have a long history of meeting the health needs of their people living in areas distant from the major population centres.

However, particularly since the mid-20th century, the growth of oil and gas exploration and extraction industries throughout the world, often in remote and hostile areas such as deserts or offshore, brought with it the need to provide for the healthcare needs of these workers, and the development of remote health practitioners specialising in these industries.

One example of this was the discovery of oil and gas deposits in the North Sea and other parts of the United Kingdom Continental Shelf (UKCS) and their subsequent exploitation, which created a whole new industry for thousands of workers who found themselves working on floating rigs or fixed platforms hundreds of miles offshore. A typical production platform in the UKCS may be home and workplace to between 100 and 200 personnel, with possibly many more (>500) working on it during periods of intensive activity, these additional personnel living on specially adapted barges ("flotels") moored alongside the platform itself.

Whereas the actual distances from land are not extreme, like other parts of the world where oil and gas exploration and extraction are undertaken, the UKCS can be a harsh environment, and isolation means that communications and transport are expensive. Transport of personnel is usually by helicopter, whereas most supplies, except the most urgent, are delivered by specially designed supply boats. As well as considerable costs, both of these means of transport may also incur risks to personnel.

To cater for the demands of the offshore and similar remote working environments, distinctive work patterns have developed. Activity is unceasing, and the maximum use of (expensive) labour is achieved through shift working. Typically, these shifts comprise a twelve-hour working day over a period of 2, 3 or 4 weeks, or longer, followed by a period of leave ("field break"). Enormous onshore support in every sphere is required to maintain any offshore operation, and training is undertaken for all eventualities.

As a result of this working environment, the workforce of over 30,000 in the UKCS (HSE, 2016a) has been required to espouse a lifestyle which entails remoteness from onshore medical facilities, and to cater for their healthcare needs, a system of remote healthcare has developed, which has also been adopted worldwide for similar working environments.

Remote Healthcare and Offshore Medics

The remote health practitioners who work in support of the oil and gas industry, whether offshore or in remote areas of the world, usually have nursing or other paramedic backgrounds, supplemented by additional training to prepare them for the increased responsibilities. The traditional model of remote healthcare relies on the supervision by a doctor of the remote health practitioners (so-called "topside cover"). However, in addition to the remote practitioners, the provision of healthcare to remote populations, including oil workers, includes certain supplementary measures to minimise the effects of a delay in accessing mainstream medical facilities. Norman and Brebner (1988) described these measures which make up a remote healthcare system as:

- Training in basic life support for all the population at risk
- Effective medical communications
- Training for both remote practitioners, and the doctors providing support from a base
- A system of medical surveillance to pre-empt or to detect at an early stage avoidable medical events

This system of remote healthcare has been adopted for offshore oil and gas installations in the UKCS, but can also be applied to any situation where access to mainstream healthcare is delayed, either through distance, or other obstacles, such as weather or transport issues. Similarly, the practice of providing "topside cover" by a medical practitioner has also been widely adopted worldwide.

The location's isolation and the logistics of transport are major factors for the remote health practitioner when there is a need to transfer a patient for further evaluation or treatment, either as an urgent or non-urgent case. The process might involve considerable cost (especially in the case of dedicated helicopters), disruption, and possible risk to the patient and others. The term "medevac" (medical evacuation) has been coined for this process and, although it conjures up images of life-saving rescue operations, the majority of medevacs are for non-life threatening reasons. Often this is because the person may not be seriously unwell, but their condition renders them unable to perform their duties and they need to be replaced. This is especially the case on offshore installations where beds are invariably at a premium, and factors such as shared cabins are not conducive to the rest and quiet required for recuperation.

Remote health practitioners working in the UKCS have come to be known as "Offshore Medics" or simply "Medics". Initially, training in first-aid was sufficient to fulfil the role, but the qualifications required by medics on an offshore installation with a minimum number of personnel was changed in the UK by the passing into law in 1989 of the Offshore Installations and Pipeline Works (First-Aid) Regulations 1989, as amended in 1993, 1995, 1999 and 2015 — abbreviated as "OFAR 1989". The legislation's Approved Code of Practice (ACOP) provides advice to comply with the requirements of the regulations, and it addresses issues such as the role, responsibilities and competencies of offshore medics and offshore first-aiders.

Registered nurses and ex-military medical technicians were initially the obvious source for these medics, and training programmes were developed to prepare them for working offshore, as were periodic refresher programmes.

OFAR 1989 stipulates the length of training, the syllabus for both initial and refresher courses and the duration of practice certificates for offshore medics. Initially, candidates with an acceptable professional background of nursing or with military medical qualifications must undergo an initial training consisting of 20 working days, including clinical attachments of 5 days each to a General Practitioner (GP) and a hospital's Accident and Emergency department. Thereafter, licensed offshore medics must undertake a refresher course of 10 day's duration not less than every three years.

OFAR 1989 (regulation 5(10c)) also requires that arrangements are in place for the work of offshore medics to be supervised by a medical practitioner based onshore in the UK, who is also available to give advice on the management of cases of illness or injury (the "topside cover" previously mentioned). Sometimes this is a doctor employed directly by the operating company but, more often, because of the 24/7 on-call requirement, specialist medical services providers are contracted to fulfil this role.

Whilst the stipulations of OFAR 1989 are a legal requirement for installations operating in UKCS waters, they have also often been adopted in other remote working environments throughout the world, unless local law, which will always take precedence, exceeds the requirements (e.g. Norway stipulates that offshore medics must be registered nurses).

In the UK, the Health & Safety Executive (HSE), a government agency, is responsible for approving and monitoring the syllabus, equipment, environment, and staff of establishments which offer both the initial and refresher training for offshore medics.

However, although establishments which offer the training for offshore medics must be approved by the HSE and undergo regular monitoring, no central database exists of personnel who hold the offshore medic certificate (Elliott, 2004). Individual training establishments hold their own records, and it is the responsibility of employing organisations to ensure that employees are appropriately qualified. Consequently, no centralised record exists of the number or profile of offshore medics, and this has been recognised as a major obstacle in efforts to regulate offshore medics.

As well as the training requirements, the professional background of personnel who wish to undertake the initial training is stipulated in the HSE guidance (HSE, 2000). Suitable backgrounds are:

- A Registered General Nurse with at least 3 years of post-registration experience,
- Royal Navy — Leading Medical Assistant (LMA) or above / Royal Marines Medical Assistance (at Corporal or above),
- Army — Combat Medical Technician Class 1 (CMT 1 RAMC) Corporal and above.
- RAF — Royal Air Force Medical Assistant (at Corporal or above)

However, there is some discretion allowed on the part of training establishments to accept other backgrounds, e.g. Paramedics, Operating Department Assistants. Along with the absence of a central register, this diversity of backgrounds and experience has proven to be a major difficulty in establishing professional recognition and identity for medics.

This lack of professional recognition has led to some dissatisfaction amongst remote health practitioners about the role. An article by Bonnar (1994) raised questions about the offshore medics' role and was critical of the under-utilisation of nursing skills and experience. Doctoral research by Ruddick-Bracken (1989, 1990) explored offshore medics' roles and their perceptions of the role, and found the attractions included high salaries and autonomous work whilst disadvantages of the role included lack of promotion prospects, little mental stimulation, work-life balance issues, non-medical administration duties, and professional isolation. Many respondents felt that they were viewed as non-productive and not held in high esteem by management.

Remote Health Practitioners in The Oil Industry: Scope of Practice

Now in its fifth decade, the UKCS offshore oil and gas industry is in its mature phase. However, whilst some aspects such as technology have developed enormously, how has the role of the offshore medic changed?

The answer is that no one really knows, and there are undoubtedly major variations in the role between different employing companies and areas. However, there are some indicators; firstly, there is the change in healthcare needs, and there have indeed been some major changes in the patterns of illness and injury in the UKCS.

Safety management has been one of the major factors in reducing the number of injuries, and, particularly after the Pipe Alpha disaster in 1988, there have been tremendous changes in the offshore health and safety regimes.

In the UK, under the Reporting of Injuries, Diseases and Dangerous Occurrences Regulations 2013, injuries resulting from work related incidents have to be reported, but only if they result in an absence from work of seven days or more (previously three days), or certain categories of injury (such as a fracture), or death (HSE, 2013). Data for such injuries and fatalities are published annually, but the threshold for reporting means that much ill health caused by, or related to, work is unreported to the regulator, the HSE.

Figures 1 and 2 present the trends for all reported injuries, and reported major and specified injuries in the period 2007/8–2016 (HSE, 2016a) and both categories show an overall decline in these events, particularly since the introduction of the Step Change for Safety (SCS) initiative.

Historically, several studies have attempted to examine the pattern of illness in the offshore industry. In the 1980's and 1990's, retrospective and prospective surveys (Norman et al., 1988; HSE, 1998) spanning a decade of medical evacuations from offshore installations in the UKCS highlighted the altered pattern in reasons for medical evacuation of workers, in particular, a reduction in injury and increase in illness (Figure 3).

Source: RIDDOR

p = Provisional

For RIDDOR, a number of system and legislative changes have occurred over recent years, making comparisons difficult with previous data. See:
www.hse.gov.uk/statistics/riddor-notification.htm

Vantage population data, used to derive the rate per 100,000 full-time equivalent workers (FTE), was subject to some variability in its estimation process until 2010.

• • • Series break (fiscal year to calendar year)

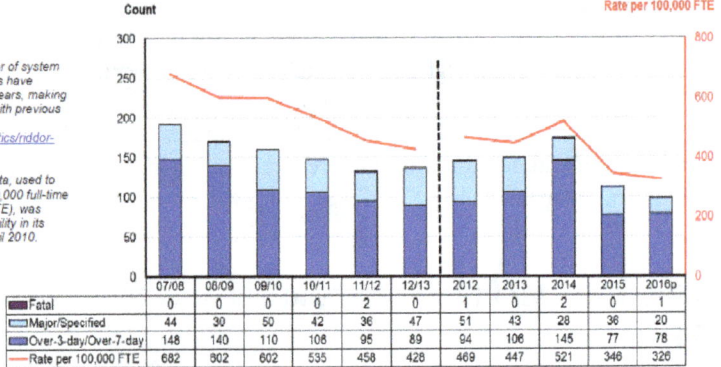

	07/08	08/09	09/10	10/11	11/12	12/13	2012	2013	2014	2015	2016p
Fatal	0	0	0	0	2	0	1	0	2	0	1
Major/Specified	44	30	50	42	36	47	51	43	28	36	20
Over-3-day/Over-7-day	148	140	110	106	95	89	94	106	145	77	78
Rate per 100,000 FTE	682	602	602	535	458	428	469	447	521	346	326

Figure 1:   All Reported Injuries Offshore 2007/8–2016

Source: RIDDOR

p = Provisional

• • • Series break (fiscal to calendar year)

- - - Series break: The category of 'specified injuries' replaced the previous 'major injury' category in October 2013. For more information, see:
www.hse.gov.uk/statistics/riddor-notification.htm

Vantage population data, used to derive the rate per 100,000 full-time equivalent workers (FTE), was subject to some variability in its estimation process until 2010.

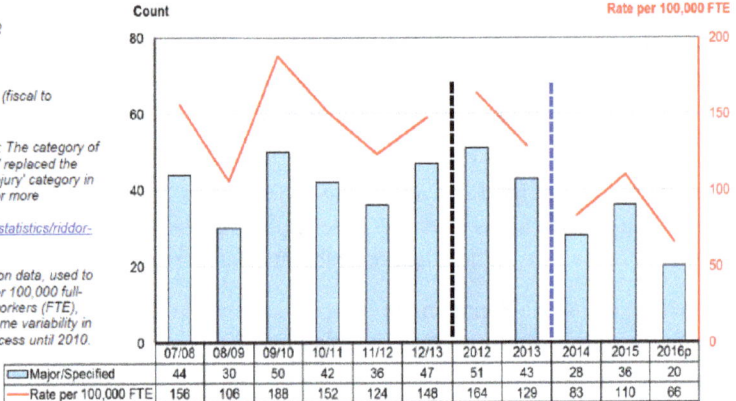

	07/08	08/09	09/10	10/11	11/12	12/13	2012	2013	2014	2015	2016p
Major/Specified	44	30	50	42	36	47	51	43	28	36	20
Rate per 100,000 FTE	156	106	188	152	124	148	164	129	83	110	66

Figure 2:   Reported Major/Specified Offshore Injuries 2007/8–2016

However, these studies relied on voluntary reporting by offshore medics and used the inclusion criterion of "evacuation for medical reasons" which was open to interpretation. Nonetheless, despite these weaknesses, several major areas of ill health were highlighted by these surveys. For example, in the retrospective survey (Norman *et al.*, 1988) dental health was shown to be one of the main reasons for workers returning onshore for treatment, and had implications for the training of medics and screening of the workforce; indeed, certificates of dental fitness were introduced for a period following the publication of the survey results.

Pre-deployment and periodic screening of the workforce is one of the tenets of a remote healthcare system as described by Norman and Brebner (1988).

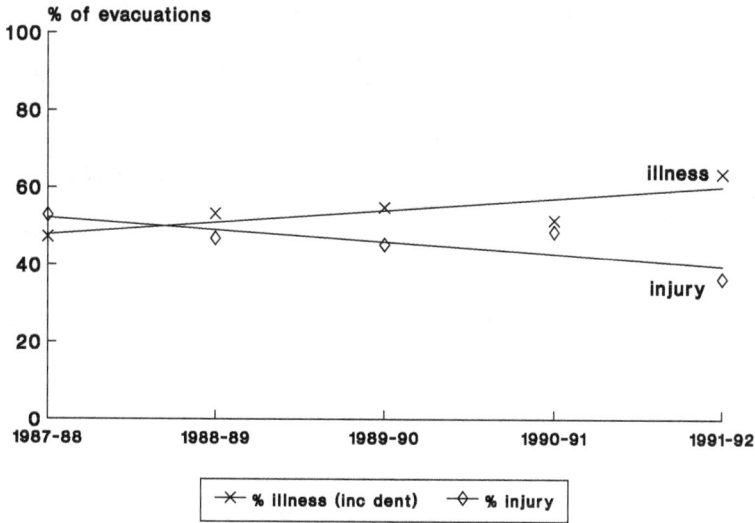

Figure 3: Reported Evacuations 1987–1992: Illness and Injury Trends (HSE, 1998)

A systematic and regulated system for screening personnel who work offshore or in other remote areas is another factor in reducing the risk of major ill health amongst the remote working population. In the UK, those wishing to work offshore have to undergo two-yearly (or in some cases more frequent) medical screening and meet the criteria for medical fitness. These criteria exclude certain conditions considered as unsuitable for the remote offshore environment (e.g. poorly controlled epilepsy or insulin-dependent diabetes). However, the medical screening is limited in scope, and it cannot detect some hitherto undiagnosed conditions such as latent heart disease, so the potential for the remote health practitioner to be faced with life-threatening cases remains a realistic prospect, and this is therefore a high priority in their training. Nonetheless, it is generally accepted that the majority of cases of ill health seen by an offshore medic will fall into the minor category — colds, upper repository tract infections, skin problems etc.

A dataset of over 11,000 presentations by workforce personnel to installation medics (O&GUK, 2018) found that 'coughs and colds', skin problems, 'aches and pains', digestive complaints and headaches were the most commonly encountered medical conditions. Almost 15% of the consultations were referred to the "topside" doctor for advice, and almost 4% resulted in a medevac.

These data support the findings of a previous project which explored the role, scope of practice and educational needs amongst offshore medics (Horsley, 2005) which found that the incidence of serious ill health or injury, and the frequency of performing advanced life support were all low.

Remote Health Practitioners Training

In the same survey (Horsley, 2005) some respondents also raised concerns about the educational preparation for the role, principally the adequacy of the current maximum of three years between refresher training, and of a perceived variation in standards between course providers. In keeping with Ruddick-Bracken's doctoral thesis findings (1989, 1990), there was also some evidence amongst respondents of a perceived low status, role overload, and a desire for increased professional recognition amongst offshore medics.

In part, this may be explained by the relative dearth of research into actual medical encounters experienced by offshore medics, and the wide range of potential medical conditions that may be encountered. Both these factors have led to difficulties in establishing the most appropriate training to equip medics for the role. The broad scope of the medical role — potentially having to manage everything from minor complaints to life-threatening emergencies — presents a dilemma for training providers whose emphasis has to be on the emergency situations, whereas such cases may, in fact, be a once-in-a-lifetime career event for most remote health practitioners working in the oil and gas industry.

Historically, the implications for medical services of the rapid expansion of activity in the UKCS was quickly recognised by the British Medical Association (BMA) which established a working party to undertake an assessment of the medical aspects of the offshore industry (Anon. 1975). One of these aspects was the variability of standards amongst offshore medics, at a time when the minimum qualification was a first-aid certificate.

The syllabi for both the initial training and subsequent refresher training for offshore medics was subsequently outlined in the guidance to OFAR 1989 (HSE, 2016b; MacNeil, 1987), although very little research has been undertaken on the appropriateness of the content. One such study (Brebner et al., 1995) used referrals from offshore installations to an A&E department over a nine-year period and established the prevalence of fractures, or suspected fractures, particularly involving the hand. However, the changing pattern of injury and illness underlines the importance of establishing a database of injuries encountered by offshore medics as a means of determining the relevance of the medic training courses.

There are, of course, healthcare practitioners whose first responder role is similar to that of the remote care practitioner. Ambulance paramedics are often cited as an analogous group, and two studies, one in the UK (Lendrum et al., 2000) and one in the USA (Pollock et al., 1997) looked at the relationship between training and practice in ambulance paramedics. Lendrum et al. (2000) analysed emergency ambulance cases for four weeks in an urban setting, and concluded that whilst training is mainly aimed at treatment of life-threatening conditions, training in the large workload represented by patients with minor sprains, strains and head injuries was under-represented. Pollock *et al.* (1997) used a postal survey of paramedics to elicit the perceived importance of paramedic skills, and found the importance of ET intubation, defibrillation and assessment to be ranked highest, although the perceived importance exceeded the emphasis placed on them in training. A review by Graham *et al.* (2003) of five years of paramedic activity in North Ayrshire concluded that changes in practice might be due to increasing experience, but also pointed out the danger of low exposure to extended skills.

Findings from both these studies are even more relevant to the remote health practitioner, whose exposure to major emergencies might be extremely limited; endotracheal intubation has, in fact, now been replaced by other forms of airway management because of the lack of regular experience.

As well as being able to assess and treat patients safely and appropriately, a critical skill of the remote health practitioner in the oil industry is to know when to refer patients for onshore treatment. Conversely, it is equally important to be able to identify those whose condition does not require immediate evacuation, when unnecessary air transport may not only have financial implications, but also involve risks to patient and crew. Although these decisions are taken in conjunction with the topside doctor, much depends on the history taking, examination and reporting skills of the remote health practitioner. Similarly, the topside doctor needs to be skilled in conducting remote consultations and have some familiarity and appreciation of the environment.

These risks were illustrated by Hagan (1982), whose role as an offshore medic also involved flying on search and rescue missions, and whose description of his role was published posthumously following his death along with five others in a helicopter crash whilst en route to attend an injured patient in the North Sea.

As mentioned previously, the diversity of backgrounds of remote health practitioners also causes problems in their initial training for the role. Some respondents to a survey (Horsley, 2005) raised concerns about aspects of the four-week initial training for offshore medics in the UKCS. One concern centred around the adequacy to prepare someone with limited experience for the complexity of the role; one respondent commented:

> *offshore medics who haven't worked without doctors, who haven't been trained to diagnose and prescribe, i.e. nurses ... struggle in their first 6 months offshore. ... I always wonder what would happen if a serious illness / incident happened in the first trip?*

Another concern was raised about what some respondents viewed as variations in standards between training providers. One especially critical comment from a respondent was:

> Currently, there is "factory mentality" where personnel are tested for competency ... some medics' skills, knowledge and behaviours are disgraceful, and there is no safeguard for clients. I believe that some medics allowed to practise are dangerous.

This highlighted the tension between course providers' commercial interests and the maintenance of standards. Although the range of topics to be addressed in the training programmes is articulated in OFAR 1989, the scope is wide and open to interpretation.

Similarly, whilst the training providers are regularly monitored by the HSE, there is some anecdotal evidence of variations between training providers and that standardisation of training is not regarded as a high priority. Some attempts to rectify this have been made by the Institute of Remote Healthcare (IRHC), a not-for-profit body established in 2008 by Professor Norman in an attempt to create a professional membership organisation dedicated to improving the healthcare of those living and working in remote and isolated environments.

Skill Decay

Among respondents from Horsley's (2005) study, it was estimated that injury accounted for fewer than 10% of consultations, and an issue recognised by many respondents was skill decay.

Skill decay concerns ambulance paramedics, offshore medics, and all emergency personnel who require to maintain their emergency skills, but is particularly relevant in situations where exposure to experience is limited, such as remote health practitioners in the oil industry.

An important review of factors that influence skill decay and retention by Arthur et al. (1998) involved 189 independent data points extracted from 53 articles. This quantitative meta-analysis confirmed that infrequent opportunities to perform or practise acquired skills led to skill deterioration and that the majority of skill decay occurs early after training. Periodic refresher training and re-certification are common methods of maintaining skill levels (Gus, 1987; Zautck et al., 1987). However, research by Chamberlain et al. (2002) into different methods of teaching CPR and their effects on skill decay provided evidence of only modest value in re-training. Alternatively, Kovacs et al. (2000) found in their randomised controlled trial of airway management that independent practice combined with periodic feedback was successful in maintaining skills.

Technology

The advent of the internet and video conferencing has undoubtedly helped reduce the isolation of remote health practitioners, and the development of the UKCS oil and gas fields was initially viewed with enthusiasm as possible areas for using telemedicine (Maclean *et al.*, 1995) and decision support (Armstrong *et al.*, 1996). The other potential application in relation to offshore medics was using teleconferencing technology to assess skills. As well as the ability to send photographs and scanned ECGs, some medical service providers use web-based databases to monitor the quality of their remote health practitioners' consultation records. However, besides a lack of consistency between medical service providers there has also been a failure to realise some of the potential which advances in technology promised; some major medical service providers still have as their mainstay for topside cover a reliance on the telephone for remote health practitioners to request advice and assistance, with all the potential problems associated with such a basic service.

Secondary Roles and Potential Role Conflict

Whilst the main role of the remote health practitioner is medical, in many cases when the caseload is limited it is generally accepted that, in addition to their medical duties, remote health practitioners perform other tasks. These additional roles are determined by employers, and they vary according to company policy and operational circumstances. In the UK the concept of such additional roles is accepted by the regulatory body, the Health and Safety Executive.

However, whilst it is recognised that these secondary roles should complement the offshore medic's main function, guidance is given also on what might be considered unsuitable roles, such as radio operators, helicopter landing officers or stewards with cleaning duties (HSE, 2002a). In the UKCS the most common types of secondary roles are administration, Industrial Hygiene (IH), and Health & Safety duties.

Administration duties commonly involve acting as "Heli-admin", i.e. managing helicopter flights and cabin allocation. Such a role is only feasible when the population is relatively small and the number of flights is limited, otherwise it can conflict with the need to be available for medical duties. The role can also involve disputes about flight allocation and, especially, cabin sharing. Industrial Hygiene (IH) is also recognised as an important area because of an increasing awareness of the morbidity and mortality caused by occupational exposures — 13,000 deaths each year are estimated to be linked to past exposure at work, primarily to chemicals or dust (HSE, 2018a).

IH roles include coordinating the management of:

- Hazardous substances (COSHH)
- Radiation, mobile and fixed sources, and normally occurring radioactive material (NORM)
- Potable water (especially Legionella management)
- Hand Arm Vibration prevention programme
- Noise management
- Display screen equipment
- Manual handling

There is a large training requirement for these roles and they can impose a significant time burden on the remote health practitioner, although there is the advantage of not being as time critical as Heli-admin duties, and not as potentially conflicting with availability for medical duties. IH management also has the advantage of adding to the knowledge and skillset of the medic, and providing a more fulfilling role.

The reduction in injuries, and the drive for economy, have led to a growing trend for the roles of offshore medic and Health, Safety and Environmental Advisor (HSEA) to be combined. Indeed, there is a degree of overlap between the two roles, especially in the area of occupational health.

However, there are also potential conflicts of interest. These include (Horsley, 2009):

- appropriate preparation and qualifications
- problems of combining the therapeutic role with, sometimes, a disciplinary role
- ethical issues of medical confidentiality
- time constraints and time management and ensuring neither role suffers
- emergency response roles, medics also in a safety role need to be very clear about their emergency roles, and ensure systems are in place to accommodate this

In the UKCS the title "medic" has, unfortunately, acquired some unfavorable historical baggage linked to the low profile and perceived unproductive nature of much of the role. Having a secondary role with increased visibility can help in rectifying negative perceptions. As one medic who was also responsible for the management of industrial hygiene commented

there was always that perception that all a medic did was sit upstairs in the sickbay...
just waiting for someone to come in and dish out Lemsip. And that's what people
believe that we do, because we weren't very public about the sorts of things that we
do, but what we're doing now from an occupational health perspective is we're very
public in the things we're delivering and people can see what we do.

In addition to these concerns, from a sociological perspective, another area of
potential role conflict relates to those tensions which can occur between professions
and bureaucracies. The term "bureaucratic" would apply to most large commercial
organisations, such as oil and gas operators. The tensions and potential for conflict
between bureaucratic organisations and individuals belonging to a profession
have long been recognised and described; the German sociologist Max Weber
(1964) is credited with possibly the most influential analysis of the bureaucratic
administration. He examined organisations in the context of the system of controls,
and listed six characteristics which make up his "ideal" bureaucratic organisation:

- specification of tasks
- hierarchy of authority
- system of rules
- impersonality
- employment based on technical efficiency and constituting a career
- efficiency

Similarly, Millerson (1964) isolated the following characteristics of a model
profession, without insisting that all professions display every characteristic. These
include:

- skill based on theoretical knowledge
- an extensive period of education
- the theme of public service and altruism
- the existence of a code of conduct or ethics
- insistence upon personal freedom to regulate itself
- the testing of the competence of members before admission to the profession

When separate, the two roles of offshore medic and HSEA are closely aligned
to professionalism and bureaucracy and, as such, demonstrate areas for
potential conflict. Theoretically, this conflict may relate to the differing views of
organisational control. In a bureaucratic organisation, the professional will be
obliged to accept the authority of a non-professional. Similarly, professional ideals

involving the special client–practitioner relationship may conflict with the more specific aims of the organisation. Four main areas of conflict have been described:

- the professional's resistance of bureaucratic rules
- their rejection of bureaucratic standards
- their resistance of supervision
- their loyalty to the organisation may not be total

An example of such an area of potential conflict might involve medical confidentiality where a nurses' professional body, the Nursing and Midwifery Council (NMC), requires that a code of ethics be adhered to. In the case of medical details, disclosure may only be made with the informed (written) consent of the client, or where required by law (NMC, 2018). To a manager, who sees his only responsibility as the efficient running of the organisation, such ethical constraints might be viewed as an unnecessary hindrance if he were required to investigate the reasons behind sickness or injury. Other sources of conflict might include the workers' access to the medic, a situation where some organisations seek to control access by workers, e.g. requiring permission from supervisors.

Safety Management

As inferred previously, safety management is one of the roles that is often combined with that of medic and, given the appropriate environment and support, and despite the potential for conflict as outlined above, the two roles can indeed complement each other. The subject of safety management is enormous and the following is only intended to summarise the main points from the perspective of the remote health practitioner.

The popular perception of the oil and gas industry, and particularly offshore installations, is of a highly dangerous working environment. This perception actually confuses hazard (anything that may cause harm,) and risk (the chance that somebody could be harmed by the hazards). The oil and gas industry is indeed a high hazard environment; hydrocarbons are inherently hazardous, and the remote environment constitutes a further significant hazard. However, whilst the potential for major hazards is ever present, in general the level of control exerted over all aspects of work and life in these industries means that, in fact, the oil and gas sector can be one of the safer working environments around.

In 2017 there was no fatalities recorded in the UKCS, and the industry's three-year rolling average non-fatal injury rate per 10,000 workers was reportedly half that of construction and transport (O&GUK, 2017).

The following figures provide a stark contrast with recorded fatal and non-fatal injuries for onshore industries in the UK; 144 workers killed at work in 2017/18, and 609,000 estimated non-fatal injuries to workers according to self-reports from the Labour Force Survey in 2016/17 (HSE, 2018b).

However, despite the year-on-year decline in work-related onshore fatalities (Figure 4, HSE, 2018c), a constant feature has been that two sectors — construction and agriculture & forestry (the latter two counted together) have always accounted for over half of the annual number of deaths. The simple reasoning behind this is that these two sectors are recognised as being highly hazardous, involving heavy machinery, lifting operations, working at heights etc., but (with some exceptions) are also acknowledged to have low levels of control.

In contrast, and again with exceptions, the oil and gas industry, and particularly offshore installations is also a high hazard environment, but it is characterised by an extremely high degree of control. This control is evident in three main areas:

- Control of hazards at source: inspection, certification and planned maintenance of plant and equipment
- Control of work
- Control directed at individuals through behavioural safety programmes

Inspection and certification of machinery can be traced to the early 20th century and the loss of vessels at sea due to explosions caused by caustic cracking around rivets in steam boilers.

This led to compulsory periodic inspection of boilers, and the Factories Act 1961 dictated fixed intervals of 14 months for steam raising equipment. The Flixborough

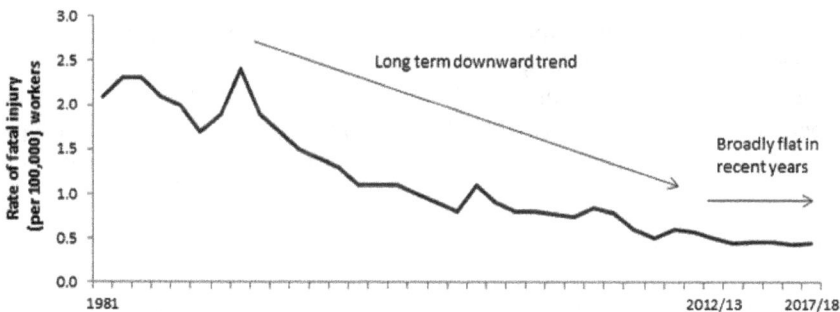

Figure 4:   Rate of Fatal Injury Per 100,000 Workers (Onshore)

chemical plant disaster subsequently led to a change in legislation for pressure systems from fixed terms to 'goal setting' (Jackson, 2014).

As with other safety processes, inspection systems evolved from proscriptive regimes to risk-based systems, using both qualitative and quantitative methods. Along with planned maintenance, computing power has enabled sophisticated programmes to be developed which can be linked to planning and scheduling systems. The other major change has been the introduction of non-invasive techniques for inspection (e.g. ultra-sound, radiography) which avoid the need to shut down equipment and processes. An important part of inspection is that it should involve a third party and a mechanism for independent verification.

The second control — control of work — is largely achieved through permit-to-work (PTW) systems, but in themselves permits are only one part of a work organisation. Central to the organisation of work is the hierarchy of individuals who play a role. Although simplified, an example of such a hierarchy is (names and permissions may differ according to the organisation):

- Site Controller: the only individual able to authorise work permits
- Area Authority (AA): visits the proposed worksite and performs initial scrutiny of work permits and releases permits to the Performing Authority
- Performing Authority (PA): creates draft permits and "accepts" authorised permits. PAs can sometimes oversee several work scopes, but are ultimately responsible for the safe working practices of the tasks

PTW systems were originally paper-based, but electronic Integrated Safe System of Work (ISSOW) programmes are now ubiquitous. ISSOW systems integrate PTW, Risk Assessment and Isolation Management under a single electronic system, providing many benefits, including efficiencies, traceability and ability to store lessons learned from previous work (Olliff, 2008).

Whereas process safety, through inspection, planned maintenance, and work management is about "keeping the oil and gas in the pipes", personal safety is about preventing accidents through the actions of individuals. Behavioural safety programmes focus on proactively motivating and empowering workers to adopt safe behaviours, rather than reactively relying on punishment for those caught working unsafely.

A key process in behavioural safety programmes is often represented as ABC:

- Antecedents: the causal event or trigger preceding the behaviour
- Behaviour: the observable thing that someone does or doesn't do

- Consequences: the outcome of the behaviour for the individual that influences the likelihood that the behaviour will be repeated

A research (HSE, 2002b) report provides more detail and examples on implementing a behavioural safety programme. However, Leathley (2016) points out two criticisms: (1) when the focus is on worker behaviour, but ignoring the antecedents and consequences rooted in management and leadership conduct, and (2) the risk that they are used as a substitute for providing a safe workplace and a safe system of work.

One safety tool linked to behavioural safety which is common in the oil and gas industry, although originating in the onshore chemical industry, is the behavioural safety observation reporting system. This tool goes under several guises, but essentially encourages everyone to participate in having conversations about good or poor behaviours. A conversation regarding a good behaviour (e.g. someone using good manual handling techniques) would result in a "commendation" for the individual. Conversely, an observation regarding a poor behaviour (e.g. someone not wearing the appropriate PPE) would ideally result in an agreement from the individual to always wear the correct protection in future. Anonymity is an important feature of such programmes, to avoid a culture of "naming and shaming". Observations are collated and, given sufficient data, trends can be identified which, in theory, can allow proactive interventions to be initiated.

One perennial criticism of safety regimes, particularly among contractors whose existence depends on securing work from larger operators, is that they encourage, either actively or passively, concealment and, potentially, the development of a culture where only good news is allowed to travel up to senior management. Sometimes a reason for this is the impact a poor safety performance has on the organisation's reputation and their success in tendering for contracts, where safety performance is one of the factors assessed in the process. Additionally, safety incentives targeted at individuals or teams can, if poorly managed, contribute to such concealment. This is especially the case when large financial or other inducements are offered which can constitute an incentive for individuals or teams not to report incidents, accidents or near misses.

This can be an area of potential conflict for remote health practitioners when accidents occur; although the practitioner should always act in the best interest of the patient, there is always the risk that conscious or subconscious bias can be experienced to avoid jeopardising the organisation's safety performance.

There is no legal requirement for formal training or certification to call oneself a safety advisor, but, in practice, the Institution of Safety and Health (IOSH) has become the recognised body for safety professionals. IOSH offer a graded structure for their members, which is linked to academic qualifications, or experiential learning demonstrated by portfolio. The categories in 2018 are:

- **Associate Member:** accredited level 3 qualification required, but no health and safety experience is necessary
- **Technical Member:** accredited level 3 qualification and health and safety experience required
- **Graduate Member:** accredited qualifications or a cognate degree
- **Chartered Member:** graduate membership and successful completion of the Initial Professional Development portfolio and peer interview

References

Anon. 1975. Medical aspects of North Sea oil. *Br Med J* **3**: 576–580.

Armstrong IJ, Haston WS and Maclean JR. 1996. Telepresence for decision support offshore *J Telemed Telecare* **2**: 176–177.

Arthur W Jr, Bennett W, Stanush PL and McNelly TL. 1998. Factors that influence skill decay and retention. A quantitative review and analysis. *Hum Perform* **11**: 57–101.

Bonnar A. 1994. Offshore medic or offshore OHN? *Occupational Health* **46**: 24–25.

Brebner JA, Norman JN, Page JG and Ruddick-Bracken H. 1995. Research based training for the nurse practitioner. *Accident and Emergency Nursing* **3**: 92–94.

Chamberlain D, Smith A, Woollard M, Colquhoun M, Handley AJ, Leaves S and Kern KB. 2002. Trials of teaching methods in basic life support (3): comparison of simulated CPR performance after first training and at 6 months, with a note on the value of re-training *Resuscitation* **53**:179–187.

Elliott RC. 2004. *Personal communication.*

Graham CA, Kumaravel M and Stevenson J. 2003. Ambulance paramedic activities in North Ayrshire: a five-year review. *Eur J Emerg Med* **10**: 279–282.

Guss DA. 1987. Airway management training and skill decay. *Emerg Care Q* **3**: 7–10.

Hagan J. 1982. Offshore nursing: offshore-hospital. *Nurs Mirror* **155**: 21–22.

Health care and first aid on offshore installations and pipeline works Offshore Installations and Pipeline Works (First-Aid) Regulations 1989 Approved Code of Practice and guidance; 2nd Edition (2000); Health and Safety Executive, London.

Health & Safety Executive (HSE). 1998. Study of medical evacuations from offshore installations. Five-year report 1987–1992. *Health & Safety Executive*, OTO 98 171.

HSE. 2002a. Offshore Division. Operations Notice 55. Suitable secondary roles for offshore medics. Available at www.hse.gov.uk/offshore/notices/on_55.htm [accessed September 2018].

HSE. 2002b. Strategies to promote safe behavior as part of a health and safety management system. Contract Research Report 430/2002. Available at http://www.hse.gov.uk/research/crr_pdf/2002/crr02430.pdf [accessed September 2018].

HSE. 2013. Reporting injuries, diseases and dangerous occurrences in health and social care. Guidance for employers. Available at http://www.hse.gov.uk/pubns/hsis1.pdf [accessed September 2018].

HSE. 2016a. Offshore Statistics & Regulatory Activity Report 2016. Available at http://www.hse.gov.uk/offshore/statistics/hsr2016.pdf [accessed September 2018].

HSE. 2016b. Healthcare and first aid on offshore installations and pipeline works. Offshore Installations and Pipeline Works (First-Aid) Regulations 1989. Approved Code of Practice and guidance. Available at http://www.hse.gov.uk/pubns/priced/l123.pdf [accessed September 2018].

HSE 2018a. Work-related ill health and occupational disease in Great Britain. Available at http://www.hse.gov.uk/statistics/causdis/ [accessed September 2018].

HSE 2018b. Health and Safety Statistics. Available at http://www.hse.gov.uk/statistics [accessed September 2018].

HSE 2018c. Workplace fatal injuries in Great Britain 2018. Available at http://www.hse.gov.uk/statistics/pdf/fatalinjuries.pdf [accessed September 2018].

Horsley HD. 2005. An exploration of the role, practice and educational needs of offshore medics in the United Kingdom Continental Shelf. University of Aberdeen: MSc dissertation.

Horsley HD. 2009. An exploration of the synergy and conflicts involved in combining the roles of offshore medic and health and safety advisor. University of Strathclyde: MSc dissertation.

Jackson P. 2014. Risky business. *Safety & Health Practitioner* 32: 44–47.

Kovacs G, Bullock G, Ackroyd-Stolarz S, Cain E and Petrie D. 2000. A randomized controlled trial on the effect of educational interventions in promoting airway management skill maintenance. *Ann Emerg Med* 36: 301–309.

Leathley B. 2016. Behavioural safety. *Safety & Health Practitioner* 34.

Lendrum K, Wilson S and Cooke MW. 2000. Does the training of ambulance personnel match the workload seen? *Pre-Hospital Immediate Care* 4: 7–10.

Maclean JR, Brebner JA and Norman JN. 1995. A review of Scottish telemedicine. *J Telemed Telecare* 1: 1–6.

MacNeil M. 1987. Offshore medic training: a university initiative. *Occup Health* (Lond) 39: 306–307.

Millerson G. 1964. *The Qualifying Profession*. London: Routledge & Keegan.

Norman JN and Brebner JA. 1988. Remote medicine: delivery of care to remote communities especially rigs in the North Sea. *Occup Health* (Lond) 40: 598–600.

Norman JN, Ballantine BN, Brebner JA, Brown B, Gauld SJ, Mawdsley J, Roythorne C, Valentine MJ and Wilcock SE. 1988. Medical evacuations from offshore structures. *Br J Ind Med* **45**: 619–623.

NMC. 2018. Nursing and Midwifery Council Code of Professional Conduct. Available at https://www.nmc.org.uk/standards/code/read-the-code-online [accessed September 2018].

O&GUK. 2017. Oil & Gas UK Health & Safety Report 2017. Available at http://oilandgasuk. co.uk/wp-content/uploads/2017/07/Health-Safety-Report-2017-Oil-Gas-UK.pdf [accessed September 2018].

O&GUK. 2018. Oil & Gas UK Guidelines for Medications & Medical Equipment on Offshore Installations, Issue 2.

Olliff S. 2008. All systems go. *Safety & Health Practitioner* **26**: 46–51.

Pollock MJ, Brown LH and Dunn KA. 1997. The perceived importance of paramedic skills and the emphasis they receive during EMS education programs. *Prehosp Emerg Care* **1**: 263–268.

Ruddick-Bracken H. 1989. The offshore medic: professional position and status. University of Aberdeen: PhD thesis.

Ruddick-Bracken H. 1990. The role of nurses offshore. (Brief research report). *Nurs Times* **86**: 52.

Weber M. 1964. *The Theory of Social and Economic Organisations*. New York: Free Press.

Zautcke JL, Lee RW and Ethington NA. 1987. Paramedic skill decay. *J Emerg Med* **5**: 505–512.

https://doi.org/10.1142/9781786347510_0014

Chapter 14

Hyperbaric Medicine and Diving

J Nelson Norman

Introduction

Man has been interested in the effects of atmospheric pressure on health for many centuries. Indeed, the efficacious effects of a sea voyage on health led Henshaw, a clergyman in rural England in 1664 to adapt the bellows of his church organ into a pressure chamber using high pressure to treat conditions of an acute nature and low pressure for those of a more chronic nature. Lord Nelson's mistress, Lady Hamilton, also latched on to this form of therapy and drove a pressure vessel mounted on a carriage drawn by two black chargers around the streets of Paris, offering cures for a variety of diseases (Norman, 1964).

In more recent times, the concept of the use of high pressures of oxygen in medicine was researched by Boerema in Amsterdam and Illingworth and Smith in Glasgow. In Glasgow, the main motivator was the possibility of its use as an adjunct to cardiac surgery and the possibility of prolonging the safe period of permissible circulatory arrest as an aid to cardiac and neurosurgery. This was based on the possibility of storing increasing volumes of oxygen in physical solution in the plasma as the atmospheric pressure is raised. An additional 2.5 ml oxygen per hundred ml blood are dissolved in physical solution in the plasma when oxygen is breathed at 3 atmospheres pressure and that is sufficient to provide basic oxygen needs without the use of haemoglobin (Boerema *et al.*, 1960).

Although the basic motivator for building hyperbaric units in Amsterdam and Glasgow was their possible value in neuro and cardiac surgery, hyperbaric techniques were soon replaced by the development of cardio-pulmonary bypass techniques which were safer. Other positive uses for hyperbaric oxygen therapy were, however, demonstrated. In Amsterdam, Boerema showed considerable value in its use in anaerobic infections (Brummelkamp *et al.*, 1963) while Smith in Glasgow demonstrated its value in the management of carbon monoxide poisoning (Norman and Ledingham, 1967). The basis of its use in carbon monoxide poisoning is that when oxygen at two atmospheres absolute pressure is breathed, sufficient oxygen is dissolved in physical solution in the plasma to bypass the blocked haemoglobin mechanism thus providing immediate relief of the hypoxia. In addition, the level of carboxyhaemoglobin falls twice as rapidly as when the most efficient conventional resuscitation gas — 5% carbon dioxide in oxygen (carbogen) is used. Equally, there is no advantage in using oxygen pressures higher than two atmospheres absolute for this purpose.

Hyperbaric chambers are expensive and not in common use in urban practice nowadays but they are frequently found in remote places where diving operations are being conducted — both in the area of sport diving and commercial diving. In these circumstances carbon monoxide poisoning sometimes occurs from exhaust fumes. If a pressure chamber is available it can be life-saving — provided those operating it know that the preferred treatment regime is oxygen at two atmospheres pressure for 30 minutes.

In Glasgow and Aberdeen, much important basic clinical and physiological work took place which was of value subsequently when the main use of hyperbaric techniques was required by industry operating in remote places — namely diving and tunnelling (Norman, 1976). Some of these still require further research, such as the toxic effect of hyperbaric oxygen on aerobic micro-organisms (Irvin et al., 1969). Pseudomonas pyogenes is particularly sensitive to increased oxygen pressures and Pseudomonas infection occurs not infrequently in the ears of saturation divers and has been responsible for dive abortion in the past since the organism thrives in the environment of saturation chambers and the progressive and very painful infections are not always controlled adequately with Gentamycin. Indeed, it is wise to screen divers' ears before a saturation dive of significant duration to prevent or at least delay the occurrence of the infection. The use of oxygen during a saturation dive is not possible since the oxygen tension within the chamber has to be precisely controlled to prevent oxygen poisoning. It was suggested at one time that the oxygen tension within the earphones used by divers at leisure could be increased to therapeutic levels without contaminating the main chamber but this has not been further researched.

Tunnels and Mines

The use of hyperbaric techniques in tunnels and caissons to balance the pressure of water in the subsoil and so to exclude it from the workings has been practised since the early days of the 19th century. The pressure used varies with the circumstances but if it is greater than 2 atmospheres, absolute decompression techniques need to be used and care taken to avoid decompression sickness — and treated if it occurs.

Part of the problem is logistics since a large workforce is usually employed and some may be exposed to different atmospheric pressures for different periods of time, making the decompression schedules complex. Careful logs and records must therefore be kept together with the work cycles of the personnel since some may have been exposed to high atmospheric pressure more than once during a twenty-four-hour period and this must be taken into account in determining decompression rates. It is possible that this logistics problem accounts for the high incidence of osteo-necrosis found originally in compressed air workers in tunnels, together with the lack of knowledge or concern about the condition in many of the workers.

Diving

Though interest in hyperbaric medicine stretches back into the past, it only became of real interest to remote healthcare practitioners in the 1970s when the new technique of saturation diving (scarcely out of the laboratories of the navies of the world) was required to fix the structures built into the sea bed to allow oil exploration and production to take place in the North Sea. For several years the medical problems of diving dominated offshore medicine but the solution of many of the problems by research and the introduction of remote operating vehicles (ROV) has reduced the importance of diving medicine for remote healthcare practitioners. Nevertheless, though diving medicine is now largely handled by specialised personnel, it is important that remote healthcare practitioners should have a working knowledge of diving medicine if they are in charge of an installation where diving takes place. Sport diving is a growing area of activity that, together with harbour diving and diving by fishermen, takes place in remote and rural areas so it should be part of the knowledge base of the fully trained remote healthcare practitioner (Bennett and Elliott, 1975; Strauss, 1976).

Like sport diving, commercial diving has become increasingly common in recent times and usually takes place in remote and often inaccessible places. The healthcare of divers is thus an important part of remote healthcare. There are various techniques used in diving and what is chosen depends on the particular task to be performed, its complexity, the depth of the water and the duration of the work.

Free swimming divers

These divers may be sport divers, commercial divers in harbours, fishermen or military divers in such operations as the removal of fouling from propellers, the defusing of mines or underwater attacks — such as that on the German Battleship Tirpitz, in a Norwegian Fiord during WWII. In the attack on the Tirpitz they carried their 'Self-contained Underwater Breathing Apparatus' (SCUBA) with them and breathed oxygen to avoid tell-tale bubbles of exhaled gas.

While there are well defined training standards and safety regulations which well organised diving clubs follow, there are many self employed divers fishing for clams in remote lochs, who may be self-taught and who may not follow the rules in such areas as repetitive dives, and subsequently get into trouble in remote places. Problems happen from time to time also in well regulated groups such as those diving in Scapa Flow in Orkney on the Kaiser's scuttled Grand Fleet. It lies at a depth of around 150 feet which is marginal for the air range of diving and enthusiastic amateurs sometimes tempt fate, disobey rules and even indulge in repetitive diving. A further problem with sport diving is that they may travel home after an episode of recreational diving and present to a GP at a considerable distance from the sea thus confusing the diagnosis. A further problem may be caused if they indulge in flying home before the safe time interval for flying after diving has elapsed. It is important that these problems are known because delay in treating the dysbaric illnesses can have serious consequences, particularly if the central nervous system is involved.

Bounce divers

A bounce dive is one in which the diver descends to the worksite, performs a task and then returns to the surface. The effect on his body depends on whether his body cells have equilibrated with the gases breathed. The cellular gas load depends on the depth of the dive and its duration. Rapid ascent may result in release of gas into the micro circulation of various organs blocking the delivery of oxygen to the cells and leading to the eventual death of the tissue supplied unless the blockage is relieved. This is decompression sickness.

In commercial diving the diver is usually compressed to the simulated pressure of the worksite in a surface compression chamber and transported to the worksite in a diving bell. After performing his task, he returns to the bell which transports him back to the surface pressure chamber where he is decompressed. In deep diving a short spell of work may require an exceedingly prolonged period of decompression. The decompression tables are subject to individual variation and this form of diving was thus seen to be both dangerous and uneconomical for the extensive deep diving required in the Northern North Sea to fix the required structures to the sea bed. For this reason, saturation diving was introduced.

Saturation diving

What is known as the point of saturation is reached when all the tissues of the body have become equilibrated with the gases breathed at a particular depth and can accept no more. No matter how long the diver remains at that depth his decompression time will be the same. Therefore, long periods of work can be undertaken with one slow and safe decompression at the end of the work cycle.

In saturation diving the diver remains at the simulated depth of the worksite in a compression chamber for his whole work cycle. This may be one, two or three weeks long. At the end of each work shift he is taken from the worksite in the diving bell to a pressure chamber complex mounted on the deck of the support vessel or structure. He is then maintained there at the simulated depth of the worksite until he returns to the worksite for his next shift the following day.

Saturation systems usually consist of a series of interconnecting pressure chambers. Some of these are used for sleeping and others for living accommodation. The atmosphere in the chambers is continuously and precisely monitored, and the divers are constantly observed using television cameras. They are cared for throughout their work cycle by highly trained diving supervisors, most of whom are retired divers.

Commercial saturation diving was pioneered during the early 1970s in the northern North Sea and this is now the technique used routinely in commercial diving operations since it is regarded as the safest system.

Effects of atmospheric pressure on the body

At sea level the atmosphere exerts a pressure of 14.7 lb. on every square inch (1.03 kg on every square centimetre) of the body surface. The surface area of an average man is 18.6 square ft. (1.73 square m) and the atmosphere thus exerts 176.6 tons on the surface of the body. The man does not feel a great oppressive weight, however, because the gases in the atmosphere enter the air containing parts of the body, such as the lungs, and come into equilibrium with the body fluids. There is therefore an outward pressure equal to the inward pressure, and they cancel each other out.

Underwater there is an increase of pressure because of the column of the water above the body. This amounts to an extra atmosphere of pressure for every 33 feet (10 m) of seawater. Commercial diving in the North Sea often takes place at depths of three or four hundred feet and thus at pressures in excess of 11 atmospheres.

The changes which take place in the body as the diver descends in the water are largely related to the effect of the increasing pressure of the gases he breathes. This is because the volume of a gas is directly related to the pressure to which it is exposed (Boyle's law). The volume of gas dissolved in a fluid is also related to the pressure of the gas to which the fluid is exposed (Henry's law).

Gases in the body

Pressure changes are thus considerable in diving. As a diver ascends or descends in the water the volume of the gases contained in the air containing areas of the body (lungs, sinuses and ears) varies with depth.

The diver is not normally aware of these volume changes. When the volume of gases contract or expand air passes in and out of his body through the normal passages to make up for the losses or gains.

Sometimes obstructions, such as mucus, develop which prevent the passage of air into or out of the body. This trapped air will then be compressed during diving, and expanded during decompression on returning to the surface. Damage or injury caused by changes in volume of the trapped gases is known as barotrauma or pressure injury.

Gases are in the blood

As the diver descends in the water the pressure of the gases in his lungs increases and as he ascends it decreases. The quantity of gas dissolved in the blood also increases or decreases in proportion with depth. This takes place rapidly in the lungs and air spaces but more slowly as the quantity of gas dissolved in the various fluids within the cells of the body also increases or decreases with depth. The rate at which equilibrium is achieved between the gases dissolved in the blood and tissues of the body depends on the type of tissue. Because the proportion of the various tissues (e.g. fat, muscle) is different in different individuals, the time taken to achieve tissue equilibrium, or saturation, varies from one individual to another. The speed and quantity of removal of the gases from the various tissues during decompression or ascent to the surface also varies in different individuals. It is this which makes it difficult to design decompression tables to suit large numbers of people with different body composition.

If the decompression or ascent takes place too rapidly the effect is similar to removing the top of a lemonade bottle too quickly. An excess of the gas suddenly appears from the circulating blood. This may cause an 'air lock' in a blood vessel, cutting off the supply of blood or oxygen to the cells supplied by that blood vessel. The effect of cutting of the blood supply to part of the body is decompression sickness. The various types of decompression sickness are determined by the position in which the block occurs and the tissue which that blood vessel supplies with oxygen.

The Dysbaric Illnesses

There are two main forms of illness associated with pressure change known collectively as the dysbaric illnesses:

1. Barotrauma which is caused by the change in volume of gases with pressure (Boyle's law).

2. Decompression sickness which is associated with the changing quantities of gas which, with pressure, become dissolved in the body fluids (Henry's law).

Barotrauma (pressure injury)

Barotrauma occurs when a gas in an air containing part of the body such as the lungs become trapped and expands as the diver ascends or contracts as he descends. This may cause damage to organs because the external pressure squeezes the wall of the air containing tissue during compression or forces its way through the wall of the tissue during decompression. The danger of barotrauma depends on which body cavity the gas is trapped. The danger to the diver's life does not always correlate with the amount of pain he suffers. The cavities or tissues of the body which are commonly affected by barotrauma are:

1. Middle ear
2. Sinuses
3. Cavities in decayed teeth
4. Lung

Symptoms and treatment of barotrauma:

1. Middle ear

The middle ear is a semi-closed cavity within the ear which is connected to the mouth by a very narrow tube called the Eustachian tube. This often becomes blocked when one has a cold, and the area around its opening swell. Anyone who has travelled in an aeroplane while suffering from a cold, will have experienced the intense earache which occurs as the pressure increases and thus the volume of the trapped gas expands when the aeroplane descends to land. The 'popping' of the ears, experienced when descending steep hills rapidly in a motorcar, is caused by the gas in the ear expanding and escaping down the tube to the mouth. The ears can be cleared in this way by inducing 'popping'. This can be done by making swallowing movements or chewing movements with the jaw.

If the Eustachian tube becomes blocked during diving and the ears cannot be cleared the eardrum will rupture, with intense pain. This is unlikely to be fatal but the pain may distract the diver, causing a life-threatening accident. Middle ear barotrauma occurs rarely in experienced divers who know how to clear their ears. But an upper respiratory infection, such as a cold, causing inflammation around the tube commonly causes the problem to develop unexpectedly. The main symptom is intense pain; blood may also be seen in the ear.

The best treatment is to stop compression or decompression until the ears have cleared. The patient should rest and painkillers can be given. Decongestants may be useful if the blocked tube is due to a respiratory infection. The patient should not dive again until the infection has cleared. But if his eardrum has ruptured, medical clearance is needed before he can dive again. Healing can take up to 6 weeks.

The condition sometimes causes perforation of the eardrum in experienced drivers saving the life of a colleague by undertaking rapid compression. Occasionally also the drum may rupture without much pain. A perforated eardrum should be suspected if the diver cannot hear well or when blood is seen in the external ear.

2. Sinus

The sinuses are cavities in the skull just behind the nose. They are connected to the nose by narrow passages. If this passage becomes blocked, for example, when the diver has a cold, air will be trapped in the sinus. As the pressure changes during diving this trapped air causes severe pain in the sinuses. There may also be slight bleeding into the nose or throat.

The best treatment is rest. A painkiller may be given if necessary. Decongestants may be useful to clear the blocked passages. The casualty should not dive again until the pain has gone and the respiratory infection is cured. Medical attention is not necessary and there will be no long-term damage.

3. Teeth

If there is a cavity in a tooth, pressure changes may cause the tooth to cave in when the diver descends, or explode when he ascends. Gas spaces at the roots of infected teeth next to fillings may also cause pain if air is trapped in them under pressure.

Painkillers can be given and the patient sent for dental treatment. All divers should have regular dental check-ups. Most divers do have regular dental examinations and injuries to the teeth caused by pressure are now rare.

4. Lungs

Barotrauma in the lungs is dangerous and can cause death. Pulmonary barotrauma or burst lung usually occurs suddenly during decompression often without warning. It can occur at any depth even in small pressure changes.

Pulmonary barotrauma occurs when air is trapped in the lungs during decompression. If the air cannot get out along the normal passageways when it expands it tears its way through the lung tissue and enters the pleural cavity.

This may be associated with a lung defect. The defect may result from trivial lung disease or be a structural defect with which the diver was born. The diver may also have a minor abnormality such as a cyst in the lung which causes no pain. Alternatively, he may have a minor lung infection causing secretions which block a small portion of lung tissue, or he may have asthma, which causes the air passages to narrow.

Medical examination of the lungs should be very thorough before a man is allowed to dive, especially if he has had any illness involving the lungs. Because of this scrupulous check-up, burst lung is uncommon, with one case occurring every two years in the North Sea when the population was approximately 1000 divers. Despite its rarity, all divers and their medical attendants should become well acquainted with the symptoms and treatment of burst lung — failure to do so could result in the death of a colleague. There are three types of burst lung depending on where the air is trapped in the lungs during decompression:

a. Pneumothorax
b. Mediastinal emphysema
c. Cerebral arterial air embolism

a. Pneumothorax

Pneumothorax occurs if the lung bursts on its outer surface, allowing gas to escape into the space between the lung and the chest wall (the pleural cavity).

The diver is usually aware of a sudden sharp pain in the chest and will often become breathless. Further decompression causes the volume of gas trapped between the lung and the chest wall to expand. This collapses the lung and forces the heart against the other lung. The diver then becomes very breathless.

If decompression is not stopped the diver will die. The air should be removed from the diver's chest by a medical practitioner passing a large needle attached to a non-return valve into the air containing space allowing the trapped air to escape through it. A diver with pneumothorax in a pressure chamber cannot be decompressed until this has been done. The diver who has reached the surface before pneumothorax is diagnosed should be treated by chest puncture and not recompressed. Recompression would only be necessary if the casualty was in acute distress and it was not possible to release the trapped air.

Pneumothorax is one of the most serious emergencies in diving. It should always be suspected when a diver complains of chest pain, particularly if the pain is accompanied by breathlessness. Decompression should be stopped immediately until the cause of the pain has been precisely diagnosed. Pneumothorax can be diagnosed by taking an x-ray across the porthole of the pressure chamber and by auscultating the chest using an electric stethoscope which penetrates the hull of the chamber by means of an insulated electrical penetrator.

Provided the casualty is kept at the same pressure, he will usually come to no harm while waiting treatment. It is always best for a doctor or a qualified remote healthcare practitioner to undertake the treatment for pneumothorax. If the patient is becoming very breathless, he should be placed in a sitting position which gives the remaining lung tissue maximum oxygen transferring capacity. Increasing the pressure of oxygen breathed should be done with caution depending on the simulated depth because oxygen poisoning may occur. It may be increased if the patient is suffering from the effects of oxygen lack however, (he may turn blue or lose consciousness,) but under the direction of the diving supervisor.

Tension pneumothorax

This is an uncommon complication of pneumothorax in which the patient becomes progressively worse even though the pressure is not changed. This is caused by a flap-like valve forming at the point where the lung ruptured which, with each breath, allows more gas to enter the pleural space. This forces the remaining lung towards the other side.

Under these circumstances the remote healthcare practitioner should pass an appropriate needle into the casualty's chest to relieve the air pressure as a matter of urgency.

Following emergency treatment, the pneumothorax patient should be sent to hospital to recover. He may not be allowed to dive again because his lungs will have been weakened and there may be adhesions between the lungs and the chest wall which would make diving dangerous.

b. Mediastinal emphysema

When this occurs the lung bursts during decompression on the side next to the heart. Mediastinal emphysema is somewhat more common than pneumothorax. In this condition the lung does not collapse but air from the lung passes into the mediastinum rather than the pleural cavity. Properly managed and treated, it resolves over a period of up to 6 weeks.

The symptoms are chest pain and breathlessness though there may be no pain. If the diver is upright, gas in the chest may rise into the neck. It can then be felt as a crackling sensation when the fingers are passed lightly over the neck. If the diver is lying down, gas may pass down his back. The pain caused may be confused with backache or indigestion.

It is important to recognise mediastinal emphysema and to distinguish it from pneumothorax because the treatment is different. If the diver has the symptoms of mediastinal emphysema the pressure should be held constant and he should not be decompressed before the diagnosis has been made — once again by taking an x-ray through the porthole of the pressure chamber and auscultating the lungs by means of an electronic stethoscope passed across the hull of the chamber.

If the condition takes place at depth the casualty should be kept at that pressure for several days to allow the lung leak to seal. He can then be decompressed very slowly under x-ray control. If decompression takes place too quickly the gas bubble may enlarge and it may then press on the heart or rise into the neck and press on the large blood vessels there reducing the oxygen supply to the brain and cause loss of consciousness. Immediate recompression to relieve these symptoms may be necessary.

If, however, the diver is decompressed fully and successfully before the diagnosis is made there is little point in recompressing him. It will not help and may create problems in subsequent decompression. He should be admitted to hospital and kept under observation until the gas has been absorbed into the blood. An investigation of the cause of the barotrauma should then be made. Frequently no cause is found but some lung weakness will have occurred and the diver should be advised to consider his future options.

c. Cerebral arterial air embolism

This is one of the most dire emergencies in diving medicine, being a blockage of the blood vessels supplying the brain. It is often associated with very fast decompression when there is a serious structural failure of the diving system, such as the uncontrolled ascent of a diving bell to the surface when the hatch is open.

It is probably caused by the decompression stretching a wide surface area of lung tissue. Consequently, small quantities of gas are allowed to pass into the arterial blood circulation of the lungs. These bubbles merge together into larger bubbles, pass up to the brain in the arterial system and end by blocking some of the blood vessels in the brain.

When a diver comes to the surface and immediately becomes unconscious, cerebral arterial air embolism may be the cause, and it should be assumed to be so. The only hope of saving the casualty's life is to get him into a pressure chamber with the best trained attendant available and recompress him immediately and rapidly to a simulated depth of 165 feet (50 m). If he is recompressed and later found not to be suffering from cerebral arterial air embolism, no harm will have been done. If the diagnosis was correct, his life may have been saved. When in the pressure chamber he should be managed as any other unconscious casualty. He may suffer respiratory and cardiac arrest so resuscitation may be necessary.

The attendant accompanying the patient may suffer a ruptured eardrum because of the rapid recompression. The attendant should therefore not be suffering from any respiratory infection if possible.

Preventing Barotrauma

1. Those wishing to work in increased atmospheric pressures should have a careful annual medical examination.
2. No one should dive with abnormalities of the lungs, sinuses or ears.
3. No one should dive with a cold or other respiratory infection.
4. Dental hygiene should be carefully maintained. No one should dive with cavities in the teeth.
5. Divers who have sustained injuries to the chest or face should be carefully medically examined before diving again.
6. The diver must be able to clear his ears easily.
7. Barotrauma can be so painful and is so dangerous that if the diver is in any doubt that he is suffering from a condition which might lead to it he should take medical advice before diving again.

Decompression Sickness (The Bends)

Decompression sickness is common in SCUBA and bounce diving, but uncommon in saturation diving. It occurs when gas bubbles form in the body fluids during decompression. It is broadly classified into type I (not serious) and type 2 (potentially lethal) decompression sickness.

Type I decompression sickness

Generally, type I decompression sickness is not serious, though it may be extremely painful and uncomfortable. It occurs when the blood supply to a muscle, tendon or skin is interrupted by the formation of a gas bubble or 'airlock' in a blood vessel. This is the commonest form of decompression sickness. If it occurs in the skin there may be a skin rash, swelling, itching and some discomfort. If a limb joint is affected there is usually intense discomfort and pain.

Type II decompression sickness

This is a serious form of decompression sickness and if it is left untreated it will probably result in permanent damage such as paralysis or a defect in balance. A gas bubble usually lodges in the blood supply of the lung or nervous tissue.

The spinal cord is more readily affected than the brain. The first symptoms may be a small area of numbness in a limb. Another common form affects the balance mechanism in the ear and is known as vestibular decompression sickness.

Symptoms of decompression sickness

Decompression sickness may be very obvious or appear in a vague way so that even the diver does not suspect it. If it affects the central nervous system the diver's judgement may also be affected. Everyone associated with diving should be able to recognise or at least suspect the condition.

The features of decompression sickness usually relate to the tissue which is involved, and so there may be:

1. Severe pain in a limb or joint, especially the shoulder.
2. Breathlessness in lung, or pulmonary decompression sickness.
3. Some form of paralysis or sensory disturbance in spinal decompression sickness.
4. Loss of balance with nausea or vomiting in vestibular decompression sickness.

Symptoms usually appear at least an hour after the decompression has been completed; but they can occur during slow decompression from a deep dive. Because the symptoms are not always clear-cut, any unusual complaint or sign occurring within 24 hours of a dive should suggest that decompression sickness has occurred. A general feeling of unwellness may be the only symptom.

The minor type I forms of decompression sickness tend to come on earlier and are more common than the serious type II forms. Type I symptoms can also mask the early symptoms of serious decompression sickness. The most minor form of decompression sickness must therefore be taken seriously and the casualty carefully observed in case type II decompression sickness develops. Both types of decompression sickness are present concurrently in the same diver in more than 30% of cases.

Management of decompression sickness

When decompression sickness is diagnosed the correct treatment is to recompress the patient as quickly as possible to the depth at which the symptoms are relieved or the depth of the original dive. This removes the gas bubbles from the circulation. The longer the bubble remains in the blood the more likely a thick coat of fibrinogen-like material will form around the bubble; and this layer becomes thicker the longer the bubble is present. If recompression then takes place, the gas may return to solution leaving the solid material in the blood vessel where it will continue to block the circulation.

When time has been allowed for the gas bubble to leave the blood — usually about one hour, the diver should be decompressed using a treatment table, which is slower than usual. There are a variety of treatment tables and many large diving companies use their own. Most authorities use those which have been tried and designed over the years by the British Royal Navy or the US Navy. The choice of table is usually made following consultation with a diving doctor.

When a remote healthcare practitioner consults a diving doctor he will as usual communicate the full details of the history and examination as for any other condition, but particular emphasis should be placed on detailed examination of the central nervous system since this is an area upon which the diving doctor will require detailed information.

Effects on Divers of Gases at Pressure

The main gases encountered and used at pressure are:

1. Nitrogen
2. Oxygen
3. Carbon dioxide
4. Helium

1. Nitrogen

Nitrogen makes up four fifths of the earth's atmosphere. It is inert and merely acts as a carrier gas in human breathing, being inhaled into the body with oxygen and exhaled unchanged. Nitrogen makes it impossible to dive with safety deeper than 165 feet (50 m) while breathing air, because beyond that depth it acts like an anaesthetic. At depths as shallow as one hundred feet (30 m) it affects performance in the same way as a small quantity of alcohol. The effect, called nitrogen narcosis, becomes progressively more marked as depth increases. Susceptibility to nitrogen narcosis varies from person to person, but at depths greater than 165 feet (50 m) the effects are dangerous. Commercial air diving is normally restricted to this depth for this reason.

Nitrogen narcosis, like drunkenness, is characterised by euphoria, sleepiness, lack of concentration and impaired coordination. If a diver notices these feelings, he should rapidly lessen his depth. Unfortunately, the overconfidence which comes with drinking alcohol also occurs with nitrogen narcosis.

The co-diver may not experience nitrogen narcosis at the same depth as his partner. If a diver sees signs of unusual action in his co-diver he should suspect nitrogen narcosis, particularly if they are diving at approximately 165 feet (50 m), and make sure his partner reduces his depth.

2. Oxygen

Hypoxaemia may occur if there is a low percentage of oxygen in the gas cylinder or an inadequate flow rate. It may also occur following an accident, if the air supply line breaks, for example. The casualty may appear blue and become breathless or even unconscious.

Pulmonary oxygen poisoning may occur in divers given oxygen to breathe at pressures greater than 0.5 atmospheres absolute and less than three atmospheres absolute for a continuous period of 15 or 16 hours or an intermittent period of exposure lasting a few hours at a time over several days.

In order to prevent this excessive quantity of oxygen being delivered to the tissue cells and damaging them, the lung walls become thickened to reduce the rate at which oxygen is transferred into the blood. The lung walls readily return to normal when the oxygen pressure is reduced, but repeated episodes of pulmonary oxygen poisoning can cause permanent damage to the lungs. The oxygen pressure in a diving gas mixture is usually kept well below 0.5 atmospheres of oxygen and pulmonary oxygen poisoning is therefore uncommon. But it can occur if hyperbaric oxygen is used in the treatment of decompression sickness.

The symptoms are irritation of the throat leading to coughing, a sharp pain behind the sternum and an increased rate of breathing. The toxicity of oxygen depends on the partial pressure of oxygen, the duration of exposure and the diver's susceptibility. The only treatment is to reduce the amount of oxygen breathed.

Neurological oxygen poisoning may occur when pure oxygen is breathed at high concentrations over a period equivalent to that at 100 feet (30 m) depth. This may occur when a breathing set is charged with pure oxygen. It does not occur often in saturation diving but may occur in bounce diving and when decompression schedules are used. It is most likely to occur in a pressure chamber during decompression, but it may also develop during treatment with oxygen at increased pressure, for instance when treating decompression sickness.

Neurological oxygen poisoning affects the brain. It may cause a convulsion like an epileptic fit. There is wide-ranging susceptibility between divers, and the susceptibility of the same diver can also vary from day to day. The main danger is that the casualty may injure himself by falling to the ground. There are few warning symptoms, although a major convulsion may be preceded by a sensation like pins and needles or by twitching of the lips.

The oxygen pressure must be reduced immediately and the sufferer prevented from injuring himself as in the management of an epileptic convulsion. There are no residual effects provided the pressure of oxygen is reduced straightaway. Neurological oxygen poisoning can be prevented if the diver is not given oxygen to breathe at pressures greater than 2.5 atmospheres absolute.

3. Carbon dioxide

In saturation diving systems the environment is monitored very precisely so that the temperature, the oxygen pressure and the carbon dioxide pressure are all maintained at correct levels. The carbon dioxide exhaled by the diver is removed by passing the chamber gas through a scrubber containing soda lime. Divers spend a good part of their working lives breathing various gas mixtures through long and complicated systems of tubes. Because of this they may be exposed to slightly increased concentrations of carbon dioxide. Very experienced divers may be more tolerant to minor increases in carbon dioxide concentration and fail to be immediately aware of gradual increase to dangerous levels. Equally, some people are abnormally sensitive to carbon dioxide and this may be the cause of some unexplained cases of unconsciousness in new divers.

At normal atmospheric pressure carbon dioxide poisoning occurs if the concentration rises above 4%. In diving this may happen if the scrubbing system is not working efficiently, if there is inadequate ventilation or contamination of the breathing gases. The first symptoms are a throbbing headache, dizziness and confusion. The diver will be flushed, sweating and breathing deeply. Eventually he will become unconscious. He should be removed from the carbon dioxide atmosphere as soon as possible and treated for unconsciousness. Artificial respiration may be necessary if breathing is poor or has ceased.

4. Helium

For many years diving was restricted to 165 feet (50 m) because nitrogen narcosis occurred at deeper levels. The search for an alternative gas to mix with the oxygen and dilute it to suitable levels for breathing led to the use of helium. Helium is not narcotic at the pressure used in saturation diving but it is scarce and expensive. Continuing research is seeking a cheaper alternative and hydrogen has been examined.

The main problems associated with helium are the high-pressure neurological syndrome (HPNS), voice distortion and temperature control. In addition, helium poisoning can occur if pure helium is delivered to the divers in error. HPNS may occur when breathing oxy-helium mixtures at depths greater than 500 feet (150 m). The diver becomes dizzy, he may have tremors, find it hard to breathe and have difficulty in swallowing. He will eventually become unconscious. HPNS can be reduced by adding some nitrogen to the helium mixture and reducing the speed of compression. When the symptoms occur in the diver not much can be done since he is separated from his attendants by a wall of steel, and reduction of pressure at great depths may take several days.

The density of helium is so different from that of nitrogen that it causes voice distortion. This may cause problems when monitoring the diver in the water, assessing his requirements and understanding his problems. It also creates difficulties when managing illness. Fortunately, un-scramblers are now available for helium speech and have overcome this difficult problem within commercial saturation diving systems. It is of importance that divers speak precisely and their supervisors learn to understand them readily. It is also important not to try to complete an unfinished sentence for the diver. He may not be trying to say what is expected. Errors like this may cause serious mistakes in the management of an emergency. For this reason, and because the communication may pass through several hands before it reaches the diving medical adviser, important messages should always be written as well as spoken.

Temperature control is a problem when breathing helium because of its high thermal conductivity. The thermal conductivity of helium is nine times greater than that of air and as a diver goes deeper and the gas he breathes becomes progressively more dense, it becomes a better conductor of heat. The heat loss from his respiratory tract eventually becomes very great. At a depth of 1000 feet (300 m) all the heat produced by the body is lost via the respiratory tract. The deep diver loses heat at a rate related to the temperature of the surrounding environment and its density. Without gas temperature control, this would not give him long to live in very cold water. When he is in the saturation chamber the gases the diver breathes are maintained at a precise temperature level. When the diver is in the water, heat is added externally to his body by means of a hot water suit. These measures counteract the loss of heat from the respiratory tract. At depths greater than 500 feet (150 m) some additional form of heating is necessary to maintain thermal balance.

It seems likely that many of the diving accidents in the North Sea in the latter part of the 1970s were related to inadequate diver heating. Divers may not be able to determine whether their body temperature is too hot or too cold. This can lead to serious accidents, since this can affect their judgement and competence. Divers are vulnerable to environmental temperature because of the increased density of the gases both surrounding them and which they breathe. They are therefore liable to overheating if the environmental temperature is high or cooling if it is low. Particularly in the helium environment, overheating can be lethal. It is the diving supervisor's responsibility to maintain optimum environmental temperatures for his divers.

Other Diving Problems

1. Drowning. This is dealt with in Chapter 2 under first-aid.
2. Ear infection. In hyperbaric environments the harmless bacteria which normally live in the human ear cannot survive. When they have died, other more harmful pathological organisms such as the Pseudomonas pyocyaneus or Eschericheria coli can enter the ear and cause infection.

Pseudomonas infection is particularly troublesome since that organism thrives in the hyperbaric environment and the infection can often only be cured by decompression to normal atmospheric pressure.

When a diver carrying pseudomonas in his ear enters a pressure chamber the whole team is likely to become infected in 4 to 5 days. If none of the divers is carrying the bacteria in his ear the condition may not appear for about 14 days. For this reason, some diving companies take swabs of the ears of the divers before allowing them to begin a saturation dive which is intended to last for a long period.

The symptoms of infection are severe pain in the ears and this may be associated with vertigo. The pain may be so bad that the dive has to be aborted.

These infections can be minimised if:

1. The pressure chamber is kept scrupulously clean and the humidity is kept as low as possible.
2. Divers maintain scrupulous personal hygiene.
3. Divers use protective ear drops (5% aluminium acetate).

If the diver is in pain, he can be given painkillers. He will always improve when he returns to normal atmospheric conditions. The ear should be swabbed and sent to a lab for identification of the organism and advice on the possible use of antibiotics.

In normal atmospheric conditions the untreated organisms may persist in the ear without causing trouble for as long as six weeks following decompression, after the symptoms have subsided. As soon as the diver returns to saturation conditions however, the bacteria rapidly multiply and the infection begins again.

Other ear infections can occur in the cells lining the ears if they become soggy and waterlogged. In many cases yeasts are responsible for these infections. The main symptoms are severe swelling in the ear with pain and redness. Treatment is by using painkillers and antiseptic drops, such as 5% aluminium acetate drops.

It is important that neither the divers' breathing system nor pressure chamber should be contaminated with toxic materials. Compressors and filters should be maintained carefully so that the machine lubricating oil does not enter the breathing gases.

Hypoxy-resins are sometimes used in the repair of concrete underwater structures. Great care must be taken to avoid introducing these substances into a pressure chamber because they would contaminate the atmosphere and the volatile constituents could be even more toxic at increased pressure.

Management of Diving Injuries

When a diver becomes injured or ill, he must first be removed from the water and recovered into a compression chamber on board the vessel or structure which supports his diving activity. It is not easy to recover an injured diver into a bell and it is extremely difficult if he is unconscious. Problems are caused by the long narrow entrance port, the heavy equipment worn and physical strength required of the co-diver in the hyperbaric environment. These difficulties have been partially overcome by installing a system of pulleys, rather like a block and tackle, inside the rescue bell which can be used to wind the diver into the bell. When the injured diver has been recovered into the diving bell and the entrance sealed, the time taken to remove the bell from the worksite to the deck decompression chamber is generally 15 to 20 minutes.

The size of the diving bell and the equipment worn by the diver makes it difficult to perform external cardiac compression. The best the co-diver can do is usually to make sure the injured man has a clear airway and is breathing properly. If the casualty is not breathing, artificial respiration should be given if possible. Attempts to compress the heart are not likely to be successful and it may be best to concentrate on achieving adequate oxygenation.

In saturation diving the casualty may not be accessible to the supporting doctors for days or weeks because of the long decompression time required. Conditions such as burst lung causing pneumothorax or mediastinal emphysema have to be treated before decompression can begin. In some cases, the diver may have reached the surface but has to be rapidly re-compressed before the doctor has seen him — as in the case of cerebral arterial air embolism. It is thus essential that divers should be well trained in appropriate first aid, diagnostic techniques and emergency procedures. It is equally important that those in attendance have sufficient knowledge to be able to describe the injured diver's condition in a way which will be helpful to medical personnel at a distance as in other remote and rural areas.

The commonest mistake when managing an injured diver in a pressure chamber is attempting decompression too quickly. If there is doubt about what action to take with a casualty it is always best to stop decompression and do nothing until a decision can be taken on management with external advice if necessary. A diver suffering from pneumothorax will come to no harm unless the pressure is changed. Thoughtlessly continuing the decompression of an injured man may cause additional decompression problems to compound his original injury.

A case which illustrates this point occurred in the mid-1970s in the North Sea when a saturation diver was badly burned by his hot water supply. The attendant was told what treatment to give for the burned area. It was emphasised by the shore-based doctor that decompression should be extremely slow because normal decompression tables are designed for healthy divers. The advice was not followed precisely. In order to get the burned casualty to medical attention rapidly, decompression was speeded up. The following day the burn had responded well to treatment and the patient was very well. The change in the decompression schedule, however, caused decompression sickness, not in the burned casualty, but in his attendant! Because of the rapid decompression the attendant had become much more seriously ill than the diver.

A number of devices have been developed and used to aid diagnosis by passing electronic signals across the hull of a pressure vessel. Equally, it is possible to take routine x-rays through the portholes of pressure chambers using portable machines and flexible x-ray plates which can be passed through the medical locks of saturation chambers. This is particularly important in the diagnosis of chest pain as has been emphasised. It is also possible to auscultate the chest using an electric stethoscope which is passed across the hull of the pressure chamber by means of an electrically insulated penetrator. The doctor instructs a co-diver on which part of the body to apply the bell of the stethoscope and he listens from the outside.

A number of other investigations are also possible using suitably insulated penetrators. Thus, it is possible to measure blood pressure, count the pulse rate and even take an ECG from outside the pressure chamber. Because of these developments it is not always necessary for a doctor to enter the chamber to make a diagnosis. If the co-diver is trained in first-aid, he should be able to treat the injured diver following instructions from the doctor, medic or specialist as a distance, using the standard tenets of remote healthcare as in other areas. In this case, however, remoteness is largely caused by half an inch of steel!

In the early period of North Sea oil exploration there was concern about the management of trauma or serious illness in saturation chambers and a system to allow transfer under pressure was devised so that the sick diver could be transferred to a large operating chamber onshore without changing the pressure. This was achieved by transferring him into a small chamber built of titanium and just within the payload of a Sikorsky helicopter. This caused much controversy mainly related to the difficulty to provide care for the diver if he should deteriorate during transfer. In any case, the system was only used once in the transfer of a diver suffering from mediastinal emphysema at 400 feet and who required prolonged slow decompression during the critical phase of an offshore dive. Since then diving related illness in pressure chambers has been managed within the chamber at the remote site and even appendicitis is now successfully managed conservatively when it occurs.

References

Bennett PB and Elliott DH. 1975. *The Physiology and Medicine of Diving and Compressed Air Work*. London: Balliere and Tindall.

Boerema I, Meijne NG, Brummelkamp WK *et al.* 1960. Life without blood. *J Cardiovasc Surg* **1**: 133–146.

Brummelkamp WH, Boerama I and Hoogendyk LN. 1963. Treatment of clostridial infections with hyperbaric oxygen drenching. A report of 26 cases. *Lancet* **281**: 235–238.

Irvin TT, Norman JN, Suwanagul A and Smith G. 1969. Treatment of aerobic infections with hyperbaric oxygen. *Internal Medicine Digest*: 36–39.

Norman JN. 1964. The effect of oxygen at elevated atmospheric pressure and hypothermia on tissue metabolism. University of Glasgow: PhD thesis.

Norman JN. 1976. The metabolic and circulatory effects of oxygen. University of Aberdeen: DSc thesis.

Norman JN and Ledingham I McA. 1967. Carbon monoxide poisoning: Investigations and treatment. In: *Progress in Brain Research*. (Eds.) Bour H and Ledingham I McA. Elsevier, pp. 101–122.

Strauss RH. 1976. *Diving Medicine*. Grune and Stratton.

Chapter

15

Environmental Medicine: The Physical Environment — Heat and Cold

J Nelson Norman

Introduction

The human body functions best if its temperature is maintained within 0.5 degrees on either side of 98.6 degrees Fahrenheit (37 degrees Centigrade). If the deviation amounts to more than a couple of degrees on either side of 37 deg C, a potentially life-threatening condition may result. This can be difficult to comprehend when consideration is given to the knowledge that man has penetrated the highest mountains, the depths of the seas, the poles of the earth in winter and the empty quarter of the Arabian desert in summer.

The contradictory manner in which the thermally weak and sensitive human being has been able to penetrate the most thermally challenging areas of the planet has been the source of a variety of studies over the years. They are of importance if man has to move from one climatic zone to another often rapidly and perform at full efficiency and safety right away. This has special importance in a military situation where there may not be time for acclimatisation to the new climate to take place after arrival in a conflict zone. The importance of acclimatisation and how long it takes to develop is also important for oil workers who may live at a considerable distance from their worksite — often in a different country — and perform their jobs safely in frequently hazardous and dangerous situations.

Cold

Many studies have been conducted over the years on both the physical and psychological effects of cold on performance. There have been extensive animal studies but it is unwise to extrapolate these to humans since the animals have normally been exposed to extremely low temperatures for prolonged periods and in a naked state. On the other hand, man modifies his behaviour with the climate, and has the advantage of clothing and shelter if the climate is severe. In addition the extensive research carried out in the 1950s on the consequences of reducing body temperature for the purposes of cardiac and neuro-surgery cannot be directly applied to man on the side of a mountain or cold worksite, since these observations were normally carried out in the controlled situation of a laboratory or operating theatre, where biochemistry and ventilation can be readily observed and controlled.

A starting point in understanding the problems of man working in the cold comes from comparative physiological studies which reveal that there is very little mammalian species variation in body temperature. An important point, however, is that the critical temperature (the environmental temperature below which metabolism rises in order to maintain the body temperature) varies greatly between species and between environments. It is usually found to be around the coldest temperature to which the animal is expected to be exposed during winter. It was found to be +20°C to +30°C for tropical animals, 0°C for the polar bear cub and −40°C for the Arctic Fox. Thus, the metabolic economy is reasonably adapted to the particular environment to which the animal is normally exposed. The problem with man at work in remote places and particularly those associated with the oil industry, is that the environment to which he is exposed may change greatly from one worksite to another and often again his home is in one part of the world and his worksite in an entirely different environment (Scholander et al., 1950).

When studies were carried out on man to determine his critical temperature there were difficulties since man has been extensively modified by the influences of civilisation but the eventual conclusion is that the value for man is around 27°C. It must thus be concluded that since the critical temperature of tropical animals is 27°C man responds as a tropical animal. This has implications in considering the situation of acclimatisation (Erikson et al., 1956).

Acclimatisation to temperature change is an important determinant of efficiency and physical performance. There are well recognised physiological changes when man moves from a temperate zone to a hot area. On the other hand there are no indices of cold acclimatisation when he moves from a temperate zone to a cold climate. It has been argued that if man is basically a tropical animal best suited to the environment of a tropical forest it is useless to expect or demonstrate physiological changes when he moves from a temperate climate to severe cold. It has been argued that the greater part of the possible physiological change in that direction has already been made by his movement from a tropical to a temperate climate and thus any further possible change in that direction must be very small or absent (MacPherson, 1958).

The measurement of the effects of cold on man are neither simple nor do they consist entirely on the measurement of the climatic variables of the district in which he lives or works. Man uses his intelligence to protect himself from unnecessary exposure to the extremes of temperature by providing himself with clothing, artificial heating and shelter. This is an important concept for those who are responsible for providing healthcare for those who work in the extremes of temperature because it does not alter their basic vulnerability — it only emphasises man's use of his intelligence to take the narrow ranges of environmental variations which he needs with him — offshore, to Siberia or the Antarctic, to the deserts of Arabia or to the depth of the sea (Norman, 1961).

The maintenance of health in isolated communities associated with environmental cold thus demands considerable forethought in the provision of an adequate diet, together with the essentials of clothing, heating and housing. It seems essential that there should be a clear understanding of the effects which the extremes of environmental temperature may have on both performance and the occurrence of injuries and life-threatening emergencies and their management, if a workforce is to be effectively cared for and the confidence of the personnel is to be maintained (Brebner, 1990).

In the 1950s it was shown that there was an exponential drop in oxygen requirements as the body temperature was reduced. Thus, when the body temperature reaches 28°C, the oxygen requirements are about one third of those needed at 37°C. This fundamental observation, which has been widely applied to the surgery of the heart and brain, certainly holds true in the operating theatre where biochemistry is controlled, where an abundance of oxygen is provided by ventilation and where shivering is controlled by muscle relaxation, (Bigelow *et al.*, 1950).

When the condition of accidental hyperthermia was reproduced in dogs and compared to that of controlled reduction in body temperature practised in the operating theatre, it was found that when the temperature fell to between 28°C and 30°C the tissue oxygen requirements in fact doubled compared to control values due to the vastly increased oxygen needs of the shivering muscles. The increased oxygen requirement is provided by maintaining an increased level of cardiac output. The heart rate, however, falls with the decline in body temperature due to the direct effect of cold on nerve transmission. This requires stroke volume to increase considerably and indicates the stressful effect which accidental cooling has on the heart. It thus seems clear that a competent myocardium is of great importance for work with safety in the cold and this has obvious relevance for the selection and continuing care of personnel for work in cold climates (Auld *et al.*, 1980; Norman, 1986).

The management of hypothermia in the intensive care units of hospitals has been relatively clearly documented. There is still some doubt on the best form of management when it takes place in a situation far from hospital care. The Royal Navy has made a convincing case for the management of immersion hypothermia by immediate re-immersion in warm water. Since the rapid rate of cooling is likely to result in a low temperature being reached before any circulatory or biochemical adjustments have time to take place the argument is that these changes may be avoided by equally rapid rewarming. It was also argued that unless urgent action was taken to reverse the meteoric fall in body temperature it could result in a critically low temperature being reached causing the heart to develop ventricular fibrillation. This is one of the explanations of post-rescue death. Since a critically low temperature will have been reached before there has been time for metabolic and circulatory changes to take place, it seems clear that re-immersion in hot water provides the most effective management of immersion hypothermia but it must be instituted with urgency (Golden and Hervey, 1981).

The condition is more complex however, when body cooling takes place in dry cold. The poor conduction of air compared to water (which conducts heat 25 times faster than air) means that cooling is much slower and there will be time for both biochemical and circulatory change to take place before the subject collapses — an event which depends upon the interaction of the state of physical fitness, the environment, the clothing assembly worn, the state of nutrition and the motivation of the subject. In the field it suggests that it is safer that more gradual rewarming should take place and there is of course much less chance of severe 'after drop' in temperature in this type of hypothermia (Norman and Brebner, 1987).

While it is important to have an understanding of the individual physiological variations in the responses which can take place in apparently normal, healthy individuals to environmental cold, it is equally important to consider the effects which minor degrees of body cooling may have on the efficiency and mental performance of people exposed to cold. For a start, wide variations in the shivering response to cold took place among a large population exposed to moderate cold in an environmental chamber and this response was also noted in under-ice divers in the Antarctic. In the absence of shivering it is difficult for man to appreciate subjectively whether he is cold or not. The shivering response is thus an important protective mechanism to a cold climate and a poor shivering response can result in the body temperature falling more rapidly than in normal controls and leading to a dangerous level of temperature without discomfort. Whether or not minor degrees of cooling do affect cognitive function and compromise safety has not been fully resolved. A clear reduction in cognitive function in a group of men exposed for two hours in a cold chamber has been shown and they also made an increased number of errors in tests on judgement and with greater confidence. It was noted however, that this was related more to changes in skin temperature rather than in core temperature. Similar findings were noted in cognitive functions in divers and were considered to be due to the distracting effects of cold from discomfort rather than to a change in central nervous function from a falling core temperature. These arguments are not yet finally resolved but are clearly of importance for the comfort and safety of man working in cold climates (Ellis *et al.*, 1985; Light *et al.*, 1980).

Maintenance of Body Temperature

Whilst alive, the body produces heat constantly and there is a requirement to maintain its temperature within half a centigrade degree of 37°C if it is to function at peak levels of physical and mental performance. This is because cellular function is related to a mass of enzyme reactions and these are very temperature dependent. When the temperature drops a mere 2°C to 35°C the life-threatening condition of hypothermia has taken place and when it rises a few degrees to 41°C a second life-threatening condition occurs — hyperthermia or heat stroke.

Body temperature results from the balance between heat loss and heat gain mechanisms. It is simplistic to say that the entire temperature changes of the body are controlled by a thermostat situated in the brain, but such a concept makes it easier to explain and understand what happens. When the temperature of the blood passing through the thermostat in the brain rises, the skin becomes flushed as blood is deviated to the surface to allow heat to be radiated away. When the temperature of the blood passing over the thermostat falls, blood is withdrawn into the core of the body and is insulated by the surface layer of fat (Norman and Brebner, 1985). When these mechanisms are insufficient to maintain body temperature within required levels, more powerful mechanisms come into play — shivering to increase heat production and sweating to increase heat loss by evaporation of the water on the surface.

Conditions Caused by a Cold Environment

These conditions may be caused by exposure of one part of the body to cold, as frostbite or by cooling of the whole body, as hypothermia. They are all more likely to occur when a cold temperature is associated with high wind speeds.

Cold injuries can be divided into freezing and non-freezing injuries. Of these, chaps and chilblains are examples of minor non-freezing injuries, while trench foot is an example of a serious non-freezing injury. Frostnip and frostbite are of course freezing injuries.

Frostnip

In very cold conditions, such as those found in Alaska, the Beaufort Sea, Siberia or the Antarctic, cold injury of exposed parts of the body is a hazard. It does occur, however, in the homeless or drunks sleeping rough in winter in cities. Frostnip is the first level of this cold injury and is recognised when a waxy patch appears on the skin, usually over the cheekbones or at the tip of the nose. If frostnip is not treated it will destroy the affected tissue and frostbite will result.

Frostnip and frostbite are not likely to be much of a problem in the maritime environment but can readily occur if the sea freezes over, and also in areas where there is a high wind velocity associated with low temperatures. Tissue does not often freeze if the windchill factor is less than 1400 (temperature −10 to −15°C).

The time taken for these conditions to develop is variable and depends on the interaction of wind and temperature with physical fitness, nutritional state and clothing assembly worn by the worker. In severe conditions frostnip can occur in 10 to 15 minutes and frostbite in an hour or so.

Frostnip is reversible. Slowly warm the affected area by placing a warm hand (or even gloved hand) over it until colour returns. In polar or sub polar conditions, where frostnip is a particular hazard, personnel should work in pairs and inspect each other's faces and other exposed body parts at frequent intervals for the typical white, waxy appearance. Well fitting and adequate clothing reduces the likelihood of frostnip occurring.

Frostbite

Frostbite most readily affects exposed parts of the body such as nose and ears. Frostnip usually develops first and if it is not recognised and properly treated, frostbite develops, damaging the tissues irreversibly. In extreme cold, frostbite may also affect the hands and feet. This is much more likely to happen if footwear or gloves become wet because of the increased thermal conductivity of water over air.

Frostbite can be recognised as a white area on the skin which may be accompanied by blistering. The area will be tender if the frostbite is superficial but numb if the frostbite is deep and the nerve endings have been damaged or destroyed. Untreated frostbite ends in gangrene with subsequent loss of affected tissue. The aim of treatment is to minimise eventual tissue loss.

Management

- Shelter the casualty and provide warm (not hot) drinks
- Increase insulation with dry clothing
- Remove anything tight from the affected area such as gloves or rings since damaged tissue will swell and the circulation may be arrested
- Take off wet clothes and cover the frostbitten area with something dry and warm
- Thaw the affected area rapidly. This can be done in several ways depending upon the circumstances:
  o Put the affected area in a lukewarm bath (39 to 41° C) for 15 to 50 minutes
  o Cover the frostbitten face or ears with a dry gloved hand
  o Put frostbitten hands under the armpits
  o Wrap frostbitten feet in a warm blanket or sleeping bag

- Dress the affected area with a light, sterile, non-adherent dressing
- Do not rub the affected area. Do not apply direct heat because it can cause burns
- Blisters are best left to heal themselves and should not be burst

While the recommended management of frost bite is rapid thawing by immersion in lukewarm water it is often best to delay treatment when it takes place in a remote and dangerous situation where survival is the first consideration since it is possible to walk on frostbitten feet and the best management may be to await rescue or recovery into a place where treatment can be given following thawing. Judgement is needed here on consideration of the circumstances.

Cold burn

This thermal injury is caused when metal at very low temperature — usually in air temperature of −40°C or below is touched and the skin adheres to the metal. The adherent part has to be removed from the metal by force as the large mass of metal cannot be re-warmed. Thereafter the injury should be treated as a burn.

Chapped hands and lips

Heavy work in a cold damp environment often leads to chapped, cracked and sore hands and lips. Some people are more susceptible than others and the crack often found in the central part of the lower lip is said to be associated with a recurrent viral infection. These conditions can cause severe discomfort and may even require time off work on occasion. Chapped lips and fingers can be relieved by painting them with Friar's balsam (resin dissolved in alcohol). The alcohol in the balsam evaporates leaving the resin as a dressing. If this treatment is repeated three times in succession before retiring at night the layer of resin excludes air and healing often occurs overnight.

Chilblains

This minor cold injury occurs on the fingers and toes following long-term exposure to mild cold temperatures. Chilblains appear as shiny red areas like mosquito bites and itch. They usually appear when the living quarters are not properly heated and disappear when they are — no matter how cold the worksite. Most ointments for chilblains are ineffective.

Trench foot

This condition is rare in industrial workers. It is caused by the combined effect of moderate cold and water on the feet, especially if footwear is ill fitting and lets in water. It varies in severity, but there is usually swelling, redness, pain and numbness in parts of the foot. The best way to prevent it is by wearing well fitting, water resistant, dry footwear. If trench foot is recognised early and the feet are dried and warmed they will get better, but if not, it can cause continuing pain and discomfort.

Hypothermia

Hypothermia is not common in well organised industrial operations and when it does occur it is usually the result of an accident where someone has fallen into the water. It is more common in explorers and mountaineers caught up in deteriorating weather and not properly clad or in elderly people living in under heated housing.

Hypothermia occurs when the body temperature falls below 35°C. When the body begins losing more heat to the surrounding environment than it can produce, the physical mechanisms for maintaining body temperature come into operation. Blood is automatically routed from the surface area of skin to the internal organs to increase insulation and shivering begins which increases the body's warmth by muscular activity. These reflexes may be sufficient to maintain body temperature, particularly if more clothes are put on and the subject can increase muscle activity by moving faster. If these reflexes and preventive measures do not maintain the temperature, the body will slowly cool. Eventually a point will be reached when the body's compensatory mechanisms fail and temperature falls rapidly until death occurs at any temperature from 32°C down to 18°C.

Body temperature does not fall in an easily predictable way when exposed to cold. This makes it difficult to assess how long someone trapped in the cold is likely to survive.

The management of hypothermia depends on how the condition was caused.

1. Exposure to dry cold

This type of hypothermia is sometimes called exposure or exposure exhaustion. The temperature falls slowly to dangerous levels and the condition is associated with fatigue or exhaustion. Severe hypothermia of this type is uncommon in industrial situations but it is not uncommon for minor degrees of hypothermia to develop while working in cold weather or following an accident where a casualty is lying exposed to the elements before being lifted and carried to a sick bay or ambulance. This type of hypothermia can adversely affect a man's judgement, and it is thus important to be able to recognise the signs of minor degrees of hypothermia if accidents are to be prevented. This can be important for those in charge of a group working in a cold climate.

The warning signs of cold exposure are:

- A change in personality: the normally aggressive person becomes withdrawn and apathetic, while the introvert loses his temper and becomes aggressive
- Increasing slowness in physical and mental responses
- Slurring of speech
- Stumbling, cramps and shivering
- Blurred vision

If any of these symptoms occur in an uninjured man it is essential that he takes shelter and rests immediately. If this is not done the casualty's temperature will fall further and he will collapse from exposure exhaustion. He is at risk of dying any time after his temperature falls below 33°C and he is unlikely to survive a body temperature lower than 20°C.

If the event takes place in the open, handle the casualty gently and do not move unless necessary. Protect him from wind and rain and insulate him from the ground under him. Wrap him in dry clothing, blankets or a sleeping bag. Give him warm drinks if available but do not give alcohol. There is, however, some controversy about alcohol which can increase heat loss but also has a protective effect against frostbite by inducing peripheral vasodilatation. Drunks who collapse in the street on very cold nights lose heat rapidly but often have no frostbite when they survive extreme degrees of hypothermia. On the other hand, a railway signal operator who tripped and fell into a snow drift some years ago and suffered severe hypothermia recovered with the loss of both feet and several fingers.

When eventually returned to living quarters, put the casualty to bed in a warm room. Usually the uninjured victim of cold exposure will feel better after several hours, even before he has reached normal body temperature. As judgement may be affected for an hour or two, he should stay in bed for 24 hours, and may need to be off work for 48 hours.

2. Immersion in cold water

This type of hypothermia develops more rapidly than exposure to dry cold because of the increased conductivity of water over air but the symptoms are the same as for cold exposure. When a man accidentally falls into cold water it is important that he does not struggle or swim vigorously because this will replace the partially warm water trapped in his clothes with cold water which will increase the rate of cooling. Survival time following immersion is extremely variable and depends on many factors. Cases have been reported of long periods of survival following immersion in tropical waters but in cold waters — such as those of the North Sea where the temperature is around 8°C, the survival time is probably ½ to 1 hour.

So-called 'post rescue death' may follow immersion hypothermia. The casualty is successfully recovered from the water and seems to be in a reasonable state of health. A short time later he collapses and dies due to heart failure. This is because immersion in cold water puts a strain on the heart as extra oxygen has to be pumped to the shivering muscles. The heart is then put under even more stress when the casualty exerts himself to get out of the water. Another factor is that the pressure of the water assists the return of blood to the heart and this is suddenly lost when the casualty leaves the water, causing a drop in blood pressure.

The best treatment is to place the casualty in a warm bath (40 to 42°C) with his arms and legs outside the water so that his body organs are warmed first. It is not necessary to remove the clothing before treatment. It is best to begin with water at around 36–37°C and gradually to increase the temperature to 40–42°C since immediate immersion in hot water can cause severe discomfort.

Case Study 2

A presentation was given at a clinical meeting in Stromness, Orkney Islands, some years ago, where a very experienced general practitioner described the case of a man who fell into the sea and was eventually recovered suffering from severe immersion hypothermia. He was taken into a local house which only possessed one small hot water cylinder. Rather than following normal advice of initial re-immersion in lukewarm water he filled the bath with all the available hot water and plunged the casualty in. When told by a naval expert that that would be extremely painful and the casualty would attempt to jump out the very experienced, practical rejoinder was, "Of course it is and that is why you need to jump in also to hold him there because there is no other hot water." That is a further example of using experience and judgement in difficult remote situations to achieve the best possible result.

Central rewarming

It was suggested some time ago that giving the casualty warm air to breathe may warm the body organs quickly and the technique was known as central rewarming. It sounded good but in practice this technique does not seem to work because only a very small amount of heat can be passed across the respiratory tract. Only in deep saturation diving, with helium are the lungs important in heat transfer.

Conditions Caused by Heat

Most of the physiological and environmental principles associated with cold illnesses apply also to the illnesses caused by heat. The additional physical parameter which must be taken into consideration when dealing with the heat illnesses is evaporation.

Air contains relatively little water vapour before it is fully saturated. Thus, if a man is working in a dry environment such as an Arabian desert, it is possible to evaporate sweat into the atmosphere around him as soon as it appears. Provided the intake of water is sufficient, he will be more efficient at higher temperatures than if he was in a coastal or offshore location. In these latter locations, where humidity is high and the air is almost fully saturated with water and it is difficult to get more water into the air. When the sweat forms it lies on the surface since it cannot be evaporated into the fully saturated air, heat is thus not removed and the temperature rises. This accounts for the difference in the nature and the frequency of the heat illnesses encountered offshore, on the coast and in inland desert areas.

In summary, the factors which affect the efficiency of evaporation of sweat are:

- The environmental temperature
- Humidity of the atmosphere
- The wind speed

The higher the wind speed, the more possible it will be to get water into water laden air because it is constantly being replaced by new air in which there may be a little space for water. Where the relative humidity approaches 100% however, sweat cannot be evaporated and the temperature will rise. Consequences of increasing the heat load are:

- Dilation of surface blood vessels in order to radiate away heat
- Increased sweating

The Heat Illnesses

There are three main heat illnesses:

1. Heat cramps
2. Heat exhaustion
3. Heat stroke

1. Heat cramps

Heat cramps occur in people who sweat profusely and do not replace salt. The onset occurs when the salt level falls to a critical value and the condition is manifested by severe cramps in various muscles, particularly those of the legs and abdomen. It occurs most commonly in those who have recently been in a temperate or cold area and have returned to a hot climate and indulged in strenuous physical activity right away. While in the temperate zone they have probably lost their acclimatisation. Following return from such an area, sweat contains salt which can be readily tasted, whereas a few weeks later the sweat contains much less salt. Heat cramps are not uncommon in children returning from school in a temperate climate to a hot climate and who indulge in tennis and other forms of sport actively as soon as they return.

This condition is quite easily treated. The casualty should be kept indoors and given extra salt in his food and an abundance of fruit juices to drink. Tomato and pineapple juice are particularly rich in potassium salts and they are useful in this condition. It is also worthwhile giving the casualty a cup of physiological saline to drink. This can be made up by adding a teaspoonful of salt to a litre of water. Following resolution of the problem, the casualty should be advised to live quietly for a few days.

The use of salt tablets routinely in hot climates went out of favour some years ago because of the association between salt and hypertension. It has however, now been shown that workers in the Arabian desert in summer are unlikely to suffer from heat cramps if they are given salt tablets of 300 mg per day. This is required to prevent heat cramps whether they are suffering from hypertension or not and in no way causes hypertension in normal people.

Case Study 3

An epidemiological study carried out in the field areas of an oil company in the UAE revealed that twice as many men reported sick during summer as in winter and the main extra complaint was of severe pains in the limbs and abdominal muscles. This resembled the heat cramps found in mines in the past. Also, it was noted that salt tablets had been removed from the dining areas following reports of the association between salt and hypertension. There were 121 reported incidences during the month of July and when 300 mg salt per man was introduced during the month of August the number of cases fell to six. Investigating the reason for the six cases it was found that they were nurses who had refused to take the salt tablets in case they got hypertension! (Ahwal *et al.*, 2000)

---

2. Heat exhaustion

Heat exhaustion is essentially a water and salt disturbance. It occurs in people who have been working strenuously in the heat and the body has become slightly mixed up with the concentration of salts and fluids due to the considerable requirement for fluids in hot climates. It is possible during maximal sweating in 24 hours to lose (and have to replace) about 30 litres of fluid. It is thus not surprising that this condition occurs from time to time.

This is not a particularly serious condition, but it is important to recognise because if it is not recognised and managed, it can lead to much more serious disturbances, of which heat stroke is one. The problem is that heat exhaustion is not easy to recognise because it presents with vague symptoms manifested by complaints of weakness, dizziness, loss of appetite, nausea and general unwellness. The temperature is normal and the skin is usually cool and moist since sweating is taking place freely and body temperature is thus controlled. This may cause confusion when the temperature is measured with a view to diagnosing heat illness and is found to be within normal limits. On the basis of these signs and symptoms, together with the temperature of the environment and the duration of exposure, the casualty should be considered to be suffering from heat exhaustion. Treatment is quite simple. The casualty should be rested in a cool room for 24 hours with lost fluids and salt largely replaced by an abundance of fruit juices, particularly tomato and pineapple juices. This will allow the body to sort itself out. It will do so within that period of time and thereafter the casualty should be advised to take it easy for a few days. Failure to recognise the condition, however, may lead to collapse or even heat stroke.

3. Heat stroke

When heat stroke takes place, it is often the result of an accident when the casualty is short of water. This may be because he has been injured and cannot move to get water or because his vehicle has broken down and he has run out of water. Heat stroke is not particularly common in well organised industrial environments where work shifts, remote travel and fluid and electrolyte replacement regimes are supervised.

What happens is that the body runs out of water and is therefore unable to sweat. All the available water has been withdrawn from the blood and the extracellular space and some has even been withdrawn from the cells themselves. The skin becomes hot and dry. Since there is no fluid available for heat loss due to the latent heat of evaporation of sweat, the body temperature rises. Thus, there is hot, dry skin and a rising temperature.

Following these fluid shifts within the body, the blood becomes more viscous. This results in cardiac strain since the heart is required to pump around this thick blood even faster in order to provide for the increasing oxygen needs of the hot cells. The heart is thus under severe strain. When the casualty collapses and falls to the ground, heat conduction from the terrain will add to the heat load. His temperature will then rise even more rapidly causing a state of mental confusion and disorientation at about 41°C, followed by unconsciousness when the temperature rises a little higher and then death from irreversible brain damage at about 44 or 45°C.

The actual cause of death can be from one or two different mechanisms. It may occur from brain damage when the temperature rises very high in those who have a fit heart. In those who have existing heart disease, however, death may take place much earlier from the failure of the heart caused by the additional work of pumping the viscous blood around the circulation. In managing these cases, it must be remembered that since the heart is under stress, great care must be taken in handling the casualty gently.

Management of heat stroke

In the management of heat stroke, the physical relations between the body and its environment must be borne in mind.

The casualty must be insulated from the terrain (conduction), provided with shade from the sun (radiation) and fanned to increase air movement (convection). This will limit further heat gain and is an important step to take in endeavours to reduce the temperature. Since the basic problem is that the casualty is unable to produce sweat, provide him with some artificial sweat. Remove clothing to expose the greatest amount of surface area possible and sponge it with tepid water. Now fan the casualty to encourage evaporation of the water applied. This will rapidly reduce the temperature and make him feel much more comfortable if he is indeed conscious.

The next problem is based on the fact that he cannot sweat because he has no water and his tissues and blood are dry and concentrated. If he is not conscious nothing can be done about this in the field and he must be placed in the recovery position and taken to hospital where he will be given fluids intravenously. In the field, however, he must be handled very gently and attempts must not be made to rush over rough ground speedily since his heart will be in a brittle state. The casualty may however, become conscious after his temperature has been reduced by first-aid measures in which case he can be given fluids to drink. Under these circumstances, or if he was conscious when found, give an abundance of fluids to drink using as much fruit juice as is available. If fruit juice is not available then give water. Give 1 or 2 L at the outset then rest for a while before giving him a further 2 L. When the casualty begins to sweat again you may consider that a cure has largely taken place. There is no rush to move a casualty such as this. It is better to cool him and, if possible, to rehydrate him until he can sweat himself before moving him. This will be much safer from the viewpoint of the heart.

In one desert oil operation a stone bath was installed in the desert clinic and filled with cold water floating with ice cubes to receive cases of heat stroke. If they survived the rushed transportation journey they frequently succumbed as soon as they were plunged into the ice-cold water. Fortunately, this practice was terminated!

Hyperthermia Associated with Fever

In young children, the body's 'thermostat' tends to be immature and even in minor degrees of infection the body temperature may soar to high levels. The effect of this on the brain can result in the development of convulsive effects. This can be very frightening for parents. The management is the same as for heat stroke. Place the child in a darkened room and apply tepid water to the surface with a sponge, then increase air movement. This will rapidly reduce the temperature and make the child feel much more comfortable. This treatment can also be used in adults with high fever. In the past, attempts were made to reduce the temperature rapidly by placing the child in a cold bath in the same way as in certain desert clinics. This undoubtedly did much more harm than good on occasion. Equally, it is not nearly so efficient as the physiological means of cooling by replacing sweat with tepid water and it is quite possible that sudden immersion in ice cold water might cause other cardiac abnormalities — such as heart stoppage!

A final point is that when serious heat or cold illnesses develop, they tend to do so with dramatic suddenness and unless you anticipate them, the first evidence is often at the point of collapse. Almost the only premonitory sign of both heat and cold effects is changes in mental function. This should be borne in mind when working in groups or with a colleague who is normally pleasant and easygoing and who then becomes difficult, argumentative and aggressive. On the other hand, a colleague who was usually the life and soul of the party and who becomes apathetic and withdrawn, is usually showing the signs of impending danger. The danger sign is not a particular mental trait but a change in the normal personality.

References

Ahwal SH, Norman JN and Brebner JA. 2000. Heat cramps in a hot desert work-site. *Kuwait Med J* **32**: 382–386.

Auld CD, Light IM and Norman JN. 1980. Cooling responses in shivering and non-shivering dogs during induced hypothermia. *Clin Sci* **58**: 501.

Bigelow WG, Lindsay WK, Harrison RC, Gordon RA and Greenwood WF. 1950. Oxygen transport and utilisation in dogs at low body temperatures. *Am J Physiol* **160**: 125–137.

Brebner JA. 1990. The provision of healthcare in remote hostile environments. RGU, Aberdeen: PhD thesis.

Ellis HD, Wilcock SE and Zaman SA. 1985. Cold and performance: the effects of information load, analgesics and the rate of cooling. *Aviat Space Environ Med* **56**: 233–237.

Erikson H, Krog J, Anderson KL and Scholander PF. 1956. Critical temperature in naked man. *Acta Physiol Scand* **37**: 35–39.

Golden FSC and Hervey GR. 1981. The after drop and death after immersion in cold water. In: *Hypothermia — Ashore and Afloat*. (ed.) Adam JM. Aberdeen: Aberdeen University Press, pp. 37–56.

Light IM, White MA, Allen D and Norman JN. 1980. Thermal balance in divers. *Lancet* **315**: 1362.

MacPherson RK. 1958. Acclimatization status of temperate zone man. *Nature Lond* **182**: 1240–1241.

Norman JN. 1961. Man in the Antarctic. University of Glasgow: MD thesis.

Norman JN. 1986. Work in cold climates. *Int J Environ* **26**: 329–340.

Norman JN and Brebner JA. 1985. Problems caused by heat and cold. In: *The Offshore Health Handbook*. London: Martin Dinitz, pp.127–142.

Norman JN and Brebner JA. 1988. The establishment of an occupational health service for the British Antarctic Survey. *Arct Med Res* **47**(Suppl 1): 365–367.

Scholander PF, Hock R, Walters V and Irving L. 1950. Adaptation to cold in arctic and tropical animals and birds in relation to body temperature, insulation and basal metabolic rate. *Biol Bull* **99**: 259–271.

Index

www.ingramcontent.com/pod-product-compliance
Lightning Source LLC
Chambersburg PA
CBHW050537190326
41458CB00007B/1817

9 781786 347503

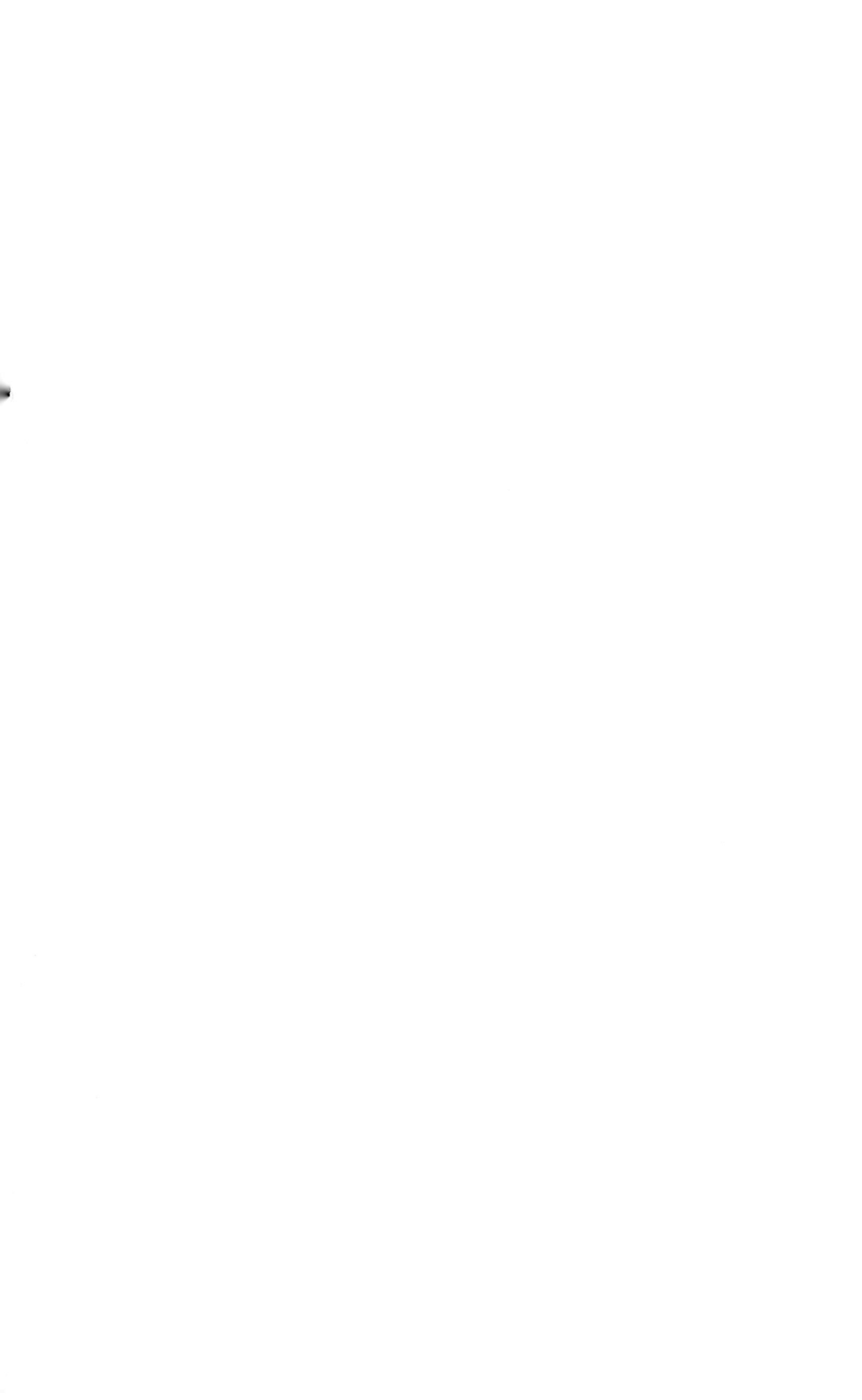

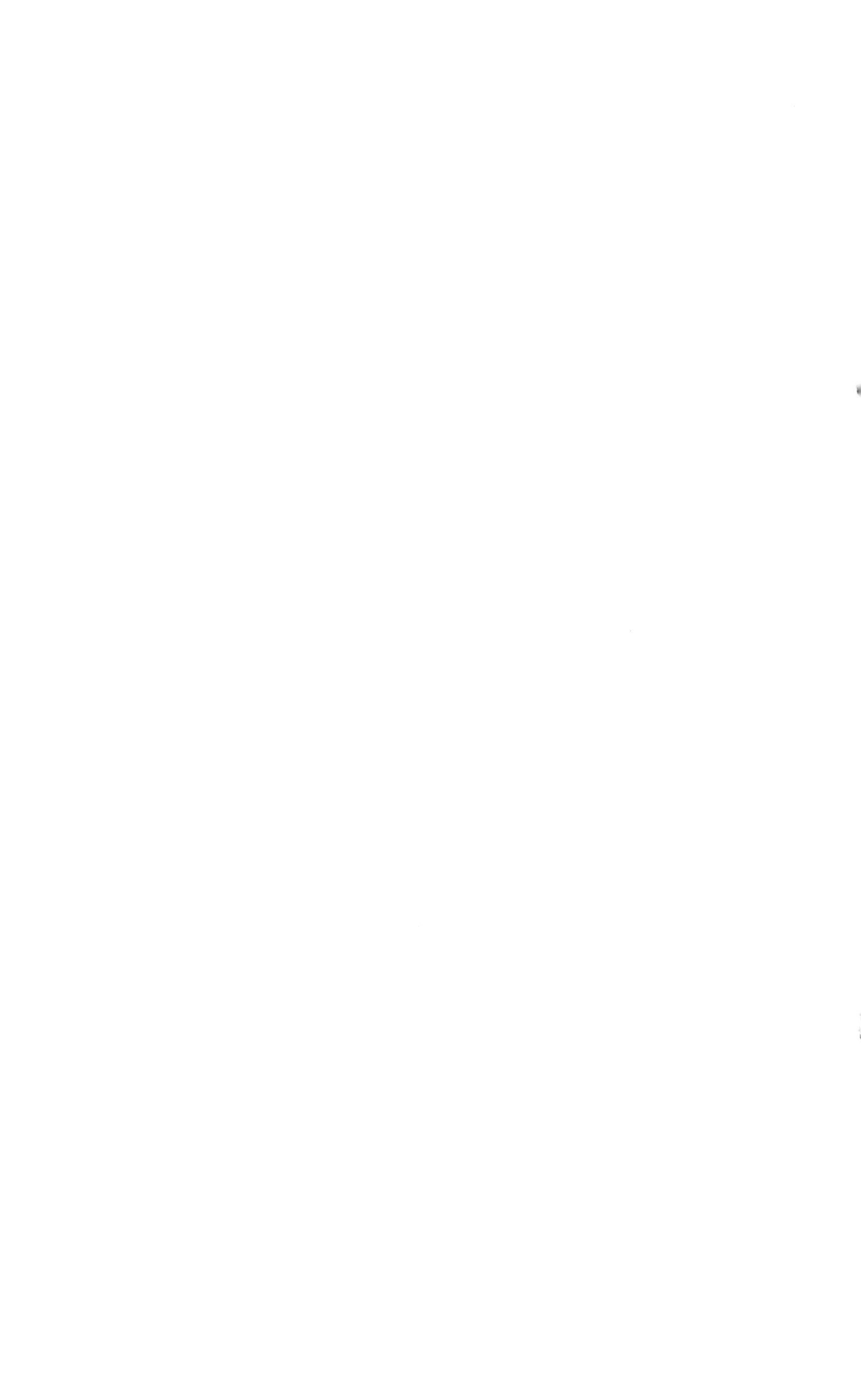